DATE DUE

FEB 24 1994	FEB 4 1997
APR 13	FEB 18.
	SEP 2 2 1996
OCT - 5 1994	NOV - 5 1999
OCT 18 1994	
NOV - 1 1994	
NOV 15 1994	
MAR 2 2 1995	
MAR 2 8 1995	
APR 11 1995	
APR 26 1995	
MAY 10 1995	
MAY 24 1995	
JUN 8 1995	
OCT 16 1995	
NOV 0 1 1995	
NOV 1 4 1995	
DEC 2 - 1995	
DEC 14 1996	

BRODART   Cat. No. 23-221

Toxic Psychiatry

OTHER BOOKS BY PETER R. BREGGIN, M.D.

Psychiatric Drugs: Hazards to the Brain
The Psychology of Freedom: Liberty and Love As a Way of Life
Electroshock: Its Brain-Disabling Effects
After the Good War (a novel)
The Crazy from the Sane (a novel)

TOXIC PSYCHIATRY

Why Therapy, Empathy, and Love Must Replace the Drugs, Electroshock, and Biochemical Theories of the "New Psychiatry"

Peter R. Breggin, M.D.

St. Martin's Press
New York

For my wife, Ginger Ross-Breggin
For helping me to love and to understand life

Production Editor: Mark H. Berkowitz
Copyedited by Sandra Dhols
Book Design by Susan Hood

Library of Congress Cataloging-in-Publication Data
Breggin, Peter Roger, 1936–
    Toxic psychiatry : why therapy, empathy, and love must replace the drugs, electro-shock, and biochemical theories of the "new psychiatry."
      p.   cm.
    ISBN 0-312-05975-2
    1. Biological psychiatry—Evaluation. I. Title.
    [DNLM: 1. Brain Damage, Chronic—etiology. 2. Electroshock—adverse ef-fects. 3. Mental Disorders—diagnosis. 4. Mental Disorders—therapy. 5. Psy-chotherapy—methods. 6. Psychotropic Drugs—adverse effects. WM 400 B833t]
RC341.B74 1991
616.89'1—dc20
DNLM/DLC
for Library of Congress   91-113

First Edition: November 1991
10 9 8 7 6 5 4 3 2 1

Warning

Do not abruptly stop most psychiatric drugs!

Most psychiatric drugs are far more dangerous to take than people realize, but they also can become dangerous when discontinued too abruptly. As described in this book, most have addictive qualities and can produce withdrawal symptoms that are emotionally and physically distressing and sometimes life-threatening. Drugs that can produce withdrawal symptoms include neuroleptics or antipsychotics, such as Haldol or Thorazine; antidepressants, such as Tofranil and Elavil; stimulants, such as Ritalin; minor tranquilizers, such as Valium and Xanax; and prescription sedatives or sleeping pills.

Stopping psychiatric drugs should usually be done gradually, and only with professional guidance.

No book can substitute for individualized medical or psychological care. However, it is important to find help consistent with one's own philosophy. The aim of this book is to present a psychosocial viewpoint. It cannot be used as a treatment handbook.

Contents

Contents

Acknowledgments

This book is the culmination of a lifetime of scientific, educational, and reform work and therefore draws insights, information, inspiration, and sustenance from many different people.

Most important is my wife, Ginger Ross-Breggin, who guided me, in the most gentle fashion, toward finding a more popular style of writing about complex technical subjects and helped edit the entire manuscript. She developed the filing system required for such a mammoth endeavor and carried on myriad back-up tasks over the years. She helped discover relevant research materials and often contributed directly to my grasp of the subjects. Yet her most important contribution cannot be described so simply. It has more to do with how she lives—with love and concern for all expressions of life and for the earth itself. She keeps me better connected to both the details and the essence of life. Our mutual feeling that there is an equal exchange between us is a blessing. During this time, Ginger also has been going to school, developing her artistic talents, delivering papers, coauthoring a book with me on conflict resolution, and being a mother to our children.

The influence of Leonard Roy Frank permeates the book. Himself the victim of electroshock and insulin coma when he was a young man, he has gone on to become a leader in psychiatric reform through his educational, organizational, and literary efforts. A constant stream of relevant books and articles has flowed across the continent from Leonard's library and files to mine. He, too, read and helped to edit the entire manuscript and, next to my wife, provided the most important input. His generosity and spiritual verve have been a constant source of encouragement. Leonard is now compiling a book of quotations, from which most of the quotations at the chapter headings of this book are drawn.

Pam Clay, an outstanding patient rights attorney, embodying the best traditions of law, has made a significant impact on the care of inmates in her state of Kentucky. She read the entire manuscript and made many valuable comments; but her main contribution has been in the regular sharing of her enormous enthusiasm and intelligence, and her inspiring devotion to the rights and well-being of those too powerless to protect themselves.

In addition to Ginger, Leonard, and Pam, several other people have read some or all of the manuscript, as well as giving me other reasons to be grateful to them. Rae Unzicker, national coordinator of the National Association of Psychiatric Survivors (NAPS), triumphed over years of psychiatric abuse to become an outstanding leader in psychiatric reform. She has regularly bestowed her extraordinary warmth on me. Jeffrey Moussaieff Masson became the first psychoanalyst to defrock himself rather than promote the self-serving cultishness of the psychoanalytic establishment. As someone who has stood up for principle at great personal cost to himself, Jeffrey has been able to provide me extra infusions of moral support and courage. He also provided important materials for the book. Another brave individual, neurologist John Friedberg, became the first physician to stand up effectively in public against electroshock, and he belongs in the medical hall of fame for bravery. He has helped educate me over the years. Robert Morgan and Bertram Karon, psychologists and authors, have persistently told the truth about psychiatric fictions in their own writings and have lent me their support. A psychologist, writer, and former president of the American Academy of Psychotherapists (AAP), Larry Tirnauer has been a regular confidant through the ups and downs of my reform efforts, often adding needed balance to my critiques. As an author, Kate Millett inspired me to reexamine my attitudes on feminist issues in the early 1970s, and more recently she has become a friend and coworker on behalf of patient rights. Psychiatrist Eileen Walkenstein, another source of personal support, has written several books critical of biopsychiatric dogma and practice and promoting a more caring, mutual approach to patients. Psychiatrist Gerald Dubin has been for many years an unfailing friend and supporter and, before he retired from psychiatry, a model of kindness and gentleness as a psychotherapist. Neurologist Robert Grimm, M.D., a marvelous physician, long-standing friend and moral support, made useful contributions to the editing, as did sociologist Phil Brown, Ph.D., and professor of social work David Cohen, Ph.D.

Over the years of reform work, I've also had useful input, help, and moral support from many other people to whom I want to express my gratitude, including psychiatrists Loren Mosher, Giovanni de Girolamo, David Richman, and Robert Seidenberg; social psychiatrist Ruth Peachey; educator Marshall Fritz; audiovisual specialist James Turney; patient ad-

Acknowledgments

vocates Bill Johnson and Mary Olympia, who are mainstays of the National Association of Rights Protection and Advocacy (NARPA); the entire
board of directors of NARPA, including Paul Freddolino and Renee
Bostick; physicians Lawrence Plumlee, Jay Salwen, and Lars Martensson;
psychologists Les Ansel, David Hill, Seth Farber, and Judi Striano; me-
diation counselor Ingrid Kepler-May; social worker Michael Weinberg;
filmmaker Beverly Jones; Ira Gruber and Sandra Kjaer of the Tardive
Dyskinesia/Tardive Dystonia National Association; and Helen Geis, the
parent of a psychosurgery victim. I also want to thank Diana James,
assistant to Gloria Steinem, for offering moral support as I have increasingly confronted the issues of male supremacy in psychiatry and society.

Many other people, too numerous to mention, have mailed me a
constant stream of news clippings and other materials from around the
world, and I want to thank them and to ask them to keep it up.

Many members of the psychiatric survivor movement were interviewed
for the book or otherwise contributed through conversations, correspon-
dence, published writings, or organizational activities. Beyond those already mentioned, I want to thank Don Weitz, Irit Shimrat, Sally Zinman,
Jenny Miller, Sandra Everett, Marilyn Rice, Fancher Bennett, John
Basham, Ron Thompson, Linda Andre, Jay Mahler, Susan Witte, Howie
the Harp, Janet Foner, Janet Gotkin, Lynda Wright, Huey Freeman,
George Ebert, Mary Ann Ebert,* Paul Dorfner, Dayna Caron, Peter
Lehmann, Karl Jensen, Lise Smedal, Caia Garupi, Maths Jespersen, and
activist attorneys Jean Matulis, Ted Chabasinski, and Carla McKague.
Among the survivors, I especially want to acknowledge David Oaks, who
gives voice to the movement through his journal, *Dendron*; Alice M.
Earl for the special reports she publishes in her *Peer Advocate*; Judi
Chamberlin, who contributes in so many ways with her keen insights
and hard work on behalf of patient rights and survivor-run alternatives;
and Dennis Nester, who has made it a personal crusade to publicize the
damaging effects of psychiatric treatments. I want to emphasize that I
have worked directly with these and many other survivors throughout the
world, and have gained immensely from them.

About two dozen of the people I've already mentioned are members
of the board of directors or advisory council of the Center for the Study
of Psychiatry, an educational and reform network of more than seventy-
five people that I founded 1971 and have directed ever since. Needless
to say, not everyone in such a large group agrees with all of my viewpoints
or all of the ideas expressed in this book; but each of them has given his
or her moral support to my work. Among those whom I have not yet
mentioned, I especially want to thank Congressman Ronald V. Dellums,

*Unlike the others in this list, Mary Ann is not a survivor of psychiatry.

Acknowledgments

Congressman Louis Stokes, and Senator Steven Symms, all of whom have been members of the Center for the Study of Psychiatry for two decades, and I want to acknowledge those who work with them on Capitol Hill and have contributed so much to my efforts, including Robert Brauer and Joe Cobb.

Richard Rubenstein, J.D., director of the Institute for Conflict Analysis and Resolution at George Mason University, where I teach, is a more recent member of the Center for the Study of Psychiatry. I am grateful to him and everyone at George Mason for providing me an exciting academic home. Jerry Miller, D.S.W., founder of the National Center for Institutions and Alternatives (NCIA), has provided special direction and support over the years.

Attorney Earl Dudley, Jr., now professor of law at the University of Virginia, has given me invaluable advice, help, and moral support at crucial moments for many years, and has exemplified for me the highest ethical standards of his profession. Ralph Temple, former director of the American Civil Liberties Union (ACLU) in Washington, D.C., and an outstanding civil rights attorney, guided me successfully through the most hazardous of recent times, helping turn an attack on me into an enormous gain for the reform movement.[1]

Two people who are not members of the Center also have played key roles in backing up my reform work and, closely related, my individual rights. Stuart Comstock-Gay, director of the Maryland ACLU, brought his organization to my support at a critical moment during the recent attack. Hubert "Hank" Schlosberg has been by my side—or only a telephone call away—almost from the very beginning. One of Washington, D.C.'s most respected attorneys, Hank first came to my aid in the early 1970s when he virtually donated his time to make sure that my efforts, and even my career, were not quickly snuffed out. The informal defense team of Temple, Schlosberg, and Dudley has proved to be most formidable. I am profoundly grateful to them.

Finally, I want to thank the remaining members of the Center for the Study of Psychiatry, the great majority of whom have gone beyond lending their name to my reform efforts. They include Kenneth Barney, M.D., Ralph Barocas, Ph.D., Melvin Belli, J.D., Linne Bourget, Ph.D., Mark Burrell, Ph.D., Phyllis Chesler, Ph.D., Lee Coleman, M.D., S. Dallas Cooley, M.D., Jonathan Ecker, M.D., C. Timothy Golumbeck, M.D., Jay Haley, Karl Hess, Keith Hoeller, Ph.D., Diane Jayson, Ph.D., Gabe Kaimowitz, J.D., David Keirsey, Ph.D., Robert D. Kephart, the late Arthur Koestler, Ron Leifer, M.D., Kim Long, M.S.W., Cloé Madanes, the late Robert Mendelsohn, M.D., Thomas Nerney, Edward Opton, Jr., Ph.D., J.D., Norman Pearl, M.D., Sharon Presley, Ph.D., Peter Prudden, M.D., Jack Raher, M.D., Kenneth Ruby, M.D., Viktor

Sanua, Ph.D., Tim Seldin, M.Ed., Milton Shore, Ph.D., Joyce Shulman, M.S.W., Ph.D., Lee Shulman, Ph.D., Richard Shulman, Ph.D., Marvin Skolnick, M.D., E. Mark Stern, Ed.D., Don Turner, M.D., Emilio Viano, Ph.D., and Robyn Zeiger, Ph.D., who is the current chair of the Center and a loved friend and colleague.

Many attorneys and advocates around the country have worked extensively with me in patients' rights and malpractice suits, and I have learned a great deal from them. They are literally too numerous to begin naming. I also want to thank the many members of the media who have covered the reform movement and who, on occasion, have stood on principle in defense of my freedom of speech. In regard to that principle, I especially want to thank Oprah Winfrey and her marvelous staff.

Over the years, several wonderful people have helped me as office and research assistants. Carol Valentine helped get the Center on its feet before there was much support in the wider world. Kelly Bangham and Kristen Magruder literally grew up around my office, adding greatly to my enjoyment of the work, and it's a pleasure to have Krissy back again. Wade Hudson made valuable contributions in helping to research several sections of this book, including psychiatry's relation to the drug industry. Another research assistant, Patrick Lufkin, helped trace the financial history of the American Psychiatric Association. Ravel Lutz, who was my assistant until recently, contributed to keeping the whole operation going, helped with editing, and made critical forays into the National Library of Medicine. Marilyn Cramer joined us as a word processor and became an editor as well, and finally Claudia DeMino has now become my do-it-all full-time assistant.

I am blessed with a superlative New York agent, Richard Curtis, who understands and supports my work, and doubly blessed with St. Martin's senior editor, Jared Kieling, who enthusiastically backed this book project. Surely that is more than an author can hope for in one literary lifetime.

Last I want to thank my children, Alysha, Benjamin, Sharon, and Linda. Not only have they shown appreciation for my reform work and my writing efforts, they have graciously accepted the competition for my time. Most recently, they have also patiently endured hours of book-title discussions.

Paradoxically, while I've had so much moral support, this book has been largely a private odyssey. Few people who are critical of psychiatric technology and biopsychiatric theories wish to spend a substantial segment of their lives studying them to become expert, nor do they necessarily want to risk the hazards of speaking out in public against them. Most of the people I have thanked in this acknowledgment have given me, above all else, the encouragement needed to proceed with this fundamentally lonely and sometimes hazardous task. Yet the writing of this acknowledgment has served to remind me that loneliness is something I need never complain of again. *That* is what I most wish to thank my many friends for.

The future of reform in psychiatry rests in large part with the psychiatric survivors themselves and the growing vitality of their movement. The survivors provide mutual support for each other, they educate the public about the dangers of psychiatric treatment and incarceration, and they are developing self-help alternatives that may ultimately supplant much of psychiatry. But like any reform or rights movement, the survivors need support from the rest of us. I want this book to honor and encourage them.*†

*The Appendixes describe how to get in touch with the psychiatric survivor movement, as well as how to stay abreast of the activities of the Center for the Study of Psychiatry.
†In all cases described in this book, unless both a first and last name are used, identifying details have been omitted or changed to protect confidentiality without affecting the substance of the story.

Introduction

What Is Psychiatry?

Many people don't know the difference between psychiatry, psychotherapy, psychology, and psychoanalysis. This book is primarily about psychiatry—a specialty within the field of medicine. *Psychiatrists* are fully qualified physicians (medical doctors) who specialize in treating people defined as having psychiatric problems. As physicians, psychiatrists have the right to prescribe drugs or electroshock, to hospitalize patients, and to treat people against their will. They are the only mental health professionals who routinely exercise these powers.* Psychiatry sets the tone and direction for the field of mental health and has been rapidly pushing it toward a more biological or medical viewpoint.

Psychotherapists are a very broad group which includes anyone helping people with problems by talking with them. Not all psychiatrists are psychotherapists or "talking doctors." As this book will discuss, many psychiatrists have little or no training in how to communicate with people about their problems. Instead they are trained in making "medical" diagnoses and giving drugs and electroshock.

Psychologists are educated in graduate schools of psychology rather than in medical schools, and they receive a Ph.D. rather than an M.D. Clinical psychologists are given training that overlaps with psychiatrists, and they often receive much more intensive training in psychotherapy

---

*Psychologists sometimes have the right to admit patients to mental hospitals. Some psychologists are also trying to obtain the training and the right to prescribe drugs. In other words, they want to obtain more of the powers traditionally monopolized by psychiatrists as medical doctors. When I give talks and workshops for psychologists, I advise them to remain as separate as possible from psychiatry. I am concerned that the public's ability to find nonmedical alternatives is becoming increasingly limited.

than do psychiatrists. Sometimes they work side-by-side with psychiatrists in mental health facilities, but they usually exercise much less authority.

In addition to psychiatrists and psychologists, many other professionals also offer psychotherapy, including clinical social workers, counselors, family therapists, some nurses, some ministers, and a variety of lay people.

Psychoanalysis is the form of psychotherapy founded and developed by Sigmund Freud and taught in his independently franchised psychoanalytic institutes. In the public's mind, psychoanalysis is correctly associated with the couch, the note pad, and the silent listener. But psychoanalysis is often incorrectly equated with psychiatry. Contrary to popular belief, Freud was *not* the father of psychiatry. Psychiatry existed long before Freud, and has been largely hostile to his teachings. Freud did not become a psychiatrist, and he warned his colleagues to beware of the medical profession.* Nonetheless, psychiatry took over and overwhelmed psychoanalysis in the United States. Very few psychiatrists have become psychoanalysts, and psychoanalysis has very little influence in modern psychiatry.

The author is a psychiatrist *and* a psychotherapist. He is not a psychoanalyst.

The main critique in this book is aimed at the medical specialty of psychiatry. Unfortunately, since psychiatry dominates the mental health profession, much of what is wrong with psychiatry is also wrong with the whole field.

---

* See Sigmund Freud, *The Question of Lay Analysis* (Norton, 1964). For a critique, see Philip Rieff, *Freud: The Mind of the Moralist* (Doubleday, 1961).

Chapter 1

Psychiatry Out of Control

A gigantic asylum is a gigantic evil, and figuratively speaking, a manufactory of chronic insanity.

—*John Arlidge (1859)*

Of all tyrannies a tyranny sincerely exercised for the good of its victims may be the most oppressive.

—*C. S. Lewis (1970)*

I am still more frightened by the fearless power in the eyes of my fellow psychiatrists than by the powerless fear in the eyes of their patients.

—*R. D. Laing (1985)*

Nothing could have prepared me for that day on the women's "violent ward," E-3. It was a cement dungeon, long and narrow, and bare except for a few boulder-size oak chairs, benches riveted to the wall, and a badly working TV in the corner of the ceiling. It looked more like an abandoned basement corridor than a hospital ward.

I was eighteen years old, a college freshman at Harvard, and I was standing in the middle of this place because a friend, Mike Dohan, had urged me to join a group of Harvard and Radcliffe students on a volunteer trip to the local state mental hospital. His brother Larry, also an undergraduate, had recently started the experiment in college volunteering. The year was 1954, a landmark in psychiatry, when the neuroleptic drug Thorazine began to flood the state hospitals throughout the nation. But the tidal wave of psychiatric medication hadn't yet broken over Metropolitan State. Met State remained an old-fashioned snakepit.

On the ward, two indifferent attendants were amusing themselves in the office and not a doctor or nurse was in sight. During the day, the patients were locked out of the barracks-like sleeping quarters. Dozens of them were herded together in gray squalor with nothing to occupy their time. Many wasted a lifetime in this place.

The first and most lasting impression was the stench. It reminded me of my Uncle Dutch's reaction to liberating a concentration camp: nausea. When I was ten, I had heard the story of his exploits as an army officer, and now they came back with renewed impact at the age of eighteen. Many of these people actually looked like concentration camp inmates —undernourished, silent, stone-faced with sunken eyes. They would sit in corners or pace about. Some talked to themselves. One gesticulated into space. Another was lying on the radiator by the filthy window. Absolutely no one socialized with anyone else. It was as if each was ashamed and afraid of the others.

A tall, lanky woman stood in front of a stolid, older lady who was sitting motionless on a bench. Then the lanky woman leaned down and smashed the sitting woman in the mouth. There was an audible thud of fist on flesh. That's all there was; not a word or glance between the two women acknowledged the event. When I reported the incident to the aides, one of them came out and checked the injured woman's teeth as if examining a horse's mouth.

The group of us from Harvard and Radcliffe spent the day trying to coax the patients into conversations. Often we succeeded, and many of them perked up considerably. When we got ready to leave, some of the women tugged on our arms, begging us to stay. In words that hardly differed among them, they would tell us, "I don't belong here." We believed them. Nobody belonged in Met State.

Then we learned that the young woman lying in the corner, as disheveled as a street person, as silent as a mummy, had been a Radcliffe student when she broke down and was committed. It seemed inconceivable that she should be in this place. It was intolerable that something better than this could not be done for her.

More than thirty-five years later, my mind easily becomes alive with vignettes from the hospital: the women begging for a chance to relate to us in any way possible, from making lewd suggestions to baking us cookies. The elderly lady taking my cherished watch from my wrist to polish it for me, and my anxiety over losing it, until she returned it later in the day, as promised, with a new shine to the case. Coming upon attendants roughing up a patient and simply bearing witness to their acts until they felt compelled to stop. The giant, maniacal-looking man who confronted me in the corridor, stared down into my eyes, and harmlessly announced, "I smoke Lucky Strike."

Sometimes the volunteers experienced the threat of the hospital first-hand. One volunteer was mistaken for a patient because she was very obese, and an aide told her she'd have to have sex with him or get transferred to the back wards. Another volunteer was left behind when our group went home and remained locked up for over an hour on a crowded back ward with no attendants; he grew terrified he'd have a breakdown and be trapped there for the rest of his life.

While the aides were sometimes menacing to the volunteers, the patients almost never were. Hundreds of students participated, and some remained alone for hours on the "violent" wards; but none were physically harmed or obviously endangered by an inmate.

Sharing the anguish of the patients and their intolerable living conditions took a toll on most of us. A single afternoon in the hospital was more than most of us could survive unscathed. We returned to Harvard and Radcliffe with headaches, upset stomachs, a stench embedded in our nostrils, and nightmares. Ahead of our time, we developed mutual debriefing methods to deal with our upset. We used dramatic techniques, such as playing the role of the patient, to reenact and to express our outrage, to fathom our despair. Sharing our emotional pain with one another helped keep us from quitting the program.

Later I learned that the woman who had become violent in such an unprovoked fashion had severe brain damage from electroshock, lobotomy, and other treatments, many long lost in her voluminous records. I began to think that the treatments had caused or worsened many of the patients' problems.

It also was apparent to me that much of the patients' upset and suffering was induced by the hospital environment itself. When working on a book about the program,[1] I wrote about this extensively; but every word was edited out by the psychiatrist who was in charge of our grant for the book project. I didn't get to tell the story of what psychiatric hospitals do to their patients until my first novel, *The Crazy from the Sane* (1970).

Asking Questions of the Uncaring

As I became a leader in the volunteer program and gained better access to the hospital and the staff, I began to ask questions. How could the staff ignore the fact that the patients suffered nearly freezing conditions in the winter and sweltering temperatures in the summer?

A staff psychiatrist told me, "Schizophrenics aren't bothered by extremes of heat and cold the way normal people are."

Even then, as an eighteen year old, this did not make sense to me. As I got to know the patients, they seemed at least as sensitive as ordinary human beings. Sometimes they seemed to be much more sensitive. Exquisite sensitivity, in fact, seemed a part of their problem. I wondered what went on in the minds of the doctors, nurses, and aides that enabled them to ignore the patients' anguish and even to compound it with the treatments.

I observed the insulin coma room, where rows of patients were purposely overdosed with insulin, causing a drop in their blood sugar, until they fell into convulsions and a coma from starvation of the brain. As I watched them writhe about on mats, near death, it seemed like a scene from hell. I watched them being fed sugar and orange juice, to awaken into a state of fear and confusion. The once difficult and unruly inmates, with their brains now permanently damaged, became gratefully dependent on their keepers after being brought back from the edge of death. Their righteous physicians called it an improvement and even a cure.

Again I asked questions.

Another staff psychiatrist told me, "Electric shock and insulin shock kill bad brain cells."

I knew from my beginning studies—although only a college student, I was already reading psychiatric textbooks—that no one had found "bad brain cells" as a cause of the psychiatric problems that were labeled schizophrenia, depression, or manic-depressive disorder. The hunt for a physical defect had been going on for centuries, with no success. Besides, how could a process as gross as shocking or starving the brain into convulsion, unconsciousness, and coma weed out the "bad cells" from the "good" ones? The cell death had to be indiscriminate.

"Why would a doctor make up stuff like that?" I asked myself. I saw no mystery in how the treatments worked. By damaging the brain and mind, they made the patients docile and passive—suitable for control within these abusive institutions.

A "Dangerous" Innovation

As the volunteer program grew in size and in ambition, the hundreds of us passing through each year began to transform the hospital. It was no longer so easy for the aides to rape or beat patients. A Harvard or Radcliffe student might stumble upon the assault. We also proved that the so-called violent patients weren't nearly so dangerous as supposed: two of us stole the keys and took half of the women's violent ward for a trip into town. We gave them money to buy trinkets in the local five-and-ten and returned them to the hospital without incident. They appreciated us and would do nothing to get us in trouble. And we realized that much, if not most, of their violence was in reaction to being abused within the state hospital. Living there was wholly demeaning and even life-threatening.

We worked hard to make the concrete fortress more livable, cleaning up and painting the wards and supervising social activities. Some of us focused on these group activities, while others of us, like myself, became more personally involved with individual patients whom we looked forward to seeing each week.

Representing the program as a college sophomore, I went to the superintendent with a simple proposal: let a dozen or more of us have one patient each, assigned for the duration of the year. We would work with the patient one afternoon a week and meet as a group with a social worker, Dave Kantor, for supervision on the same afternoon.

The superintendent was outraged. How could we dare confront him with such a proposal—college freshmen and sophomores treating back ward schizophrenics? It was my first experience with how easily the psychiatric establishment becomes threatened and how dearly it holds onto its dogma about the importance of medical and professional credentials. Only when I explained that I could transfer the entire volunteer program to another state hospital did the superintendent agree to our terms. Our program had brought the hospital its only positive coverage in the local and even the national press.

The president of the Boston Psychoanalytic Society also protested our proposal. This Freudian psychiatrist warned that without extensive professional training we would harm, even ruin, these hapless denizens of the hospital depths. His protest sticks in my mind alongside images from my first day on the wards: the woman being struck in the face, the woman urinating on the floor, the aides amusing themselves in the office. Harm them? Ruin them? With a little caring human contact?

Why would a psychoanalyst feel that his turf was threatened by student volunteers in a state mental hospital?

In my two years of work at Met State, I had never seen a psychoanalyst set foot in the place. I was discovering that psychoanalytically trained psychiatrists could defend their trade union prerogatives and professional turf as fiercely as their more biologically oriented colleagues.

Fourteen of us were begrudgingly given individual patients to work with one-on-one. Many were older, chronic patients. "Burnt-out schizophrenics" was the term used by the staff to describe many of them. Presumably, they were beyond harm—or help.

Mr. Liebowitz Goes Home

My own particular patient, an elderly man I'll call Mr. Liebowitz, was diagnosed as psychotically depressed, overcome with feelings of worthlessness and hopelessness. It was impossible to motivate him to do anything. He was afraid of people and phobic about having a heart attack. When I introduced myself to him, he tried to shoo me away like some vastly annoying fly. I thought to myself, "He'll never even talk with me!"

After a time he began to trust that I actually would show up each week and that I would be a friend to him. Like most inmates, he was absolutely friendless, and my attempts to establish a relationship must have seemed strange and inexplicable to him. Gradually he let me help him get better clothes from the dispensary and encourage him to work on some simple projects in the hospital carpentry shop. Soon he became willing to chat with me about what he might do to get out of the hospital.

Fearful at first about a heart attack, Mr. Liebowitz gradually allowed me to help him walk outdoors around the hospital, and then eventually around the hospital grounds. We became more able to talk about his actual physical condition, which was excellent, and to contrast his fears to reality. We chatted about his concerns about old age and put them in a more hopeful perspective. I am sure that the interest of a young college student did much to convince him that he still possessed some human worth.

Then I helped him select a home for older and retired people in town, where he was able to take advantage of going outdoors, shopping, and visiting in the community. It was more than a decent place to live and he was very pleased to be free of the hospital.

Other students in the program had more extraordinary accomplishments. Some worked with more grossly "psychotic" patients, those suffering from hallucinations and delusions, and helped them return to their families. While Mr. Liebowitz didn't talk much, many of the other patients became quite involved in expressing their feelings and discussing their lives with their student aides. For many of the students, this once-a-week supervision with the social worker became as intense as graduate training in psychotherapy. Nor did medication play any role in the outcome. Our patients were not yet receiving the new "miracle drugs."

The Results

By the end of the year, eleven of our fourteen patients had been released from the hospital. Only three of those eleven would return in the follow-up, which lasted one to two years. This is a far better record than that achieved by trained professionals working in programs relying on psychiatric drugs. We accomplished this "miracle" by showing our patients care and attention; by talking with them and taking them for walks, by helping them get properly fitted with eyeglasses, false teeth, or clothing, by reacquainting them with their forgotten families, or by connecting them with more humane supervised facilities outside the hospital. In some instances, where the patients had been more verbal and the students better able to communicate, the treatment had been indistinguishable from psychotherapy delivered by a trained professional.*

Growing Disillusionment

Even then, as a college student in the mid-1950s, I suspected that the "miracle drugs" weren't curing anyone. Three years of volunteering and two summers of doing research involving drugs in the hospital had impressed me more with the robotic indifference of the drugged patients than with their improvement. If anything, they seemed less reachable as people. The claims for "emptying the hospitals" were not being made yet, and in the years that followed, I would doubt their validity, long before the contradictory data began to pile up.

Again and again I found myself wondering what was the matter with psychiatry. Why wouldn't the profession adopt such a humane solution as the widespread use of volunteers? Why wouldn't it follow up our enormous success by trying the program in every hospital in the nation? Why wouldn't it commit funds and staffing to volunteer efforts? Why were drugs preferable? And why in the world wouldn't the psychiatrists see the obvious—that their treatments and their hospitals were doing far more harm than good?

As I finished my college career, I was already interested in psychiatric reform. I had barely an inkling of the forces within human nature, society, and psychiatry itself that would make reform in psychiatry seem beyond reach.

The New/Old Psychiatry

I had learned as a college student that love and care, and supporting the patient's self-determination, were the most effective elements in helping people, even in rehabilitating "lost souls" on the back wards of state mental hospitals. I also was learning that many of these inmates were simply homeless—disheartened poor people with no place to go. But after I entered my medical and psychiatric training, I would never hear another word about the importance of love in helping people

---

*The program proved so successful that I was able to convince psychologist Robert White, the chairman of the Department of Social Relations at Harvard, to turn our volunteer project into an official undergraduate course. It was probably the first time undergraduate students gained credit for a seminar in which they worked therapeutically with individual patients. Andy Morrison, who became a psychiatrist, led the experimental seminar as a college student.

through their helplessness and despair. Even supporting the patient's sense of self-determination and personal responsibility would rarely be mentioned. And problems of poverty and homelessness would be wholly ignored. Instead I was taught that the patients had "diseases," like schizophrenia, major depression, and manic-depression or bipolar affective disorder. They needed pills instead of people; shock instead of social reform.

The so-called revolution in psychiatry was beginning as early as 1963, when I began my first year of residency training at the Massachusetts Mental Health Center, where I was a teaching fellow at Harvard Medical School. I had gone there because of Harvard's reputation as a psychosocially oriented program with extensive one-to-one contact with patients and with psychologically oriented supervisors. But the program already was changing, and I was told that I could work with only one or two patients individually and that I would have only a limited amount of supervision in psychotherapy. By 1966, when I had finished my training and become a full-time consultant at the National Institute of Mental Health (NIMH), psychiatry was well on the way toward its wholesale conversion to biochemical and genetic theories and to technological interventions, such as drugs and electroshock.

Ironically, the "new psychiatry" was not at all new to me, because it resembled nothing so much as the old state mental hospital psychiatry, where patients were considered biologically and genetically defective and subjected to degrading, damaging treatments. Tragically, what was once the psychiatry for the poor—biopsychiatry—was now becoming the psychiatry for everyone.

In the past there had been a double standard. In the state hospitals and public clinics, the vast majority of patients had always been treated as objects, without concern for their feelings or for the human causes behind their helplessness and despair. They were blunted with drugs, insulin coma, electroshock, or lobotomy—the surgical mutilation of the highest centers of the brain. But a relatively small number of better-off people, especially those in major urban centers, sometimes received a more humane psychotherapy. Even though psychoanalysts never made up more than 10 percent of the profession, most educated people mistakenly equated psychiatry with psychoanalysis rather than with the always much more dominant biopsychiatry. Now the disparity between the rich and poor was being eradicated and everyone was being diagnosed with genetic aberrations and "biochemical imbalances" suitable for drugs or shock.

The Modern Psychiatrist

Many people continue to think of the psychiatrist as the wise, warm, and caring person who will help them tackle their problems. But the modern psychiatrist may have no interest in "talking therapy." His or her entire training and commitment is more likely devoted to "medical diagnosis" and "physical treatment." He or she may look at you with all the empathy and understanding of a pathologist staring through a microscope at germs, and then offer you a drug.

The same is true if you are seeking help for a member of your family, such as your elderly mother who's getting more difficult to care for at home, or your son who's become supposedly hyperactive, difficult, or uncomfortable in school. You may want advice on how to be more helpful to your mother or your son; but the psychiatrist will explain that their problems are biological and treatable with drugs, electroshock, or hospitalization. You may be relieved at the prospect of having the difficulty prescribed away by an expert. But beware—you are creating effects from which your mother or your child may never recover.

Because this may be hard for you to believe, let me put it another way. The next time you go to a psychiatrist, you may find yourself in the office of someone who has never been taught how to talk with you about your problems or those of your family. Nor has he or she been trained to understand personal and family conflicts. Instead the doctor will listen, make some observations, jot down some notes, make a medicalized diagnosis, and prescribe a physical treatment. He or she may even draw blood and listen to your heart. Not your metaphorical heart; your flesh and blood heart. But as we'll see, attempts to substitute physical interventions for human services often are doomed to cause more harm than good.

Recently, while teaching a seminar at a mental hospital, I asked the assembled psychiatrists, psychologists, social workers, and nurses if their recent training had dealt at all with the issue of caring about or loving their patients in the process of helping them heal. Among the fifty participants, only one person, a nurse, raised her hand.

The Decade of the Brain

President George Bush signed a congressional resolution declaring 1990 the first year of the Decade of the Brain. This has become psychiatry's main promotional theme, aimed at selling biological and hospital psychiatry to the public and at garnering more money for research into the brain as the seat of personal, social, educational, and political problems.

This new/old biopsychiatry has so taken over the profession that in some psychiatric training programs, such as Johns Hopkins University School of Medicine, psychotherapy is no longer a required course, and in most others it gets short shrift. As the medical and biological wing of the profession has taken over, compassionate psychologically oriented psychiatrists have been replaced by biochemists and lab researchers as department heads. Major journals devote nearly all their space to studies on the brains, blood, and urine of psychiatric patients—without so much as a passing mention of patients as people with thoughts and feelings relevant to their condition and their recovery.

People suffering from what used to be thought of as "neuroses" and "personal problems" are being treated with drugs and shock. Children with problems that once were handled by remedial education or improved parenting are instead being subjected to medical diagnoses, drugs, and hospitals. Old people who used to be cared for by their families are being drugged in nursing homes that find it more cost effective to provide a pill than a caring, stimulating environment. Increasing numbers of elderly women are being given electroshock.

Thus far the media have largely embraced and even promulgated the new biopsychiatric public relations line that many forms of human unhappiness are hereditary and best treated with drugs and shock and, in the future, genetic engineering. Dozens of mass-market books misinform the public that a "broken brain" or "biochemical imbalance" is responsible for personal unhappiness.

Yet the only biochemical imbalances that we can identify with certainty in the brains of psychiatric patients are the ones produced by psychiatric treatment itself.

Purging Psychiatry of Psychology and Psychotherapy

Some leading psychiatrists now propose to eliminate psychotherapy entirely from the basic training of psychiatrists, something that already has occurred in individual programs. At a 1987 symposium on "Training Psychiatrists for the 90s: Issues and Recommendations," Gary Tucker's presentation was dramatically entitled "Psychotherapy Will Not Be Central in Psychiatric Education." Tucker, an influential psychiatrist, applauded the general decline in teaching psychotherapy to young psychiatrists and came out flatly against teaching psychiatrists to be "expert in psychotherapy." He urged that "our residency training program curricula should reflect this newfound theoretical freedom from domination by the psychotherapeutic model."

In his presidential address to the Society for Biological Psychiatry, Wagner Bridger went so far as to declare that personality is in no way affected by childhood. In a report in the July 1989 *Clinical Psychiatry News** he declared, "There seems to be no relationship between early experience and adult outcome" in the human life cycle. According to Bridger, even a "horrible" parentless or institutionalized childhood has "no effect on later personality development." All that matters is genetic predisposition and current life influences. The past isn't prologue; it is nothing.

British psychiatry, if anything, has outpaced America in adopting bio-psychiatry as all of psychiatry. In the July 1983 *British Journal of Psychiatry*, B. A. Farrell surveyed "The Place of Psychodynamics in Psychiatry" and found that "mainstream" psychiatrists now believe that psychological approaches are of "no use" in their thinking or their actual work. The same is true in most European countries.

Popular books by psychiatrists promote the new anti-psychotherapy model of psychiatry. Nancy Andreasen helped formulate the American Psychiatric Association's (APA) official *Diagnostic and Statistical Manual of Mental Disorders* (DSM-III, 1980). In her popular 1984 book *The Broken Brain: The Biological Revolution in Psychiatry*, she writes, "*The major psychiatric illnesses are diseases*. They should be considered medical illnesses just as diabetes, heart disease, and cancer are" (p. 29). Later in the book she describes the ideal new psychiatrist as someone who no longer takes his or her time listening to patients' problems but who methodically asks questions to make a diagnosis, in the manner of an internist or neurologist. She offers convincing illustrations of brain scans allegedly demonstrating shrinkage in the brains of "schizophrenics" caused by their "mental illness."†

In *The New Psychiatry* (1985), psychiatrist Jerrold Maxmen confirms that "there has been a revolution in psychiatry" and that psychiatrists no longer concern themselves with what Freud or Jung had to say or with the nuances of various psychological theories. Meanwhile, he observes, the public still thinks of the psychiatrist as a psychotherapist, and "consequently, never before has the public had such outdated views of what modern psychiatrists think and do" (p. 14).

Donald W. Goodwin warns in *Anxiety* (1986) that talking therapies

---

* Page numbers for quotations have not been cited if the quotes are from specific articles or book chapters where they may be located with relative ease. Where they are from books, page numbers will usually be provided in the text or in endnotes. To avoid cluttering the text, articles are usually cited by month and year.

† We shall find that drugs are usually the cause of shrinkage in the brains of schizophrenics (chapter 4).

are of little value and that psychotherapy can make "people feel worse; talking about the problems reminds them of them" (p. 107). This is not the reaction of an embittered patient who rejects self-understanding, but a professional pronouncement by a professor and department chair of psychiatry.

In *The Good News About Depression* (1987), psychiatrist Mark Gold declares that if you're feeling upset or depressed, "you need not wait. The biopsychiatric approach has become *the* way at many of the best psychiatric centers in the country" (p. 25).

Lewis Judd, psychiatrist and outgoing director of NIMH, traveled the country before his departure lecturing to lay and professional audiences about the miracles of biopsychiatry. Claiming that 15 percent of Americans have mental illness at any one time and that more than 20 percent will suffer from it eventually, he declared that "neuroscience" has the answers. Speaking to the American Psychiatric Association in 1990, he said, as if a fact, "There are genes that code for specific illnesses, and we intend to find them." He explained how psychiatry is now "neuroscience" and how the future efforts of NIMH would focus on brain research.

In another talk, to the Southern California Psychiatric Society on April 28, 1990, Judd stated that most psychiatric disorders are proven physical diseases and that psychiatry already has "a very good understanding of the genetics" and "pathophysiology" of manic-depressive disorder. He showed brain scans that allegedly pinpoint the source of depression in a patient's brain. In regard to anxiety or panic disorder, he declared, "We now know exactly where it comes from" in the brain. Even obsessive-compulsive disorder has a known "pathophysiology," according to Judd, who pointed to specific parts of the brain that are disordered. He claimed that psychiatry already possesses "superb models" for the "molecular genetics" of mental disorders. Finally, in the fall of 1990 an extensive advertising supplement for the Decade of the Brain was placed in major newspapers. Speaking of mental disorders, Judd says, "Two decades of research have shown that these are diseases and illnesses like any other diseases and illnesses. They just happen to involve the brain." The supplement, paid for by the National Foundation for Brain Research and assisted by NIMH, states that 20 percent of Americans suffer from these supposed diseases, a veritable epidemic of physical illness.

Is it possible that these claims have no basis in fact and that the entire promotional campaign is nothing more than that—a promotional campaign? We shall examine these questions in depth.

Psychiatrists in Despair

Sensitive, caring students are increasingly reluctant to enter psychiatry, and some already in the profession are dropping out. A young resident in psychiatry recently told me how she tried to refuse to give electroshock, only to be challenged by her department chairman, "Then why did you go into psychiatry?" She gave the treatment rather than be fired. Another young psychiatrist explained to me how he lost his job in a clinic because he refused to give everyone drugs. An older psychiatrist has told me the same thing.

One of my psychiatric colleagues—a "talking doctor" like myself—tells me, "I wouldn't do it over again. No, if I knew where psychiatry was going, I'd never have become a psychiatrist." To avoid daily confrontations with the new psychiatry, he has withdrawn from the academic community to the isolation of his private practice. Another psychiatrist spoke even more directly through his actions: he "retired" twenty years ahead of time and changed careers. He couldn't stand what's become of the profession. Still another colleague, who continues to teach psychiatric residents, explained to me, "They have changed. Young physicians going into psychiatry are more aloof, less caring, less involved with people." This confirms my own impression of the residents I occasionally instruct. They are very threatened by any suggestion that their patients suffer from psychosocial problems and that physical treatments might do more harm than good.

In the February 1988 *American Journal of Psychiatry*, Morton Reiser asks in his title, "Are Psychiatric Educators 'Losing the Mind'?" Reiser complains that opportunities for young psychiatrists to develop psychotherapy know-how are rapidly disappearing. He warns psychiatric educators not to give up the mind or to lose it by default to other mental health professionals.

In the September 1989 *Clinical Psychiatry News*, Lothar Goldschmidt laments that "opening any psychiatric journal of our time is like opening a textbook of chemistry," and "psychiatrists to a large extent have given up practicing psychotherapy and addressing themselves to emotional problems." Psychiatrists are not trained in the humanities or "even in basic psychology." He writes, "Residents in psychiatry know close to nothing about various fields that have contributed to our understanding of the human mind."

We have the opportunity to witness these changes in American psychiatry through the ideas of a psychiatric Rip van Winkle. Marcio Vasconcellos Pinheiro became a board-certified psychiatrist after sixteen years in the Baltimore area and then returned to his native Brazil in 1974. In 1987, a little more than a decade later, he returned to the United States to find psychiatry drastically changed. In the November 1989 *Psychiatry*, he wrote a viewpoint entitled "U.S.A., 13 Years Later".

Since I returned to the U.S.A. I have come across a whole new generation of psychiatrists, coming from the best medical schools, who are unable to pay attention to their patients' subjective worlds. They have been trained to look at people's outsides: behavior is what counts, in the best American, mechanistic, pragmatic tradition. In my opinion, American psychiatry, while considering itself more scientific, has returned to the unfortunate attitudes of the pre-Freudian days. . . . My hope is that, sooner or later, the distortions I perceive will be corrected and priorities will again be set placing people as the main consideration.

If you are educated in the humanities or have read a few good self-help psychology books, and if you like to think about yourself and others, you may have more insight into personal growth than your psychiatrist does; and if you've taken a few college courses or read a little in academic psychology or psychoanalysis, you might know more theory as well. If you've also shared feelings and personal problems with some of your friends, then you may well have more experience and practice in "talking therapy" than your psychiatrist.

On the other hand, your psychiatrist will have more power than you. He or she can prescribe drugs or shock, lock you up against your will, talk behind your back with your husband, wife, or parents and make plans for your future without consulting you. As a medical expert in malpractice and patients' rights suits, I have dealt with numerous cases of individuals who sought psychiatric help for routine problems in living, such as sadness over the loss of a loved one, only to find themselves swept along the path of biopsychiatry, ending up with permanent brain dysfunction and damage from drugs and shock treatment.

The Future

What will happen to the well-being and values of Americans if the 1990s become not the Decade of the Human Spirit and the Human Community but the Decade of the Brain?

- Parents and teachers increasingly will surrender their responsibility for the care and education of children to mental health professionals when problems arise at home or at school.
- Millions of children will end up on "legal" drugs or in psychiatric hospitals.

- Untold numbers of children and adults will be saddled with the false conviction that they have genetic defects and lifelong "crossed wires" and "biochemical imbalances."
- Innumerable adults with solvable personal problems will end up taking drugs, getting shock treatment, or being locked up in mental hospitals—or all three.
- Many millions of elderly people will be drugged and shocked into oblivion and hurried to a premature death, often while residing in nursing homes.
- Psychiatrists will make renewed calls for an increase in lobotomy and other forms of psychosurgery.
- Droves of homeless people will be corralled into revamped, but still dreadful, state mental hospitals.
- Organized psychiatry increasingly will become dominated by the interests of the multi-billion-dollar pharmaceutical industry as the profession becomes wholly dependent on the drug companies for its survival.
- Several million more Americans will suffer permanent brain damage from psychiatric drugs and electroshock while the profession denies that it is happening.

In fact, all of these things are going on right now. Yet how could this happen with so little awareness on the public's part? How could professionals devote themselves to such destructive programs with so little apparent concern for the truth or the rights and well-being of their patients?

Confronting Psychiatric Reality

When I first decided to become a psychiatrist, I thought that the maltreatment of patients in the state mental hospitals was an aberration within the profession—something that well-intentioned professionals ultimately could reform. Then in the early 1970s I became appalled by the return of lobotomy and newer forms of psychosurgery, and I organized an international campaign against the new wave of brain mutilation.[2] I hoped that many of my colleagues would rally against the large-scale surgical blunting and subduing of mental patients. However, when I appealed to the profession to do something about the resurgence of psychosurgery, I found almost unified opposition to any critical self-examination. I ended up devoting years to working on my own with the U.S. Congress, state legislatures, the courts, the media, psychiatric survivor groups, a few other professionals, and the general public. While I was able to prevent the wholesale return of psychiatric surgery, the experience left me with increasingly grave questions about my profession.

17

In trying to understand psychiatry's refusal to be accountable for the damaging effects of psychiatric brain surgery, I began to realize that lobotomy differs little in principle from the most potent psychiatric drugs and from electroshock. All of the major psychiatric treatments work by producing brain dysfunction, and too often they result in lobotomylike effects and permanent damage. I discovered that biopsychiatry resists criticism of any one of its theories and physical interventions because all of them rest upon the same flawed principles and harmful practices.

Part I of this book, " 'Schizophrenic' Overwhelm and Neuroleptic Drugs," will discuss the nature of so-called madness, its treatment by psychiatry, and the damaging effects of "antipsychotic" drugs on the brain and mind. In part II, " 'Depressive' and 'Manic-Depressive' Overwhelm, Antidepressants, Lithium, and Electroshock," we will examine the causes of depression and so-called bipolar disorder, and their treatment. In part III, " 'Anxiety' Overwhelm and the Minor Tranquilizers," we shall discuss panic attacks, phobias, obsessive-compulsive disorders, addictions, and eating disorders, and their treatment. In part IV, "Women, Children, the Homeless, and the Psycho-Pharmaceutical Complex," we shall document how the psychiatric monopoly abuses our most vulnerable citizens, including the widespread diagnosing, drugging, and hospitalizing of youngsters. Finally, part V, "Psychosocial Alternatives," will present caring, successful human service approaches to helping patients with a full range of difficulties, from problems in living to severe emotional upsets labeled psychotic. In addition to chapter 16, which is devoted to psychosocial approaches, there will be many opportunities along the way to contrast useful and humane alternatives to those of biopsychiatry.

Part I

"Schizophrenic" Overwhelm and Neuroleptic Drugs

Chapter 2

Understanding the Passion of "Schizophrenic" Overwhelm

The moment a man begins to question the meaning and value of life he is sick.
                    —*Sigmund Freud (1937)*

Neurosis and psychosis are modes of expression for human beings who have lost courage.
                    —*Alfred Adler (1870–1937)*

The socially visible characteristic of the psychotic person is that he becomes a stranger among his own people.
                    —*Joint Commission on Mental Illness and Health (1961)*

An elderly black woman at St. Elizabeths, a local state mental hospital, was refusing to take her psychiatric drugs, and her attorney sought my help in gaining her release. During my interview with her, she told me, "I won't take those devilish pills. You can't doctor a soul with pills." I made a note to tell the judge that her position was reasonable for a religious person to take. She might have a legal right to refuse medication under the hospital's own rules in support of religious objections.

She next told me, "They want to force me to take drugs to make an example for the other patients. I show the other patients they shouldn't take those terrible pills. That's why they're trying to force drugs into my body —to shut up my mouth."

Her attorney agreed that she was indeed being made an example. So again, nothing was far-out about her remarks.

"Them doctors, they never treat no one with no respect," the woman said.

My experience with inhuman conditions in state hospitals confirmed what she was saying. I nodded once more.

Then, in a hushed and confidential voice, she said, "The staff, they don't want to believe that *I'm God*. But I am. They'll see. I'll have my revenge. An eye for an eye, like I said in the Bible."

In a flash, I saw her losing her case in court. She'd never cover up her true feelings, even if winning her case, or saving her very life, depended on it. As much as I still believed in her right to refuse toxic psychiatric drugs, the judge would dismiss her protests the moment she announced that God was sitting in the witness chair.

The seemingly deranged person's preoccupations, even when they aren't so overtly religious, typically focus on his or her place in the universe, often in an exalted or at least central role that seems highly unrealistic. This is an aspect of what I mean by the *spiritual* focus of what becomes labeled schizophrenia—its attempt to deal with the largest problems of personal identity and the meaning in life.

People diagnosed schizophrenic often seem in crisis over the meaning of their lives and their personal identities. At the same time, they seem to think irrationally and to act ineffectively. Frequently they have stopped taking care of their basic survival needs for food or safe shelter. When someone threatens to lock them up in a mental hospital, they often escalate the very communications that are getting them in trouble. In the end they may not be able to escape dependency on their parents or to keep themselves out of a locked ward.

Angela, a woman in her thirties, was seeing me for a medical consultation because she had a devastating neurological disorder produced by psychiatric drugs. The hospital records and her family made clear that Angela was at one time very disturbed, but that in recent years she'd been free of so-called hallucinations and delusions. During her interview with me, she showed signs of brain damage from the drugs, such as inappropriate laughing, rambling, and difficulty focusing her attention; but she said nothing that sounded "crazy."

As we were finishing the consultation, Angela mentioned that she watched television a great deal.

"Well, I'll be appearing on a local talk show tomorrow, so don't be surprised if you see me."

"Oh, that's nice," she said, "but please don't say anything to me while you're on the TV."

"Don't worry, I would never do that," I reassured her.

"Why wouldn't you talk to me on the TV?" Angela retorted. "Dan Rather and all the others do. Everybody knows it: you watch the television and the television watches you."

Because she trusted me, Angela let slip her beliefs or fantasies about her personal relationship to the TV. She had covered them up with other doctors, not because the medication "helped" her, but because she wanted to keep from being drugged against her will.

Biological psychiatrists—nowadays *most* psychiatrists—are fond of saying "You can't talk to disease." The communications of so-called schizophrenics make no sense at all to these doctors who want to control "symptoms," such as hallucinations and delusions, with drugs, electroshock, and incarceration.

The idea that these extremes of irrationality are due to a disease is inseparable from the survival of psychiatry as a profession. If schizophrenia is not a disease, psychiatry would have little justification for using its more devastating treatments. Lobotomy, electroshock, and all of the more potent drugs, including the neuroleptics and even lithium, were developed at the expense of locked-up people, most of whom were labeled schizophrenic. The search for biochemical and genetic causes keeps psychiatrists, as medical doctors, in the forefront of well-funded research in the field. The notion that patients have "sick brains" justifies psychiatry's unique power to treat them against their will. It also bolsters psychiatry's claim to the top of the mental health hierarchy. In short, if irrationality isn't biological, then psychiatry loses much of its rationale for existence as a *medical* specialty.

"60 Minutes" Dramatizes Psychospirituality in "Schizophrenics"

On July 27, 1986, "60 Minutes" produced a show entitled "Schizophrenia." It was based on biopsychiatric theories, and one of their experts declared, "We know it's a brain disease now. It's like multiple sclerosis, Alzheimer's disease." On the show, vignettes of patients were presented to impress the audience with the bizarre quality of their communications, and hence the absurdity of any psychological meaning or underpinning to their "disease."

The first "60 Minutes" patient, Brugo, bolsters his identity with spirituality, as well as religion, and declares that he's "not extinct": "And I'm Croatian Hebrew, which is Adam and Eve's kin. And I have been Croatian Hebrew for centuries and cent—upon centuries. And I'm a Herto-erectus man, and I'm also part Neanderthal, and I mean to keep that heritage, 'cause I'm not extinct."

Packed into these few remarks is symbolism about his desperate need for personal value and dignity, his identification with religion and humanity, and perhaps his awareness of primitive impulses stirring inside himself, as well as his fear of personal extinction. Here is more than enough material to stimulate anyone's desire to communicate with him.

The second patient, Jim, is dismissed by the interviewer because he is "convinced he was shot to death when he was a baby." Yet his brief remarks seem like a metaphor for child sexual abuse by a male: "I had my head blown off with a shotgun when I was two years old. And—and before that, things happened in my crib. I remember all these things and stuff, but I just remember, you know. I remember all this stuff."

A therapist with experience in listening to people immediately would wonder about what lies behind Jim's direct hints about terrifying memories from early childhood, not to mention the symbolism of the crib in relation to his present trapped condition. More than one patient of mine has begun with just such anguished fragments of memory before discovering the agony of his or her abusive childhood and its relationship to current entrapments.

Another "60 Minutes" patient, Ronnie, clearly is struggling with his own identity and his separateness or isolation from other people. He, too, talks in psychospiritual terms, again with undertones of possible sexual abuse: "I thought everybody's bodies was connected to mine, and their—their spirits were—I was—I was laying in bed and I played—you know how we live, where, you know, like you're smashing some air for yourself? Well, like, I was smashing every spirit next to me, and the—all kind of bad things were happening."

Still another patient, Lynn, directly identifies herself with God and with being "different," and clearly tells us that her "wisdom" is more than she can handle. She's practically inviting us to ask her about the inner knowledge she cannot bear: "I've got the wisdom of God in me, and I have to learn how to cope with it. Nobody seems to think you're supposed to survive when you're different. [*Crying*] But I know—as—like the words in Job said, all I can say was, 'Have pity on me, my friends. I've been touched by the hand of God.' "

Brain Disease or Psychospiritual Crisis?

The patients' quotes were selected by "60 Minutes" to demonstrate that so-called schizophrenia is a biochemical disease rather than a crisis of thinking, feeling, and meaning. Yet people with real brain disease—such as Alzheimer's, stroke, or a tumor—don't talk symbolically like these people do.

Instead of metaphors laced with meaning, brain-damaged people typically display memory difficulties as the first sign that their mind isn't working as well as it once did. They have trouble recalling recently learned things, like names, faces, telephone numbers, or lists. Later they may get confused and disoriented as they display what is called an organic brain syndrome. In fact—and this is very important—advanced degrees of brain disease render the individual unable to think in such abstract or metaphorical terms. The thought processes that get labeled schizophrenia require higher mental function and therefore a relatively intact brain. No matter how bizarre the ideas may seem, they necessitate symbolic and often abstract thinking. That's why lobotomy "works": the damage to the higher mental centers smashes the capacity to express existential pain and anguish.* As we'll find out, it's also why the most potent psychiatric drugs and shock treatment have their effect.

Objects or Beings?

How are we to approach people who get labeled schizophrenic? Do we think of them as troubled humans struggling in a self-defeating style with profound psychological and spiritual issues, usually involving their basic worth or identity? Or do we view them as if they are afflicted with physical diseases, like multiple sclerosis and Alzheimer's disease, in which their feelings, thoughts, anguishes, and aspirations play no role? Do we try to *understand* them, or do we try to physically *fix* them? Do we look for profound hurts and failed psychospiritual efforts in their lives, or for biochemical aberrations in their brains? Do we wonder about what meanings and values they are seeking—and how they became so helplessly mired down in the process—or do we search for the biochemical imbalances that have twisted their brain processes?

If people who express seemingly irrational ideas are best understood mechanistically, then these people are broken, disordered, or defective devices. If we take the viewpoint that they are persons, beings, or souls in struggle, then an infinite variety of more subtle possibilities comes to mind for understanding and helping those who seem mad, crazy, or deranged.

If we are beings rather than devices, then our most severe emotional and spiritual crises originate within ourselves, our families, and our society. Our crises can be understood as conflicts or confusion about our identities, values, and aspirations rather than as biological aberrations. And as self-determining human beings, we can work toward overcoming those feelings of helplessness generated by our past spiritual and social defeats.

---

*In volume two of the 1959 *American Handbook of Psychiatry* lobotomist Walter Freeman writes:

What the investigator misses the most in the more highly intelligent individuals is the ability to introspect, to speculate, to philosophize, especially in regard to the self. . . . Creativeness seems to be the highest form of human endeavor. It requires imagination, concentration, visualization, self-criticism, and persistence in the face of frustration, as well as trained manual dexterity. . . . On the whole, psychosurgery reduces creativity, sometimes to the vanishing point. (Pp. 1526, 1534, 1535)

By contrast, the typical modern psychiatrist—by disposition, training, and experience—is wholly unprepared to understand anyone's psychospiritual crisis. With drugs and shock treatment, the psychiatrist instead *attacks* the subjective experience of the person and blunts or destroys the very capacity to be sensitive and aware. No wonder the treatment of mental patients often looks more like a war against them. It often is.

Psychospirituality Combined with Helplessness

The notion of madness or derangement has many connotations, mostly negative, such as grandiosity, emotional extremism, willfulness, irresponsibility, and irrationality. Yet we also associate these people with sensitivity, creativity, and prophetic preoccupations with the meaning of life. They often express passionate, painful emotion through psychological or spiritual metaphors wrapped in symbolic elements of suffering and martyrdom. From the ancient Greeks and Hebrews to modern times, "mad" people have been viewed as endowed with special psychospiritual, creative qualities. We know that many great minds have suffered, endured, or perhaps even drawn their creativity from what others call their madness.

I have chosen the word *psychospiritual* to denote the special awareness and concerns of people who get such diagnoses as schizophrenia, bipolar or manic-depressive disorder, and major depression. The word is similar in meaning to "psychological" before it acquired a more mechanical, pseudoscientific definition in modern times. The 1856 *Webster's Dictionary* defines psychology as the study of "the human soul or the doctrine of man's spiritual nature." By psychospiritual I mean pertaining to the self, identity, or personality of the individual, including his or her striving to live a better, more fulfilling or meaningful life. I intend no specifically religious connotation. The emphasis is on the human tendency to live by principles and ideals—however rational or irrational, and however loving or loveless, these may seem to be to others.

So-called schizophrenics, especially during their initial crisis, almost always are preoccupied with the meaning of life, God, love, and their own personal identity, often with cataclysmic implications about the end of the world or the disintegration of their own personalities. I recall one of the first people diagnosed schizophrenic whom I treated. She was a young, recently married woman from a sexually oppressive background. Unable to bear her feelings when touched by her husband, she believed instead that she'd been physically touched by the hand of God while praying in church. In our talks she was overcome by doubts of whether she was a sinner or a saint. Such burning psychospirituality involves a search for the meaning of one's own life, and often it is fueled by overwhelming feelings of guilt, shame, or anxiety.

In those people labeled "chronic schizophrenic," their psychospiritual preoccupations become lifelong, with seemingly irrational beliefs coexisting alongside unusually perceptive insights. They may grow increasingly helpless and lapse into vague feelings of being persecuted. Over time, the beliefs can lose their vigor and originality and become compulsive and routine. However, we shall find that with or without treatment most people labeled schizophrenic tend to improve over the years and to lose their overt symptoms.

Being Labeled

How is it that some spiritually passionate people become labeled schizophrenic and find themselves being treated as mental patients? How is it that a spiritual crisis becomes diagnosed as a disease? The outcome depends greatly on the cultural setting. In Russia, for example, political dissidents are diagnosed as "sluggish schizophrenia" and then locked up and drugged.[1] In most Western countries, however, the diagnosis usually is determined more by one's lack of personal power and self-determination, often as reflected in homelessness, than by one's political convictions. It also is determined by the tolerance for deviance among one's family, friends, associates, or local authorities.

Most people who get labeled psychotic have failed to take charge of their mental processes in a rational way or failed to live important aspects of their lives effectively. Frequently the stubborn repetition of bizarre ideas gets them into terrible trouble. When confronted about their failure to take control of their minds or their lives, they compulsively reiterate their most irrational positions, such as "I can't stop the radio waves from giving me these feelings" or "The space people are talking to me on the intercom at work." Often great efforts must be made to convince, encourage, or help them to take care of simple everyday needs, such as eating, bathing, or remembering to make a phone call. In everyday language, they often seem grossly irresponsible; but more specifically, they lack the ability or willingness to control or determine the course of their lives. They typically lack self-control and self-determination in regard to their mental processes and their actions. Often they feel that they are evil and worthless, thus encouraging self-neglect.

This combination of psychospiritual passion and overwhelming helplessness is characteristic of almost all of the people we tend to label mad, crazy, or insane, including people diagnosed by psychiatrists as psychotic, schizophrenic, manic-depressive, or even severely anxious or depressed. Each is an example of *psychological overwhelm* or, at the least, hazardous stumbling along life's path.

Anton Boisen's Spiritual Crisis

In 1920 Anton Boisen underwent a severe emotional crisis and psychiatric hospitalization, then went on to devote himself to writing and to reform work. His book *The Exploration of the Inner World: A Study of Mental Disorder and Religious Experience* (University of Pennsylvania Press, 1971), first published in 1936, remains one of the most original and profound ever written on the subject of madness.

As a young man Boisen experienced "a violent delirium" filled with "a terrifying idea about a coming world catastrophe." Ahead of his time, he attributed the coming disaster not merely to a revelation of "strange and mysterious forces of evil," but also to abuse of the world's natural resources. Boisen displayed the typical extravagant extremes of self-evaluation and identity found in madness: "I myself was more important than I had ever dreamed of being: I was also a zero quantity."

He was diagnosed as "catatonic dementia praecox," an older term for schizophrenia, and his family was told that his case was hopeless. But after three weeks of terror and overwhelm in which he lost thirty pounds, "Then I came out of it much as one awakens out of a bad dream." He felt as if he had descended into one world and abruptly come out into another; and like so many others, he brought back new spiritual awareness with him, while getting no help whatsoever from the organicist, or biological psychiatrist.

The doctors did not believe in talking with patients about their symptoms, which they assumed to be rooted in some as yet undiscovered organic difficulty. (P. 5)

Unchanged in mainstream psychiatry since 1920, and indeed since 1820, is the way in which biopsychiatrists have continually predicted a soon-to-be-found biological origin of personal distress.

Spiritual Triumph or Spiritual Defeat

Boisen was discharged and eventually returned as a chaplain to do research on madness in psychiatric hospitals. To understand "how the situation looks from the point of view of the individual himself," he recorded and categorized the communications of 179 hospitalized patients.

Most of the patients expressed a profound sense of the "mysterious" in life, probably due to "some eruption of the subconscious which is interpreted as a manifestation of the supernatural." Boisen found that "very commonly it is as if the conscious self had descended to some lower region where it is no longer in control but at the mercy of primitive and terrifying ideas and imagery which throng upon it." Under these pressures, a new psychospiritual "solution" was "inevitable."

Boisen's view of madness is very close to William James's view of the mystical religious experience. James believed that mysticism was an expression of the deepest personal yearnings reaching toward unity with a Higher Power. The famous American philosopher and psychologist recorded his observations in *The Varieties of Religious Experience* (1902) two decades before Boisen's mystical madness.

Boisen's patients also endured a sense of "peril," often with a premonition of some great, impending world change, usually a disaster. Frequently they anticipated playing a key role in these earthshaking events. Equally often, the peril originated from something threatening to erupt from within. These two themes—the mysterious and the perilous—are the stuff of a psychospiritual journey.

But the journey in each case had led to overwhelm and helplessness and these failed prophets tended to shift blame or responsibility away from themselves. Many heard accusing voices. Others believed they were influenced or controlled by outside forces, such as electrical currents.

For Boisen, there wasn't any fundamental difference between these patients and the "religious genius" that had been dear to him in his education and reading.

Who am I? Why am I in this world? What's the matter? What is going to happen to me and to my friends? How can I save the situation? How can I make atonement for my mistakes and sins? How can I bring about a realization of the possibilities that ought to be? These are generally the questions in the focus of attention both in hospital experiences and in those of the men of religious genius. Probably those questions are central in any philosophy of life. (P. 80)

For the person in psychospiritual crisis, "Philosophy and theology are no longer theoretical and abstract problems. They are matters of life and death." The "psychotic" episodes are radical explorations of solutions to severe identity threats: "The sufferer is facing what for him are the great and abiding issues of life and death and of his own relationship with the universe."

Boisen means what he says—that it is wrong to think of these experiences as illnesses. "The fact that a person hears voices indicates that the deeper levels of the mental life are stirred," he tells us. "This in itself is neither good nor bad. Paul of Tarsus heard a voice on the road to Damascus and that fact is hardly to be regretted" (p. 311).

Even though the patients had trouble taking care of themselves from day to day, Boisen rejected demeaning them with diagnoses. The issue is one of "spiritual defeat and spiritual victory." This is the key to Boisen's lesson for us: a psychospiritual crisis that fails to resolve creatively is not an illness, but a spiritual defeat.

Biopsychiatry, with its use of mind-blunting techniques, almost guarantees defeat. Had Boisen himself been hospitalized a decade later in the 1930s, after the advent of the various shock therapies and lobotomy, he probably would have been crushed by routine psychiatric treatment. Today, the neuroleptics or electroshock would abruptly terminate his search into the meaning of his confusion and despair, leaving him dulled and confused.

Boisen's book received little attention within psychiatry. Although many of his articles were published in *Psychiatry* and elsewhere over several decades,[2] they had no significant impact. Acceptance of a psychospiritual approach would have put much of psychiatry out of business. It still would.

Nonetheless, approaches to schizophrenia as a spiritual crisis continue to surface occasionally in the psychiatric literature. In the December 1971 *Archives of General Psychiatry*, Arthur Deikman describes the so-called schizophrenic person as a failed mystic:

Both mystical and psychotic states have arisen out of a situation in which the individual has struggled with a desperate problem, has come to a complete impasse, and given up hope, abandoned the struggle in despair. For the mystic, what emerges from the "cloud of unknowing" or the "dark night of the soul" is an ecstatic union with God or Reality. For the psychotic person, the world rushes in but does not become integrated in the harmony of *mystico unio* or *satori*. Instead, he creates a delusion to achieve a partial ordering or control.

R. D. Laing and "The Politics of Experience"

In *The Politics of Experience* (1967), psychiatrist R. D. Laing gave madness a ringing endorsement and heaped criticism on organized psychiatry.

According to Laing, "schizophrenics have more to teach psychiatrists about the inner world than psychiatrists their patients." To paraphrase him: the mad are inarticulate poets; psychiatrists are articulate know-nothings.

Mad persons are victims of a corrupt upbringing: "Behavior that gets labeled schizophrenic is *a special strategy that a person invented in order to live in an unlivable situation*" (p. 115). What's wrong is not "in the patient," but in his family and in society. The problem is also in the psychiatrist who diagnoses and treats the patient, thereby increasing his or her confusion and self-doubt. If guided with kindness and understanding the schizophrenic experience could become a transcendental journey of death and rebirth toward a new, more positive meaning in life: "Madness need not be all breakdown. It may also be breakthrough. It is potentially liberation and renewal as well as enslavement and existential death" (p. 133).

Laing had much to say of worth in his early work, but he romanticized people who get labeled schizophrenic by largely ignoring the psychological overwhelm and helplessness undergone by many of them. Often the journey into the unconscious takes place by default. Overwhelmed by their past and present life, their identity or selfhood shatters, they fail to distinguish between inner and outer, dream and reality. Whether or not there is an element of conscious choice in taking these psychospiritual leaps usually is impossible to tell; but the great question is, "How hard will he or she work to make something creative out of the experience?" Tragically, antipsychotic drugs and electroshock may prove too drastic a handicap, as psychological helplessness is compounded by brain dysfunction.

Separating the Crazy from the Sane

My friend Sarah was sitting in church one day when a young man burst into the middle of the sermon and howled, "The church is a whore!" The helpless fellow was dragged off to the local mental hospital, while Sarah sat still, thinking, "He's right! But I've been afraid to say it!" One person's schizophrenia is another's revelation.

Many people go through terrible periods of psychospiritual overwhelm before going on to new levels of living. Albert Schweitzer comes to mind. After World War I he became seriously despondent and was called depressed, and then went on to a renewed dedication to both his jungle hospital and his philosophy. Eventually he wrote eloquently of his central theme—reverence for life. Walter Freeman, a psychiatrist who performed five thousand lobotomies,* also described going through a deep despondency as a young physician, but he came out lobotomizing people.[3] He would write with eloquence about how mental patients were better off without so much brain function. During a taped interview in the archives of the American Psychiatric Association Library, Freeman is asked about criticism of his mentor, Egas Moniz, who lobotomized Portuguese state hospital patients. With a wry laugh, Freeman quips, "Oh, there's plenty of Portuguese." On spiritual journeys, there's no guarantee of the quality of the outcome. As my friend Leonard Frank has reminded me, there's no way to label Freeman's victims "insane" or "irresponsible" while exonerating the dean of lobotomy as "sane" and "responsible."

Passion of Everyday Life

Psychoanalyst and psychiatrist Robert Seidenberg has pointed out to me that many experiences that may seem psychotic are readily accepted by the public, including reports of prolonged encounters with extraterrestrials, out-of-body experiences, and recollections of prior lives. He himself believes that these are unconscious expressions of what Freud called "primary process" thinking and that so-called schizophrenics learn this way of thinking from their parents.

It's clear that the line between what gets called psychotic and more accepted human experiences is thin and that it is moving all the time. Indeed, the distinction has nothing to do with medical or psychiatric diagnosis. People get labeled when they become helplessly overwhelmed by their psychospiritual passions or when they become troublesome or when they run afoul of the authorities.

Romantic love, for example, has much in common with what clinicians call mental illness, leading many to conclude that passionate lovers are crazy people. In *Sexuality and Medicine,* edited by Earl Shelp (1987),

---

*Freeman provided this figure in a telephone conversation with me in approximately 1970. Later I was asked to be the expert witness in the first malpractice suit against him, but he died before it could be completed. A letter written by Freeman to the patient in the suit warned her to go to a hospital, because in checking on his postlobotomy patients around the country, he found that many of them had committed suicide. He never published those observations. The patient in this case suffered from severe dementia—the global loss of intellectual and emotional functioning—as a result of Freeman's lobotomy. Freeman—who used an ice pick inserted through the eye sockets—would mutilate many patients in one day as he swung through various state hospitals. He did not use sterile technique, and he sometimes showed off by stabbing the patient through both eye sockets at once with an ice pick in each hand. Not a pariah among his colleagues, he was awarded honors and was director of neurology and psychiatry at George Washington University in the District of Columbia.

my chapter on sexual dysfunction as a spiritual disorder cities the opinions of professionals who demean love by equating it to insanity. In the 1980 edition of his *Principles of Clinical Psychiatry*, for example, psychiatrist Arnold Ludwig systematically compares romantic love, which he calls "love mania," to other forms of so-called mental illness. Freud thought that love was an aberrant expression of narcissism and warned against indulging in it. William James labeled romantic love a "monomania" and wrote clinical vignettes that ridiculed it. Yet, as already noted, James's descriptions of a mystical union with God often sound exactly like falling in love or going mad.

Anger and Rebellion

People undergoing psychospiritual crisis—romantic love, adolescence, the peak experiences described by Abraham Maslow, religious ecstasy, and mysticism—are frequently rebellious and sometimes revolutionary. They commonly find themselves in conflict with one or another authority, from parents and police to religious and educational institutions. This happens because they frequently tend to put their immediate spiritual needs and priorities above the demands of authority, and because they often handle their conflicts with authority in an ineffective, self-defeating, or helpless manner.

Rebelliousness often involves conduct that seems irresponsible by conventional standards. Where passionate, spirited encounters with the meaning of life take place, ordinary concepts of responsibility often get left behind. Sometimes it seems as if people must temporarily reject or throw off responsibility in the process of reaching new plateaus. That they become exceedingly difficult to live with does not make them "mentally ill" or diseased.

The comparison to romantic passion is, again, striking. Romeo and Juliet, for example, defy the authority of their feuding families, and they pay the price when they prove incapable of organizing their escape. Yet the moral of the story is that love transcends clannish prejudices and eventually unites the feuding families. Romeo and Juliet's ideal of love survives beyond their deaths.

People often are labeled schizophrenic during their teen years. Adolescence, with its struggle to form identity in the face of unleashed passions, easily gets called "mental illness." Whether adolescents become labeled mentally ill often depends mostly on the love, patience, and tolerance of the adults who surround them.

After passionate people get psychiatrically labeled, they become especially vulnerable to defeat and disaster. Psychiatrists commonly force treatment on them, then claim that they must be "mentally ill," because they resent and resist being diagnosed and treated.

The Family

Overt outrage and hatred toward their parents is a frequent characteristic of most people who get labeled crazy. Often they attack their parents emotionally, and frequently their communications portray their parents in a seemingly irrational fashion as agents of the devil, the FBI, or other feared authorities. With obvious metaphorical meaning, they literally may describe seeing horns growing out of their parents' heads.

In turn, the parents too often tend to reject responsibility for their children's emotional anguish. This phenomenon may well explain the positions taken by the National Alliance for the Mentally Ill (NAMI), a national organization of 100,000 parents of disturbed offspring, whose informal rallying cry can be characterized as "We are not to blame." NAMI supports genetic and biological research, involuntary treatment, state hospitals, drugs, and electroshock. It attempts to stop federal funding for psychosocial investigations of schizophrenia. It also tries to muzzle advocates of the psychosocial position. In two cases I am aware of, professionals with opposing views have been met with harassment, attacks on their jobs, and disruptive activities when speaking publicly.

By trying to exonerate themselves of responsibility for the emotional suffering of their children, by supporting the most oppressive biopsychiatric technologies, and by attempting to crush dissent, NAMI has become an institutional embodiment of the kind of parents who can drive a child into helpless despair.

The alleged motive for this, of course, is "It's for your own good." But as Alice Miller describes in her book *For Your Own Good* (1984), many mad people have been physically, sexually, and emotionally abused within their families. As we shall see in chapter 14, "Suppressing the Passion of Women," Freud knew, but ran from, the truth that most of his female patients had been sexually abused. And in the chapters on children and on women, we'll look more specifically at how child abuse affects later life.

The families of mad people often frustrate progress toward selfhood being made by their children. Therapists who deal with these families often feel the need to work together in teams to preserve their own emotional stability. In *Schizophrenia and the Family* (1965), Theodore Lidz, Stephen Fleck, and Alice Cornelison describe how these families often sabotage the therapy process, as if fearing the maturation and ultimate departure of their offspring.

A series of British studies in the 1970s showed that relapses among patients labeled schizophrenic were related to "Expressed Emotion," or EE—the intensity of negative communication (criticism, hostility) and the degree of emotional overinvolvement on the part of their parents. Studies found that relapse rates were 50 percent in high-EE homes and only 15 percent in low-EE homes. Research has shown that schizophrenics with high-EE families did better when they had little contact with them. By contrast, patients from families rated high on expressions of warmth did better. These studies, summarized by Julian Leff in "Factors in Schizophrenia," in the October 1989 *Psychiatric Annuals*, were replicated in the United States in white, black, and Hispanic cultures.

Another group of studies, also reviewed by Leff, has shown that the patient's future can be improved through family therapy aimed at teaching better ways of communicating. This, in my view, strongly substantiates a familial origin for so-called schizophrenia.

In *Stressful Life Events* (1989), editor Thomas W. Miller has put together a series of studies confirming that stressful life events, such as family and personal conflict, as well as combat, can precipitate episodes of schizophrenia or lead to its reoccurrence. Leff and Christine Vaughn begin their chapter citing studies that show "it has now been established that life events play a part in the precipitation of episodes of depression and of schizophrenia. There is also good evidence that the emotional atmosphere in the home generated by the patient's key relatives exerts a significant influence on the recurrence of schizophrenia."

In the same book, David Lukoff and his coauthors discuss how "research over the past 30 years has documented several socioenvironmental factors that affect the course of the illness." Not only do family attitudes influence relapse, but life stresses in general influence the onset of schizophrenia. In addition to EE, another factor, labeled AS—a measure of "directly observed critical, guilt-inducing, and intrusive statements made by parents"—is related to the precipitation of schizophrenic episodes. Still another factor that plays a role in the development of schizophrenia is CD, which includes "disruptions, language anomalies, and lack of clarity and closure in parental interactions." The Lukoff review concludes that all three factors within the family—EE, AS, and CD—"help predict the onset of schizophrenia spectrum disorders."

Still in the book *Stressful Life Events*, Bruce Dohrenwend and Gladys Egri review studies of the relationship between stressful events and the onset of schizophrenia and conclude, "Stressful life events whose occurrences are outside the control of the subject play a part in the causation of schizophrenic episodes."

Ironically, while organized psychiatry promotes schizophrenia as a genetic and biological entity, actual research increasingly substantiates its environmental origins. In the next chapter we shall see that the research confirming biological and genetic factors, compared to that confirming environmental ones, is almost nonexistent.

The Plight of the Passionate, Sensitive Offspring

In my experience, not all families with children in spiritual despair are obviously abusive, but there is almost always a severe psychospiritual incompatibility between the labeled patient and one or both parents.

Parents of disturbed offspring commonly observe, "She was different from the others from the beginning—too sensitive. That's what she was, overly sensitive." Another sentiment frequently expressed by these parents: "Oh, she was different from the start. She didn't seem to respond to us. She wasn't willing to be held. She was always less social than her brothers and sisters." This withdrawal response represents a normal sensitivity to the anxieties, tensions, lovelessness, bad feelings, negative vibrations, fears, and so on emanating from the parents.

Youngsters who are going through psychospiritual overwhelm are almost always more aware of the lovelessness and quiet despair within the family than are their parents or their seemingly more normal brothers and sisters. They struggle more with questions, such as the meaning of life and love, the existence of God, the need for creativity in their lives, or the suffering of others in the wider world. Among the younger women, feminist issues are often the focus of attention. Among the men, male identity is a primary concern, as the tortured youngster struggles with the contrast between his own inner sensitivities and the more acceptable macho male image. In this age of pop psychology, many young mad people also are acutely aware of the disastrous outcomes of their upbringing. They try to get their parents to read books about childhood. Talking with the designated patient is often far more interesting and exciting than talking with the rest of the family, who typically cannot relate to psychospiritual issues on the same level as the member who's been diagnosed as mentally ill.

Envy and Shaming in the Family

Envious feelings often motivate the hostility directed toward the wounded member of the family. The story of Cinderella expresses how the most beautiful, sensitive, and spiritually shining child can become the butt of ridicule and abuse. It is difficult for a mother, father, or older brother or sister to accept that someone has arrived in their circle with unique sensitivity, passion, or awareness. They feel put to shame by the new member. In turn, they shame him or her.

Many of the symptoms associated with so-called schizophrenia are blatant attempts to compensate for humiliations experienced while growing up. I'm reminded of the fifteen-year-old frail, frightened boy who came into the hospital declaring that he was a boxing champion. He even could describe his main bouts. His true story was one of being physically abused at home and dominated by bigger boys at school. With regularity, therapists see young men who attempt to bolster their self-esteem by declaring they are somebody extraordinarily important, when deep down they feel humiliated and worthless.

Adults who feel that others are laughing, talking, and plotting behind their backs probably experienced these humiliations earlier in the family. People who hear voices saying "You're a jerk" are telling us something about their past personal experiences. The young woman who declares she is a famous scientific genius may feel humiliated by her mother's subservience to a domineering husband and by her mother's failure to become a person in her own right.

Humiliation frequently leads to outrage. The person who is shamed into feeling impotent and worthless wants to strike back in anger and even in hate. The outrage of these despairing people should not be dismissed as "mental illness," however extreme it gets. The more extreme it is, the more we must hold ourselves open to evidence that great pain, in the form of humiliation, has been inflicted upon them.

Psychologist Alfred Adler was among the first to notice the role of humiliation in what gets labeled schizophrenia. As obvious as it is, it goes largely unnoticed in psychiatry. Happily, there are now a number of popular books that give shame itself adequate recognition, including John Bradshaw's *Healing the Shame that Binds You* (1988) and Gershen Kaufman's *The Psychology of Shame* (1989).

Tragically, psychiatrists tend to further provoke these outraged people with drugs, restraints, and isolation rooms, reenacting and reinforcing the original humiliations experienced in the family. Outrage in a person should lead us to search for its sources. The inquiry, in the case of the profoundly overwhelmed, will require patience and a willingness to understand metaphorical, oblique, and disguised references to past trauma and deprivations. Madness, like our dreams, is filled with hints.

A therapist working with a young person's parents often can help them find better ways of relating that are free of humiliation and far more tolerant. This opens the way to more loving communication. When this happens, the youngster's helplessness and irrationality may subside in a matter of days or weeks, although long-term problems typically will remain for parents and child alike.

Humiliation and Overwhelm

By saying that mental helplessness and profound feelings of humiliation are central to what gets called schizophrenia, I don't mean to suggest that people bring spiritual defeat upon themselves or that they choose their helplessness in some perverse way. Nor do I believe they are born with it, ever.

Mental, psychological, or learned helplessness*—I use the terms interchangeably—can be inflicted on a person very early in life, before the beginning of verbal awareness, conscious choice. Infants, for example, may withdraw if deprived of maternal care. They may cease to reach out effectively to new individuals who offer sustenance and love, and instead wither and die. Older children will become depressed if they lose their parents. Children exposed to emotional, physical, or sexual abuse almost always tend to develop psychological helplessness.

Even among adults subjected to extreme psychological stress, many will tend to become helpless. In Nazi extermination camps, large numbers of people—Jews, gypsies, and Soviet army officers alike—developed a robotic, selfless existence. Only a few managed to maintain sufficient self-determination to plan successful escapes or to survive captivity. I have met some of them, and they are exceptional. Similar collapses into helplessness were observed among American soldiers subjected to the systematic brutality of prisoner-of-war camps in North Korea and Vietnam. The term *brainwashing* was applied to these forms of carefully orchestrated physical and emotional torture.

Lesser degrees of mental helplessness frequently surface during and after stressful experiences, leading to the commonly made diagnosis of Post-Traumatic Stress Disorder. All people probably suffer from one degree or another of mental helplessness in their routine lives. They need to collect their wits or regain their composure before proceeding with some difficult task. That is, they need to become rational and self-determined, and not helpless, despite their fears.

While most people are driven into extremes of mental helplessness by

---

*The concept of psychological helplessness which I elaborate in *The Psychology of Freedom* (1980) is similar to that of learned helplessness proposed by Martin Seligman in *Helplessness* (1975).

childhood experiences, it's up to them as adults to choose to work on overcoming it. The adult can decide, "I can start to overcome these feelings of helplessness right now." Naturally it can take time to practice and to learn a new approach to life, but the decision to start opens the gates to enormous personal growth.

Blaming

People overcome with humiliation often tend to blame others. This is in contrast, as we shall see, to depressed and guilt-driven people, who tend to blame themselves. The blame goes out to seemingly inappropriate targets because the abuser (the parent) cannot be safely called to account. The ashamed individual feels controlled by outside forces, from TV programs and radio waves to extraterrestrials. Sometimes famous people will be blamed, even though there's never been any personal contact. Sometimes real people in the person's life may be blamed, but with a farfetched accusation, such as a wife or husband is poisoning the food.

The assignment of blame outside oneself always expresses a kernel of truth: "I've been damaged by others; I've been hurt in ways I cannot explain; my childhood experiences horribly damaged me; I'm at the mercy of others; I feel so humiliated, I want to disappear from the face of the earth." Metaphorical accusations colored most of the communications by the patients in the vignettes from the "60 Minutes" program mentioned earlier. Such helpless blaming leads to the individual being labeled schizophrenic, and others do indeed take over his or her life.

People undergoing psychospiritual crises express the most intense degrees of shame and humiliation I have ever witnessed. Some of my patients' faces have seemed on the verge of bursting with shame when reliving severe humiliations from the past. At the core is a feeling of being utterly worthless, humiliated, or meaningless. At the same time, they often feel enormous anger or hate, because when blame is shifted outward, so is rage.

The tendency to feel humiliated and to become blaming in a compulsive manner is very common in severe conflict with others and is seen, for example, in most couples that come for therapy. It is interpreted as a sign of schizophrenic paranoia only when the blaming seems grossly irrational to the observer. But a human failing does not become a disease simply because it is extreme.

Feeling ashamed is closely related to mental helplessness. Extreme shame is the emotional expression of feeling overwhelming worthlessness.

Shame, then, is the expression of a particular kind of helplessness—that associated with core feelings of inconsequence and powerlessness. *

Should Parents Feel Guilty?

Guilt is also a helpless, self-defeating reaction—a distracting and damaging emotion. The core feeling of guilt is that we are very bad, harmful, and undeserving of life. Guilt differs from the insignificance and impotence of shame, because guilt-ridden persons feel that they do have significance and power—but an evil, damaging kind. Remorse, a feeling of regret that motivates us to change or to make amends, is distinctly different from guilt. What most people call guilt smacks of helplessness and plays little or no useful role in our lives.

When a parent reacts with overwhelming guilt to injuring a child, the parent will want to hide from the truth of what actually transpired. Feeling like a bad person makes us want to reject responsibility for the damage we have done to others. It encourages us to wallow in self-pity and self-hate. Ironically, resenting the pain of guilt can even make us angry at the person we have injured, leading us to do more injury.

Genuine remorse is another matter. If remorseful, we can get past hating ourselves and instead seek to reform ourselves, to undo the damage where possible, and to make sure we never repeat it. Increased parental honesty and responsibility, and not parental guilt, is what's needed.

Parents who freely acknowledge the harm they have done can experience enormous moral relief and rediscover their potential to positively influence the lives of their offspring. In my practice I sometimes see parents who decide late in their lives to ask forgiveness and to make amends, and their grown children are almost always grateful, joyful, and eager to build a better relationship. Parents almost always maintain this capacity to influence their children's lives for the better. I know one mother who relented on her deathbed and opened her heart to her son, uniting them at the end and bringing joy to both.

The Course of "Madness"

Much of what I have said about psychospiritual despair and overwhelm applies most accurately to the acute, flamboyant experience usually found in younger people. Few people continue to blaze with psychospiritual

---

* Although an imperfect theory, I find it helpful to think of fear and helplessness as the root of all negative emotions, with shame, guilt, and anxiety as derivatives with different qualities.

passion indefinitely; as noted earlier, most people, after several or many years, will tend to "mellow out." If they become labeled "chronic schizophrenics," their seemingly more irrational communications tend to become rote, and one sees naught but the smoking embers of the spiritual fire. They tend to respond most favorably to psychosocial support, such as a friend or ombudsman, and to help in finding a job and a decent place to live. Nonetheless, one often can find a warm, rich personality lurking beneath the facade of even the more withdrawn long-term patient. What is labeled "withdrawn" in hospitals is sometimes an emphatic refusal to communicate with one's jailers.

Psychiatry often presents the impression that a large percentage of people called schizophrenic will undergo deterioration. Manfred Bleuler, in *The Schizophrenic Disorders* (1978), reported on 208 patients followed for more than twenty years. He found that most people diagnosed as schizophrenic go on to make more than a marginal social and economic adjustment, with 60 percent able to support themselves.

In the *British Journal of Psychiatry* in 1980, Luc Ciompi reported on "The Natural History of Schizophrenia in the Long Term," with a group of 289 patients studied over an average of 36.9 years. He found that almost half had a "favorable" outcome—27 percent with a complete remission and another 22 percent with "minor residuals." Rather than symptoms of schizophrenia, most suffered from poor social adjustments. Only 40 percent were living with their families or by themselves, while the remainder were in community facilities or hospitals.

Both Bleuler and Ciompi found that treatment had little to do with the outcome: patients from the first three decades of the century did no differently than patients from the 1940s and 1950s, the era of "modern" treatments. Patients had a better outcome if they had been stronger emotionally prior to the onset of the psychospiritual crisis and if they had had a more acute, florid, and transient onset. As the patients grew older, they tended to become more calm and to improve.

Ciompi's report also noted that negative family attitudes and stressful life events were important in bringing about a poor outcome. He concluded that "doubtless, the potential for improvement in schizophrenia has for a long time been grossly under-estimated. In the light of long-term investigations, what is called 'the course of schizophrenia' more closely resembles a life process open to a variety of influences of all kinds than an illness with a given course."

As reported in the June 1, 1985, *Science News,* a follow-up of "chronic" patients in the Vermont state hospital system disclosed surprisingly good outcomes for many of them thirty years later. "Most displayed slight or no schizophrenic symptoms, had one or more moderately to very close friends, required little or no help in meeting basic needs and led relatively full lives." Although averaging age sixty-one, 40 percent had full-time employment.

In a recent review in the May 1987 *Hospital and Community Psychiatry*, Joseph Zubin and John Strauss confirmed that long-term follow-up studies were correcting "the clinician's illusion" that most so-called schizophrenic patients do poorly. They observed, "Given a more complete picture, the number of patients who significantly improve or recover is much greater than is now expected by most clinicians." The outcome seemed most influenced by social factors, such as attitudes toward the patient's recovery on the part of family members and professionals. They encouraged recognition of the limits of psychiatric treatment and urged that treatment "remove the obstacles that stand in the way of the natural self-healing process." I am reminded again of my experience with Met State, where it first became obvious to me that the treatments themselves were impediments to the patients' making any progress.

Recent cross-cultural studies by the World Health Organization (WHO) have found that the course of schizophrenia, with recovery rates over 50 percent, is often better in developing countries than in the industrialized, urban West. Psychiatric interventions, more available in the modern countries, are a negative factor, while the greater social support available in the developing countries is a positive one. In reviewing the studies, psychiatrist Giovanni de Girolamo concludes that "the integration of patients in a natural social environment, and the restriction of medical interventions to an indispensable degree may provide an optimal care strategy."*

We shall look more closely at effective psychosocial alternatives in chapter 16, including studies showing the superiority of nondrug approaches.

Psychiatry's Responsibility for "Poor Outcomes"

Psychiatry, of course, intervenes mightily in the psychospiritual crisis with huge doses of toxic drugs and sometimes electroshock that cause many patients to deteriorate markedly over the years. The presumption that these patients have a "mental illness" has discouraged the provision of psychosocial supports, such as supervised living in decent housing and other human services, including psychotherapy. On more than one oc-

---

* From Giovanni de Girolamo, "WHO Studies on Schizophrenia: An Overview of the Results and Their Implications for the Understanding of the Disorder," in *Psychotherapy and the Psychotic Patient*, ed. Peter Breggin and H. Mark Stern (Haworth Press, forthcoming). It will appear as both a hardcover book and a double volume of the journal, *The Psychotherapy Patient*.

casion I have met a supposedly intractable case of chronic schizophrenia in a state hospital whose record nonetheless documented considerable improvement during those brief months when a counselor was giving one-to-one attention. Usually the counselor was passing through for training and soon departed, leaving a gaping hole in the inmate's life.

Recently I was interviewing a "mute" black inmate who had been locked up in St. Elizabeths in Washington, D.C., for more than forty-five years. After much effort on both our parts, he was able to acknowledge to me the tragic story of how he had first been raped in the institution as a seventeen-year-old boy nearly five decades earlier. This man—supposedly unable to show feeling—grew sad in front of my eyes and was able to acknowledge it by repeating the word *sad* beneath his breath. He left our talk looking perked up, if only for a few minutes. But I knew he had become a sexual slave, still subjected to rape in his older and more frail years.

The Public Defenders Office was seeking his release after this interminable and abusive confinement. His dedicated attorney, Michael Ryan, had asked me if I could explain why his client had abruptly deteriorated and become a chronic inmate days before he was scheduled for release those many years ago. The old chart showed that the outgoing, likeable young man had, abruptly, become confused, disoriented, "paranoid," guilt-ridden, withdrawn, and terrified of going to bed—never to recover again. It was apparent to me that he'd been sexually assaulted the night before his condition precipitously deteriorated. Eventually we were able to piece the story together.

As a teenager before the assault, he had never seemed "crazy" or been diagnosed as psychotic. After being admitted to St. Elizabeths for evaluation following a relatively minor crime, he had been found free of any severe mental disorder; but his discharge had been delayed for several months, perhaps through inertia and perhaps because he was a useful worker in the understaffed wartime hospital.

After the assault, the doctors assumed that an innate schizophrenia had surfaced. Even though inmate rape always has been rampant on state hospital wards, there's no hint that the doctors suspected that anyone had victimized the young patient in any way. Instead of discharging him or protecting him against further violence, they surmised that it was lucky for the patient that his schizophrenia showed up before he was sent into the community again. Meanwhile, the sexual abuse continued.

Eventually the doctors gave him electroshock and then many years of toxic drugs. The unrelenting sexual abuse and the ongoing psychiatric assault over the years had led to his utter mental and physical dilapidation. He was now a bent, fragile-looking figure who scurried endlessly about the ward as if in flight.

In June 1991 a jury of his peers returned a verdict of "no mental illness," allowing his release after a lifetime of abuse. A safe haven is now being arranged for him.

This man's shattered life illustrates both the need for human companionship on the wards of a typical state mental hospital and the need for protection from vicious forms of violence that can destroy the integrity of the individual. But more than that, his tragic life demonstrates the need to abolish involuntary treatment and state mental hospitals.

A self-fulfilling prophecy of failure dominates the professional outlook toward schizophrenia, leading to therapeutic neglect and to a continuing disregard for the basic needs and safety of inmates. Both this man's doctor and the nurses admitted to me, rather casually, that yes, he was still a victim of sexual abuse at the hands of younger, stronger males; but they seemed to take it for granted as something that weaker inmates must endure. Attitudes have changed little since my volunteer days at Metropolitan State thirty-five years ago.

On Being an Inmate

Many people who seem "crazy" by ordinary standards never get labeled mentally ill. They not only stay out of hospitals, they become great creators or leaders—or eccentrics. Similarly, many people who are put into mental hospitals actually suffer from personal and social problems that have little or nothing to do with being irrational.

The main characteristics of state mental hospital inmates, we shall find, are poverty, homelessness, and lack of family or community support. Surely, many psychiatric inmates seem grossly irrational—but many do not. And irrational or not, they end up in the hospital for reasons other than their mental condition. Powerlessness is the key to becoming a psychiatric inmate.

The Need for Havens

Many people could benefit from a haven or retreat in which to be safe while working through their psychospiritual crises. Many would seek such an alternative if they did not have to fear involuntary treatment and toxic drugs.

At present, psychiatry provides no safe havens, although a number have proven successful in the past. We look at those that have proven themselves in chapter 16. Meanwhile, every psychiatric facility I know of in the country now routinely uses medication and subjects the individual to the risks of involuntary incarceration and coercive treatment. Each subjects the patient to rituals of humiliation that are demeaning and suppress personal growth.* Each neglects the psychological and spiritual needs of the individual.

Individual Responsibility

Ultimately, every individual must choose whether or not to overcome any hardship or oppression inflicted by the family, society, or psychiatry. Human beings retain a measure of free will as long as they remain conscious. Indeed, without the exercise of that flickering will, there is no hope for people; and it is the helper's role to encourage every hint of self-determination.

I frequently collaborate in patients' rights activities with former psychiatric inmates who share their life stories with me. Psychiatry's pessimism about the people they have labeled schizophrenic is proven wrong by my experiences with numbers of them throughout the United States, Canada, and Europe, many of whom lead interesting, exciting, productive, and satisfying lives. Some are among my dearest friends as well as being colleagues in the patients' rights movement.

Often these individuals—who call themselves survivors of psychiatry —reached a point during their spiritual crisis when they faced the need to take charge of their minds, their bodies, and their lives. With that they began their climb out of irrationality and despair, often into a far more enlightened and self-determined state than prior to the breakdown. Sometimes they seemed to recover almost wholly under their own steam; more often they were helped by others, and especially by others in the survivor movement.

Reaching out to others often becomes the first step back to human reality. When someone then responds with love and care, the recovery process is on its way. But this rarely happens in the psychiatric system. When the patient reaches out, the psychiatrist puts a pill in the hand.

Is there such a thing as schizophrenia? Yes and no. Yes, there are people who think irrationally at times and who attribute their problems to seemingly inappropriate causes, such as extraterrestrials or voices in the air. Yes, there are people who think they are God or the devil and repeat the claim no matter how much trouble it gets them into. But no, these people are not biologically defective or inherently different from the rest of us. They are not afflicted with a brain disorder or disease.

* The humiliating nature of hospitalization in the best facilities is described in D. L. Rosenhan's famous study, "On Being Sane in Insane Places," *Science*, January 19, 1973, pp. 250–58. It will be described in chapter 13. Also see my novel *The Crazy from the Sane* (New York: Lyle Stuart, 1970), which dramatizes the experience of patients on a Harvard teaching service, as well as in a state hospital.

They are undergoing a psychospiritual crisis, usually surrounding issues of basic identity and shame, and typically with feelings of outrage and overwhelm. They communicate in metaphors that often hint at the heart of their problems. The only reason to call them schizophrenic is to justify the psychiatric establishment and its treatments. By refusing to diagnose or to label people who already feel rejected and humiliated, we welcome them back to the human community and promote humane, respectful, and loving attitudes toward them. And we help to prevent the rampant abuses we are documenting.

Yet the reader has heard a whole different story in the press and on TV, and perhaps directly from psychiatrists. The story is that schizophrenia is a genetic and biochemical disease subject to treatment with drugs. We turn now to those claims.

Suppressing "Schizophrenic" Overwhelm with Neuroleptic Drugs: Medical Miracle or Chemical Lobotomy? The Effects of Haldol, Prolixin, Thorazine, Mellaril, and Other "Antipsychotic" Drugs

My concern is that people are having their minds blunted in a way that probably does diminish their capacity to appreciate life.
—*Jerry Avorn, M.D.*, Boston
Globe, *November 25, 1988*

It's very hard to describe the effects of this drug and others like it. That's why we use strange words like "zombie." But in my case the experience became sheer torture.
—*Wade Hudson, testimony before the Senate Subcommittee on the Abuse and Misuse of Controlled Drugs in Institutions (1977)*

People's voices came through filtered, strange. They could not penetrate my Thorazine fog; and I could not escape my drug prison.
—*Janet Gotkin, testimony before the Senate Subcommittee on the Abuse and Misuse of Controlled Drugs in Institutions (1977)*

Frequent Effects: sedation, drowsiness, lethargy, difficulty thinking, poor concentration, nightmares, emotional dullness, depression, despair. . . .
—*Dr. Calagari's* Psychiatric Drugs *(1987)*

Although antipsychotic drugs have been termed "major tranquilizers," their principal treatment effect is to organize psychotic thinking.

Antipsychotic agents may treat delusions, hallucinations, and other thought disorders. . . .

> —*American Psychiatric Press,*
> Textbook of Psychiatry (1988)

Alexandria sat in my office filled with fright—as much fright as she could feel through the dose of the psychiatric medication. The teenager's face was flat in expression, her body sagged, she moved as if mired down. She looked profoundly depressed. And yet she wasn't feeling at all depressed; she was terrified. She looked depressed because she was suffering from what we psychiatrists call "psychomotor retardation"—the enforced paralysis of mind and body that routinely results from treatment with neuroleptics, the drugs most frequently given to patients labeled schizophrenic.

A few weeks earlier, Alexandria had begun to see and hear things that weren't there and to mutter incoherently about God and death. The parents of this sensitive, poetic teenager at first thought she was going through a phase, maybe even playing a role from one of her beloved novels. That was until she stopped coming out of her room. When they tried to coax her out, she screamed hateful things at them about how they came from the devil and wanted to hurt her. Alexandria's parents saw an ad on TV promoting a local private psychiatric hospital for "the caring treatment" of adolescents, and they found hope in it. She was "acting crazy" some of the time, they later told me, but she was still herself when they left her in the hospital the first day. She was full of vitality and completely alert. When they said good-bye, she hugged them and cried. Her mother cried, too.

When they visited again the next day, they hardly recognized their daughter as she trudged toward them with shuffling steps and bent shoulders. She had been injected with Haldol. Alexandria's parents took her out of the hospital and brought her directly to me.

Now I talked alone with Alexandria while her parents sat nervously in the waiting room. Out of the corners of her eyes, she looked inquisitively around my office. She touched a gleaming crystal and patted a model of a fawn. It was as if she couldn't believe she was in such a bright and cheery room filled with wonderful distractions. I saw her eyes shift toward a small carved duck that was nearer to me, and I handed it to her.

She said, "Exactly."

I wondered what lay behind that cryptic and seemingly inappropriate remark, but I said nothing. She seemed to be relaxing.

She fondled the duck for awhile. "It's so colorful," she said.

"It's one of my favorites, too. I love birds. Do you like the Audubon prints?"

She turned slowly in her chair to see them. "No," she said. "He shot birds."

"Yes, I understand that," I agreed. "I don't like that either."

After a pause, she said, "What's happening to me?"

"What do you mean?"

"My mind. I can't think. I can't feel."

"Tell me some more."

"Like those poor ducks . . . the ones in the photographs. The awful black-and-white photographs."

I had no photos of ducks in my office, only the model she was holding, and it took me a moment to realize what she was talking about. Newspaper photos came to mind.

"The ducks in the oil spills?"

"You noticed those pictures, too?" She perked up. "I feel like that, like a duck, my feathers all matted down and stuck together."

I gestured to indicate her arms, which lay heavily on the chair, stiffened by the drug effect.

"Not just my arms . . . my mental wings," she explained to me. "My mental wings and feathers . . . matted down and stuck together."

"It's the medication," I said. "It does that to everybody in the doses you've been given."

"The medicine?" A small smile flickered across her face. "It's not me?"

"No," I said, "It's not you."

"Oh, God," she said, "I thought I had finally lost my mind."

"No, it's nothing like that," I reassured her. "It will wear off."

Alexandria had been on the medication for such a short time, only a few days, that it was safe to stop it abruptly. I promised never to force her to take any medication.

After talking with Alexandria long enough for her to gain some confidence in me, she agreed to inviting in her parents. Then I explained to her mother and father how I would approach their crisis as a family problem. I would help them to relate better to this sensitive, spiritual young woman who was going through such a difficult time, and help all of them to better understand, support, and love one another. Sometimes it would be painful, I said, especially when Alexandria expressed the feelings of hurt and pain that caused her to speak so hatefully to them. But it would open up the opportunity for growth and ultimately for better relations in the family. I added that I liked Alexandria and that in our few minutes together I already sensed that she and I shared many feelings, values, and attitudes. I hoped to help her come through her part of the family crisis with a new and better understanding of herself and a great ability to express her anger in more productive ways and to live effectively in the world.

Once Alexandria found someone she could communicate with, she felt less frantic and more hopeful. The need to flee from reality was no longer so pressing. Through our work together, her parents learned to be more patient with her and to look more honestly at the negative impact of their own attitudes, especially their overinvolvement with her in a negative, critical fashion and their difficulty in expressing unconditional love.

Alexandria would have long-term personal and family difficulties to handle; but she was through the worst of her crisis in a matter of weeks. Indeed, her most difficult problem was recovering from the medication. It took more than a month before she felt in touch with her finely tuned feelings and before she could think with her usual clarity.

It was relatively easy to help Alexandria with her acute "schizophrenic" crisis because it was her first experience with such overwhelming helplessness and fear and she was highly motivated. She understood her urgent need for finding a meaningful way of life and had the courage to pursue her ideals. Of equally great importance to this young person, her parents also were motivated to make changes in her best interest. They were willing to look at their own contribution to Alexandria's crisis and to learn new ways to understand and to love her.

It also was relatively easy to help Alexandria because she had not been driven into hiding by years of psychiatric treatment. The longer a person has been subjected to the humiliation of being diagnosed and misunderstood by professionals, and the longer a person has been subjected to psychiatric drugs—the harder it is to make progress.

Neuroleptic Drugs

The agents inflicted upon Alexandria are known by a variety of designations, including major tranquilizers, antipsychotics, and neuroleptics. These words are synonyms. The original ones, including Thorazine and Mellaril, are called phenothiazines, and sometimes that term is used too loosely to designate the entire group. In psychiatry, the term *neuroleptic* is now preferred. Neuroleptic was coined by Jean Delay and Pierre Deniker, who first used the drug in psychiatry, and means "attaching to the neuron." Delay and Deniker intended the term to underscore the toxic impact of the drug on nerve cells (see chapter 4).

List of Neuroleptics

The public identifies most psychiatric drugs by their trade names—the proprietary trademarks under which the companies own and market them. With generic names in parentheses, a list of trade names of neuroleptics in use today includes Haldol (haloperidol), Thorazine (chlorpromazine), Stelazine (trifluoperazine), Vesprin (trifluopromazine), Mellaril (thioridazine), Prolixin or Permitil (fluphenazine), Navane (thiothixene), Trilafon (perphenazine), Tindal (acetophenazine), Taractan (chlorprothixene), Loxitane or Daxolin (loxapine), Moban or Lidone (molindone), Serentil (mesoridazine), Orap (pimozide), Quide (piperacetazine), Repoise (butaperazine), Compazine (prochlorperazine), Dartal (thiopropazate), and Clozaril (clozapine).*

The antidepressant Asendin (amoxapine) turns into a neuroleptic when it is metabolized in the body and should be considered a neuroleptic. Etrafon or Triavil is a combination of a neuroleptic (perphenazine) and an antidepressant (amitriptyline), and it combines the impact and the risks of both. †

The neuroleptics are the most frequently prescribed drugs in mental hospitals, and they are widely used as well in board-and-care homes, nursing homes, institutions for people with mental retardation, children's facilities, and prisons. They also are given to millions of patients in public clinics and to hundreds of thousands in private psychiatric offices. Too often they are prescribed for anxiety, sleep problems, and other difficulties in a manner that runs contrary to the usual recommendations. And too often they are administered to children with behavior problems, even children who are living at home and going to school.

The Numbers of Patients Treated

No one knows the total numbers of neuroleptic drugs taken by patients each year, but estimates are possible. While the overall number of beds in state hospitals is down, annual admissions are up from the 1950s, and most of the several hundred thousand patients admitted each year are diagnosed as schizophrenic. Nearly all of these are prescribed neuroleptics. Hundreds of thousands more are getting them through outpatient clinics. Well over a million people a year are treated with neuroleptics on the wards and in the clinics of state mental health systems.

Additional millions more are receiving neuroleptics or antipsychotics

---

*Clozaril (clozapine), the center of considerable controversy, will be discussed in chapter 4.
†Although physicians sometimes fail to realize it, many other nonpsychiatric drugs are also neuroleptics. The list includes some antihistamines, such as Tacaryl and Temaril; some antinausea drugs, such as Compazine and Torecan; and some drugs used in conjunction with anesthesia, including Inapsine, Largon, and Phenergan, which is also used as an antinausea and anti–motion sickness agent. Serpasil (reserpine), a rauwolfia derivative, has neuroleptic qualities and is used as an antihypertensive and rarely as an antipsychotic. Serpasil is one of many trade names; others include Harmonyl, Raudixin, and Sandril. In nonpsychiatric usage, the doses are usually sufficiently small to avoid producing a neuroleptic toxic effect on the brain and mind, but caution should be exercised, especially in regard to Compazine, which can cause severe neurological reactions in relatively low doses.

through sources outside the state mental hospital system and long-term clinics. Of the estimated two million patients in nursing homes, many of them are on neuroleptics. Add to these patients the tens of thousands being treated with these drugs in private psychiatric hospitals, and in the psychiatric and medical wards of general hospitals, plus the tens of thousands in institutions for people with retardation, the untold thousands in board-and-care homes, still more in prisons, and hundreds of thousands in private practice—and the total swells to many millions. Even homeless people in shelters are sometimes forced to take them.

The National Prescription Audit provided by the FDA reported twenty-one million prescriptions for neuroleptics in 1984. These figures are drawn from retail pharmacies and therefore do not include patients in institutions or patients dispensed medications directly from clinics. Of course, many patients obtain more than one prescription a year, but the figures suggest that at least several million individuals are obtaining neuroleptics from retail pharmacies each year.

That huge numbers of people are treated with neuroleptics is confirmed by the figures occasionally released by the pharmaceutical companies. The first neuroleptic was chlorpromazine, whose trade name is Thorazine. In a 1964 publication entitled *Ten Years' Experience with Thorazine*, the manufacturer, Smith Kline and French, estimated that *fifty million* patients had been prescribed chlorpromazine in the first decade of use (1954 to 1964). The figure probably was worldwide. In recent years, haloperidol, sold by McNeil Pharmaceutical under the trade name Haldol, has become the most prescribed neuroleptic. In a letter to attorney Roy A. Cohen dated August 13, 1987, McNeil's director of medical services, Anthony C. Santopolo, provided a glimpse at Haldol's escalating use. The figures for patients first treated with Haldol grew from 600,000 in 1976 to 1,200,000 in 1981.*

Overall, the estimate I made in my 1983 medical book, *Psychiatric Drugs*, of five to ten million persons per year in America being treated with neuroleptics probably remains valid today. The sheer size of these numbers should motivate us to learn everything we can about the impact of these agents on the brain and the mind.

The Clinical Impact of the Neuroleptics

Textbooks of psychiatry and review articles claim that the neuroleptics have a specific antipsychotic effect, especially on the so-called positive

*The rate was increasing by 100,000 to 200,000 per year and is probably much higher now. The figures were based on submissions to the FDA and therefore probably were limited to the United States.

symptoms of schizophrenia, such as hallucinations and delusions, marked incoherence, and repeatedly bizarre or disorganized behavior.

Meanwhile, very little is written in professional sources about the apathy, disinterest, and other lobotomylike effects of the drugs.[1] Review articles tend to give no hint that the medications are actually stupefying the patients and that life on a typical mental hospital ward is listless at best. And so we must turn to the earliest research reports on the drugs. The pioneers, eager to show the potency of their new discovery, were far more candid and graphic in describing the effects to doctors as yet unfamiliar with them.

The Nature of Lobotomy

To grasp what the pioneers said about the neuroleptic effect, it's important first to understand the lobotomy effect to which it is compared. Lobotomy usually refers to the surgical cutting of nerve connections between the frontal lobes and the remainder of the brain. The frontal lobes produce the bulge in the human forehead, distinguishing our profile from that of other animals, and they represent the evolutionary flowering of the brain. The frontal lobes are the seat of higher human functions, such as love, concern for others, empathy, self-insight, creativity, initiative, autonomy, rationality, abstract reasoning, judgment, future planning, foresight, willpower, determination, and concentration. The frontal lobes allow us to be "human" in the full sense of that word; they are required for a civilized, effective, mature life.

Lobotomy basically knocks the frontal lobes out of commission. Depending on the amount of damage done, the effect can be partial or relatively complete. In the extreme, the patient becomes obviously demented, with the deterioration of all higher mental function. The lobotomist P. MacDonald Tow wrote a book-length treatise on the effects of lobotomy entitled *Personality Changes Following Frontal Leukotomy* (1955). In it he observes, "Possibly the truest and most accurate way of describing the net effect on the total personality is to say that he is more simple; and being more simple he has rather less insight into his own performance" (p. 235). The mental impairment, he found, "is greater in the higher and more peculiarly human functions."

Tow gives insight into why so many lobotomies were performed on inmates of state mental hospitals. Lobotomized patients become more dependent and more suitable for control in a structured institution. Deprived of their autonomy, initiative, or willpower, "[their] performance is considerably better in a structured situation."

In a symposium entitled *The Frontal Lobes* (1948), Swedish psychosurgeon Gosta Rylander dramatically reports the reactions from friends and family of surgically lobotomized patients. A mother says, "She is my daughter but yet a different person. She is with me in body but her soul is in some way lost. The deeper feelings, the tenderness, are gone. She is hard, somehow." A friend says, "I'm living now with another person. She is shallow in some way."

Rylander's anecdotes give us a second insight into why lobotomy was performed. The patients become less emotionally spontaneous and passionate. They become more shallow and relatively inert, or blunted. This blunting makes them less troublesome to others and, again, better psychiatric inmates.

More modern psychosurgery sometimes attacks areas beneath the frontal lobes, in the emotion-regulating limbic system. The impact is always the same: the production of a person who is emotionally blunted and more dependent, and hence more easily controlled. In 1982 a Danish team led by Heidi Hensen published a detailed study of the impact of modern forms of psychosurgery that employ electrodes to melt selected portions of the brain. Published as a small book, *Stereotactic Psychosurgery*[2] confirms that damage to the frontal lobes and surrounding limbic system with smaller lesions continues to produce a lobotomy effect or syndrome: "emotionality fades," "contact with other people becomes more flattened and the immediate bearing more mechanical," and there is a "weakening of initiative and [the patient's] ability to structure his situation."

In a word, people become more *robotic* after damage to their frontal lobes and limbic system.[3]

The Birth of Chemical Lobotomy—Reports from the Drug Pioneers

In 1952, the first shot in the "revolution in psychiatry" was fired in Paris by the two pioneers Delay and Deniker. They published their findings on chlorpromazine (Thorazine) in French in *Congrès des Medecins Aliénistes et Neurologistes de France*. Here is the first report ever of the impact of the neuroleptics, given in relatively small doses: "Sitting or lying, the patient is motionless in his bed, often pale and with eyelids lowered. He remains silent most of the time. If he is questioned, he answers slowly and deliberately in a monotonous and indifferent voice; he expresses himself in a few words and becomes silent."

Note the straightforward description of the apathy and lack of initiative typical of lobotomy.

The first report in North America was published in 1954 in a journal of the American Medical Association (AMA), *Archives of Neurology and Psychiatry*, by Canada's Heinz Lehmann. Lehmann and a coauthor graphically describe the "emotional indifference" and specifically call it the "aim" of the treatment. Like Delay and Deniker, they found that "the patients under treatment display a lack of spontaneous interest in the environment. . . ."

Contrary to today's promotional claims, the pioneers had no illusions about specifically curing or even ameliorating the patient's schizophrenia. Lehmann and his colleague asserted, "We have not observed a direct influence of the drug on delusional symptoms or hallucinatory phenomena." In a follow-up article one year later in the official journal of the Canadian Medical Association, Lehmann declared that in some cases "chlorpromazine may prove to be a pharmacological substitute for lobotomy."

The first British report by D. Anton-Stephens came out in the *Journal of Mental Science* in 1954 and is consistent with the others. Again using doses that are small by today's standards, Anton-Stephens found that "psychic indifference" is the "characteristic psychiatric response to chlorpromazine." Patients don't lose their symptoms, they lose *interest* in them.

Throughout the 1950s, textbooks continued to tell candidly about the lobotomylike impact of the drugs. In the 1958 edition of the most widely read book, *Modern Clinical Psychiatry*, authors Arthur Noyes and Lawrence Kolb summarized, "If the patient responds well to the drug, he develops an attitude of indifference both to his surroundings and to his symptoms" (p. 654).

A Boon to Psychiatric Institutions

From the psychiatrists' viewpoint, the drugs had two advantages over surgical lobotomy and over electroshock. With the drugs, one could at least hope that the damaging effects would not be permanent. And the dose could be "titrated"—that is, it could be raised and lowered to obtain the desired effect. As an ostensibly more humane intervention, drug therapy both salved the consciences of psychiatrists and made them feel more like legitimate doctors. But in doing so, the neuroleptics opened the way to unparalleled abuses on a far more massive level involving scores of millions of patients throughout the world. In the words of psychiatrist Thomas Szasz in an article in the 1957 *Archives of Neurology and Psychiatry*, "Restraint by chemical means does not make us guilty; herein lies the danger to the patient."[4]

How the Neuroleptics Produce Lobotomy

While the neuroleptics are toxic to most brain functions, disrupting nearly all of them, they have an especially well-documented impact on the dopamine neurotransmitter system. As any psychiatric textbook will confirm, dopamine neurotransmitters provide the major nerve pathways from the deeper brain to the frontal lobes and limbic system—the very same areas struck by surgical lobotomy. Most psychosurgery cuts the nerve connections *to and from* the frontal lobes and limbic system; chemical lobotomy largely interdicts the nerve connections *to* the same regions. Either way, coming or going, it's a lobotomy effect.

Thus the mechanism of action of the neuroleptics is no mystery: *clinically* the drugs produce a lobotomy and *neurologically* the drugs produce a lobotomy.

As early as the 1960s and 1970s, many researchers had come to the conclusion that the drugs "work" by suppressing the major nerve pathways into the frontal lobes and emotion-regulating limbic system. They acknowledged it in muffled voices in the literature, voices so hushed that you could not hear the dreadful phrase *chemical lobotomy*.

For example, the 1980 American Psychiatric Association's *Task Force Report: Tardive Dyskinesia* displays an illustration of dopamine pathways in the human brain. Starting from two main trunks deep in the brain, the dopamine nerves spread out like the branches of a tree, reaching into the emotion-regulating limbic system and frontal lobes. The text explains that this dopamine tree is shut down by the neuroleptics. Yet there's no hint that this drawing could be labeled "An Illustration of the Chemical Lobotomy Produced by Neuroleptics."[5]

While American psychiatrists continue to deny the obvious reality of chemical lobotomy, I've found that European psychiatrists often acknowledge it openly, even in public and to the press. At a conference held in Sweden in the spring of 1990, I debated a number of psychiatrists. Many of them admitted that the neuroleptic effect is a chemical lobotomy. They differed with me only in denying its permanency (see chapter 4).

Addicted to Lobotomy

Neuroleptic treatment was labeled lobotomy by Peter Sterling in the March 3, 1979, *New Republic* in an article entitled "Psychiatry's Drug Addiction." Sterling was neither a psychiatrist nor a physician, but a young neuroanatomist at the University of Pennsylvania, when he wrote:

The blunting of conscious motivation, and the inability to solve problems under the influence of chlorpromazine resembles nothing so much as the effects of frontal lobotomy. . . . Research has suggested that lobotomies and chemicals like chlorpromazine may cause their effects in the same way, by disrupting the activity of the neurochemical, dopamine. At any rate, a psychiatrist would be hard-put to distinguish a lobotomized patient from one treated with chlorpromazine.

Lobotomizing Dogs and Russian Dissidents

Like surgical lobotomy, chemical lobotomy can have no specifically beneficial effect on any particular human problem or human being. It puts a chemical clamp on the higher brain of anyone. A corollary is that the drugs can be used to subdue any person or animal.

In *The Tranquilizing of America* (1979), Richard Hughes and Robert Brewin put it this way: "When used on a large population of institutionalized persons, as they are, they can help keep the house in order with the minimum program of activities and rehabilitation and the minimum number of attendants, aides, nurses, and doctors" (p. 157).

On many psychiatric wards the neuroleptics are given to 90 to 100 percent of the patients; in many nursing homes, to 50 percent or more of the old people; and in many institutions for persons with mental retardation, to 50 percent or more of the inmates. Neuroleptics also are used in children's facilities and in prisons. It becomes difficult to argue that they have a specific antipsychotic effect.

Consider the use of neuroleptics in the Soviet Union for the control of political dissidents. In *Soviet Psychoprisons* (1979), political scientist Harvey Fireside discloses the imprisonment and forced drugging of a Russian dissident poet named Olga Iofe, a nineteen year old so free of symptoms that one Russian psychiatrist was forced to testify, "A mild schizophrenia does not presume a personality change apparent to one's associates" (p. 39). She was singled out for treatment after she protested against the resurgence of Stalinism: "The massive drugs she was forcibly given were, in Dr. Norman Hirt's opinion, 'in fact a chemical lobotomy,' in light of reports that, on her release, Iofe 'appears to be permanently damaged, an altered person' " (p. 40).*

Haldol, the most frequently used neuroleptic in America, is also a favorite in the Soviet Union. Russian dissident Leonid Plyushch gained media-wide attention in the United States when he held a press conference after fleeing to the West. On February 16, 1976, *U.S. News and*

---

*Norman Hirt is a Canadian psychiatrist who testified before Congress about the Soviet abuses. Psychiatrists find it easier to criticize Russians for giving mind-blunting and brain-damaging drugs to political dissidents than to criticize themselves and their colleagues for giving them to ordinary citizens in their own countries.

World Report quoted Plyushch's reaction to being drugged in a Russian psychoprison: "I was horrified to see how I deteriorated intellectually, morally and emotionally from day to day. My interest in political problems quickly disappeared, then my interest in scientific problems, and then my interest in my wife and children."

Plyushch's political interests were the more recent and hence least firmly entrenched in his mind and brain, and so they were the first to go. By profession he is a scientist, so these more deeply embedded interests held out somewhat longer. As with almost any person, his social life, especially his family life, is even more integral to his mind and brain than his profession, and this held up the longest.

Were the Russians inundating this man with huge doses of some especially deadly drug? The February 14, 1976, *New York Times* provides more detailed excerpts from Plyushch's press conference, at which he said, "I was prescribed haloperidol [Haldol] in small doses."

The neuroleptics also are used in tranquilizer darts for subduing wild animals and in injections to permit the handling of domestic animals who become vicious. The veterinary use of neuroleptics so undermines the antipsychotic theory that young psychiatrists are not taught about it.*

The Fundamental Principle of Psychiatric Treatment

The brain-disabling principle applies to all of the most potent psychiatric treatments—neuroleptics, antidepressants, lithium, electroshock, and psychosurgery. The principle states that all of the major psychiatric treatments exert their *primary or intended effect* by *disabling normal brain function*. Neuroleptic lobotomy, for example, is not a side effect, but the sought-after clinical effect. It reflects impairment of normal brain function.

Conversely, none of the major psychiatric interventions correct or improve existing brain *dys*function, such as any presumed biochemical imbalance. If the patient happens to suffer from brain dysfunction, then the psychiatric drug, electroshock, or psychosurgery will worsen or compound it.

---

*Veterinary literature and practice has established that these drugs must be limited to short-term use only. They're too dangerous for animal consumption, except in emergencies and terminal states. Yet they are less dangerous to animals, in whom it often is more difficult to produce the permanent drug-induced neurological disorders seen in humans (see chapter 4). Recently, our frisky Shetland sheepdog was given a very small dose of neuroleptic to prevent car sickness. My daughter Alysha soon noticed that he became more obedient and "stopped barking at everything."

If relatively low doses produce no apparent brain dysfunction, the medication may be having no effect or producing a placebo effect. Or, as frequently happens, the patient is unaware of the impact even though it may be significant. Anyone familiar with the behavior of people drinking alcohol knows how easily a slightly intoxicated person may deny being impaired or even claim to be improved. Most people coming off cigarettes become abruptly aware of missing the sedative and tranquilizing effects that previously were taken for granted.

Iatrogenic (Treatment-Caused) Helplessness

Brain dysfunction, such as a chemical or surgical lobotomy syndrome, renders people much less able to appreciate or evaluate their mental condition. Surgically lobotomized people often deny both their brain damage and their personal problems. They will loudly declare, "I'm fine, never been better," when they can no longer think straight. Sometimes they deny that they have been operated on, despite the dime-size burr holes in their skulls palpable beneath their scalp. Superficially, the denial looks so sincere that prolobotomists cite it to justify the harmlessness of the treatment.

Even without the production of brain dysfunction, the giving of drugs or other physical interventions tends to reinforce the doctor's role as an authority and the patient's role as a helpless sick person. The patient learns that he or she has a "disease," that the doctor has a "treatment," and that the patient must "listen to the doctor" in order to "get well again." The patient's learned helplessness and submissiveness is then vastly amplified by the brain damage. The patient becomes more dutiful to the doctor and to the demoralizing principles of biopsychiatry. Denial can become a way of life, fixed in place by brain damage.

Suggestion and authoritarianism are common enough in the practice of medicine but only in psychiatry does the physician actually damage the individual's brain in order to facilitate control over him or her. I have designated this unique combination of authoritarian suggestion and brain damage by the term *iatrogenic helplessness*. Iatrogenic helplessness is key to understanding how the major psychiatric treatments work.[6]

There is little or no reason to anticipate a physical treatment in psychiatry that will control severely disturbed or upset people without doing equally severe harm to them. If psychosurgery, electroshock, or the more potent psychiatric drugs were refined to the point of harmlessness, they would approach uselessness. In biopsychiatry, unfortunately, it's the damage that does the trick.

Clarifying a Confusing Point

Whether or not some psychiatric patients have brain diseases is irrelevant to the brain-disabling principle of psychiatric treatment. Even if someday a subtle defect is found in the brains of some mental patients, it will not change the damaging impact of the current treatments in use. Nor will it change the fact that the current treatments worsen brain function rather than improving it. If, for example, a patient's emotional upset is caused by a hormonal problem, by a viral inflammation, or by ingestion of a hallucinogenic drug, the impact of the neuroleptics is still that of a lobotomy. The person now has his or her original brain damage and dysfunction *plus* a chemical lobotomy.

Claims for Curing Specific Schizophrenic Symptoms

But what about claims that the treatments reduce psychiatric symptoms, such as so-called hallucinations and delusions? Gerald Klerman was the major figure in transforming the image of the neuroleptics from non-specific flattening agent to antipsychotic medication. Klerman was an avid advocate of biopsychiatry from early in his career and went on to become director of NIMH. Klerman's research findings were published in various places, including Alberto DiMascio and Richard Shader's 1970 compendium *The Clinical Handbook of Psychopharmacology.**

Klerman found that the four most improved "symptoms," in descending order, were combativeness, hyperactivity, tension, and hostility. In short, the drugs subdue and control people. Hallucinations and delusions—the cardinal symptoms of schizophrenia—ran a poor fifth and sixth. †

Since drugged patients become much less communicative, sometimes nearly mute, it's not surprising that they say less about their hallucinations and delusions. Had the investigators paid attention, they would have noticed that the patients also said less about their religious and political convictions as well as about their favorite hobby or sport. There's no wild

---

*Klerman acknowledged that his NIMH research was not rigorous by scientific standards. There were no controls and the data were generated by "clinical impressions" made by psychiatric professionals who tend to be promedication. Those rating the effect of the drugs on the patients knew that the patients were receiving so-called antipsychotic medications and they could give free rein to their biases. Nonetheless, the results did not end up supporting Klerman's claim for a specific antipsychotic effect. This did not daunt Klerman from continuing to make the claim.

†While combativeness and hyperactivity were markedly reduced in 49 percent and 38 percent of patients, respectively, hallucinations and delusions were markedly reduced in only 30.5 percent and 21 percent. Other problems typically associated with mental illness were unimproved by the drugs, including judgment, insight, and emotional tone, or affect.

cheering for the home team on the typical psychiatric ward. Furthermore, the drugs cause so much discomfort (see chapter 4) that patients often stop saying what they believe to avoid getting larger doses and to bring a more speedy end to the treatment. As many ex-patients have told me, "I learned right away I'd better shut up or I'd get more of that stuff." What's astonishing is that despite investigator bias and the global inhibition produced by the drugs, communications labeled hallucinations and delusions continued to be recorded.

Klerman vociferously claimed that his research confirmed an antipsychotic effect, and few, if any, people bothered to check his data.

They Who Are Different from Us

After I described the lobotomizing effect of the neuroleptics during a 1989 debate with an internationally known psychiatrist, the opposing doctor admitted that he himself had taken "one small dose of neuroleptic" and then experienced an overwhelming and unbearable sense of "depression" and "disinterest." But he went on to say that his patients, because of their "abnormal brains," underwent no such lobotomy effect. Unlike normal people, the patients supposedly felt better because the drug "harmonized" their biochemical abnormalities. This was not the first time I'd heard this argument made by a psychiatrist.

The outrage expressed by ex-patients in the audience contradicted his assertions about the harmlessness of the medications. So does the clinical literature cited in this and the next chapter.

What does it say about professionals when they argue that their patients are so different from themselves? Biopsychiatry lives by the principle that its patients are so different from other humans that almost anything can be done to them, including surgical, electrical, and chemical lobotomy. By contrast, the ethical helping person assumes that those seeking help possess the same human sensitivities as anyone else, including the therapist.

Drugs and Adjustment

Life in a mental hospital is so inhibited, constrained, and suppressed that patients might *seem* better adjusted when heavily drugged. As already noted in chapter 2, D. L. Rosenhan describes in the January 19, 1973, *Science* that even the most highly regarded mental hospitals are humiliating and oppressive places, even for normal volunteers masquerading as patients. Typical state hospitals, where many drug studies are conducted, are intimidating and frightfully violent. In Erving Goffman's phrase, these "total institutions" also stigmatize and demean their inmates. His analysis in *Asylums* (1961) helps us understand why a drugged patient would seem better adjusted than a drug-free person in such a setting; the chemically lobotomized patient fits better into the social role of mental patient, with its obedience to authority, conformity, lack of dignity, acceptance of mundane routines, and restricted opportunities for self-expression. Similarly, books and stories by former patients in all kinds of psychiatric facilities almost always describe them as wholly suppressive and demoralizing. * To say that patients behave better in a mental hospital when they are drugged is more a commentary on the requirements of being an inmate than on the allegedly beneficial qualities of drugs.

Unfortunately, the patient may face an equally suppressive life situation after discharge from the hospital. Board-and-care homes and nursing homes are at least as boring and stifling as psychiatric hospitals. Often they offer nothing but a bed, a TV, and perhaps a local park bench. Again, it is no surprise that patients might seem to adjust better to them when drugged. Indeed, most drug-free people would want to take flight rather than to waste away in a facility that offers nothing in the way of rehabilitation, recreation, or social life.

Nor is life necessarily less stultifying when the patient returns home to his or her family. As we saw in chapter 2, the families of children labeled schizophrenic are, at their best, unable to relate to their overwhelmed offspring. At their worst they are outright abusive. Typically the parents are overinvolved and unrelentingly critical of their son or daughter. Again, it's no surprise that drugged offspring might seem better adjusted to life in these families, while drug-free might continue to be resentful, rebellious, and difficult to control.

Drug experts and psychiatric textbooks that tout neuroleptics almost never concern themselves with the living conditions to which they are asking or forcing the drugged patient to adjust.

Research Studies on Efficacy

Even considering the built-in biases favoring drugs in typical research studies, the data do not unequivocally support the use of neuroleptics.

---

* For example, see the compendium of stories and poems in Bonnie Burstow and Don Weitz, eds., *Shrink Resistant: The Struggle Against Psychiatry in Canada* (Vancouver: New Star Books, 1988); or the following autobiographical accounts: Janet and Paul Gotkin, *Too Much Anger, Too Many Tears: A Personal Triumph Over Psychiatry* (New York: Quadrangle, 1975); Judi Chamberlin, *On Our Own: Patient-Controlled Alternatives to the Mental Health System* (New York: Hawthorn, 1978); and Kate Millett, *The Loony-Bin Trip* (New York: Simon and Schuster, 1990).

In comparing hospitalization with and without drugs, the data are not even consistent. For example, a team led by Maurice Rappaport reported in 1978 in *International Pharmacopsychiatry* that patients treated with placebo in the hospital and no medications on follow-up "showed greater clinical improvement and less pathology at follow-up, fewer rehospitalizations and less overall functional disturbance in the community than the other groups of patients studied." Of the group that never received medication, only 8 percent were rehospitalized. Of the group that received medication at some time during or after hospitalization, 47 to 73 percent were rehospitalized. The worst performance was for those patients who were drugged both during *and* after. They suffered a 73-percent return rate.

Gordon Paul and his colleagues investigate long-term maintenance drug therapy for "hard core, chronically hospitalized patient groups" in the July 1972 *Archives of General Psychiatry*. These patients also were exposed to an active psychosocial rehabilitation program on the wards. One group was abruptly changed from medication to placebo without the staff knowing that a research project was going on. It was found that in the early stages of treatment, medication interfered with participation in the rehabilitation program, and that later on it had no effect, beneficial or otherwise. The authors conclude that the "widespread practice" of giving neuroleptics to chronic hospital patients should be discontinued, because the medications are unhelpful, expensive, dangerous, and interfere with rehabilitation.

Some researchers present a rosier picture for drug intervention. In the Northwick Park study published by T. J. Crow and his team in the *British Journal of Psychiatry* in 1986, 30 to 50 percent of the patients relapsed with drug therapy and 70 percent relapsed without it. Even if we accept these findings, however, they do not seem so astonishing in the light of the "natural history" of what is called schizophrenia (see chapter 2). As noted earlier, regardless of the treatment regime, one-half or more of patients diagnosed as schizophrenic eventually will make a social and economic adjustment outside the hospital, and that about one-third do well. The results of positive drug studies will seem still less impressive when we examine the high rate of drug-induced permanent brain damage, which can exceed 50 percent among long-term patients (see chapter 4). *

---

* As the American Psychiatric Press's *Textbook of Psychiatry* (1988, p. 387) recognizes, many long-term patients tend to develop increasingly negative symptoms, such as withdrawal and apathy. We will find convincing evidence that the drugs actually *produce* the negative symptoms that then become confused with chronic schizophrenia.

Casting Further Doubt

A review published in the October 1989 *American Journal of Psychiatry* raises serious questions about the validity of the most accepted use of neuroleptics—the control of acute psychotic episodes. From McLean Hospital and Harvard Medical School, Paul Keck and his associates, including Ross Baldessarini, could find only five studies on the use of neuroleptics in acute schizophrenia that used scientific controls, comparing placebo or sedatives to the neuroleptics. These five studies found that "the same overall degree of improvement was observed during treatment with all the agents tested." Specifically, Valium (a minor tranquilizer and sedative) and opium "demonstrated efficacy similar to that of neuroleptic during the first day and through 4 weeks of treatment." In other words, sedatives and narcotics performed as well as the so-called antipsychotic drugs in the acute treatment of schizophrenia. The authors suggest, "Perhaps the early effects of antipsychotic drugs are nonspecific and are largely the same as those of sedative agents."

More demoralizing to advocates of neuroleptics, Keck and his coauthors also found that in some studies, a placebo performed as well as the neuroleptics. They conclude that the apparent efficacy of neuroleptics in treating acute patients may in fact be due to other factors, such as a respite from conflicted home life.

The authors also remark that drug efficacy in the long-term treatment of chronic patients is equally unconfirmed. Significantly, Keck and his colleagues constitute a very respected research team from one of the most esteemed institutions in psychiatry, and they are well-known advocates of psychiatric medication.

Returning People to Productive Lives with the Drugs

One entrenched myth is that the antipsychotics helped to empty the state mental hospitals, thereby returning many people to more useful, better lives. The American Psychiatric Press's *Textbook of Psychiatry* (1988), for example, declares unequivocally: "The rapid decline in the number of patients in psychiatric hospitals has been among the most persuasive examples of how pharmacologic therapies in psychiatry have a beneficial impact not only on the individual patient, but on society as well" (p. 770). The overall process was given the misnomer "deinstitutionalization."

In reality, the drugs did not cause the emptying of the state hospitals, which did not begin in earnest until 1963, more than eight years after the introduction of the neuroleptics in America. At that point, the hospital population had been relatively static for many years—558,000 inmates in the peak year of 1955 and 504,000 in 1963—and admissions actually had skyrocketed. After 1963 a rapid decline in inmate population began throughout the country. In that year, "mental illness" became covered for the first time under federal disability programs, culminating in Social Security Disability (SSI). Now the patients could be sent to old-age homes and board-and-care facilities, to be paid for by their meager disability checks. The states had successfully shifted the financial burden from themselves to the federal program.

"Deinstitutionalization" is itself a misleading term, because very few of the discharged patients became independent. Most were transferred into other supervised facilities, usually with even less to offer than the state mental hospitals, which at least had expansive grounds and a few organized activities. Some of the inmates were cast out on the streets as homeless people. At the same time, the infamous "revolving door policy" began, with frequent short readmissions to drug the patients again before sending them back to their dismal, lonely surroundings.

The primary function of drugs in this process is to make it easier to ship robotic patients from one place to another. That the drugs did not cause deinstitutionalization is confirmed by the Swedish experience, where the process is only now beginning in that country, twenty-five years after the introduction of the drugs. Emptying American hospitals was a matter of social policy—moving patients out and taking fewer in —not a medical miracle.

Into Nursing Homes

The aged made up the largest portion of the old state mental hospital population, and they were the first to be thrown out during deinstitutionalization. A 1989 study by Jerry Avorn and his colleagues from Harvard, published in the *New England Journal of Medicine*, surveyed fifty-five rest homes in Massachusetts. They found that 39 percent of the inmates were receiving neuroleptics and that 18 percent were receiving two or more. Several other studies confirm the drugging of the elderly in understaffed, oppressive nursing homes throughout the country.

Private board-and-care homes are no better. Psychiatrist Theodore van Putten and his colleague J. E. Sparr wrote "The Board and Care Home: Does it Deserve a Bad Press?" in the July 1979 *Hospital and Community Psychiatry*. They describe patients lobotomized by the drugs, suffering from blunted feeling, passivity, and lack of initiative, interest, and spontaneity. Most lived "in virtual solitude."

Onto the Streets as Homeless People

A number of other former inmates have ended up as street people, but not nearly so many as are institutionalized in other settings, such as nursing homes, board-and-care homes, and jails. Furthermore, homelessness as a problem is directly attributable to economic changes. There has been a drastic decline in low-income housing, coupled with an increase in numbers among the very poor. Deinstitutionalization in Denmark, by contrast, has *not* produced rampant homelessness, because the government provides sufficiently large disability payments and enough affordable housing to keep ex-inmates off the streets.

That many American homeless do have severe psychological problems merely confirms that our more helpless citizens suffer the most acutely and quickly from economic pressures, such as low wages and high rents. Homelessness itself is undoubtedly not good for one's mental stability.

We should reject psychiatry's call to subject ever-increasing numbers of the homeless to enforced medication with neuroleptics. When it diagnoses, drugs, and incarcerates the homeless poor, psychiatry covers up the political issue—society's unwillingness to provide jobs, housing, or an adequate safety net. People victimized by socioeconomic conditions are turned over to psychiatry for further abuse. All of us then rest more easily—except for the victims.

In January 1980, the editor of *Clinical Psychiatry News*, psychiatrist William Rubin, wrote poignantly about the fate of deinstitutionalized patients:

Patients aren't warehoused in snakepits any longer. They sit instead in wretched welfare hotels and Bowery flophouses. The shopping-bag ladies and other casualties wander the streets, prey for all the vultures, until they are harmed or in some other way attract the attention of law-enforcement authorities. Then they are sent back to the state hospitals; cleaned up; pushed through the revolving door back into the community.

As most observers now agree, so-called deinstitutionalization was not a blessing to the former inmates; it was a callous abandonment. It is simply false to claim that deinstitutionalization returned thousands of inmates to productive lives in the community.[7]

Psychosocial Approaches Instead of Drugs

In their book *Community Mental Health* (1989), Loren Mosher and Lorenzo Burti describe Soteria House in California, a nondrug psychosocial treatment home that was compared to a control group of patients going through the regular psychiatric system. Using small, homelike quarters with nonprofessional therapists, Soteria outperformed the traditional mental hospital system and neuroleptic drugs. In a chapter in his 1989 book *The Limits of Biological Treatments for Psychological Distress*, Bertram Karon reviews a variety of studies showing the superiority of psychotherapy over neuroleptics in the treatment of schizophrenic patients. Karon's own psychotherapy project showed that patients did best in the long run when they received no medication or used it only during the times of worst distress. In chapter 1 we saw how effective untrained volunteers can be in helping people gain release from custodial institutions.

Loren Mosher's Soteria House project, Karon's psychotherapy research, the Harvard-Radcliffe Mental Hospital Volunteer Program, and other psychosocial approaches will be described in more detail in chapter 16.

In summary, the neuroleptic drugs are chemical lobotomizing agents with no specific therapeutic effect on any symptoms or problems. Their main impact is to blunt and subdue the individual. In the next chapter we'll see that they also physically paralyze the body, rendering the individual less able to react or to move. Thus they produce a chemical lobotomy and a chemical straitjacket. Indeed, there is relatively little evidence that they are helpful to the patients themselves, while there is considerable evidence that psychosocial interventions are much better. The drugs are also the cause of a plague of brain damage that afflicts up to half or more of long-term patients. We turn now to that drug-induced epidemic.

Chapter 4

The "Miracle Drugs" Cause the Worst Plague of Brain Damage in Medical History

. . . antipsychotic drugs have been termed "neuroleptics," in that these drugs' actions imitate a neurological disease.
> —*American Psychiatric Press*, Textbook of Psychiatry *(1988)*

It is also clear that the antipsychotic [neuroleptic] drugs must continue to be scrutinized for the possibility that their extensive consumption might cause general cerebral dysfunction.
> —*Unpublished paper coauthored in 1978 by Igor Grant and others, including Lewis Judd; comment expurgated from published versions*

Every violation of truth is not only a sort of suicide in the liar but is a stab at the health of human society.
> —*Ralph Waldo Emerson*

Roberta had been treated for several years with the "miracle drugs," neuroleptics such as Thorazine, Haldol, Mellaril, and Prolixin. My medical evaluation described her condition:

Roberta is a grossly disfigured and severely disabled human being who can no longer control her body. She suffers from extreme writhing movements and spasms involving the face, head, neck, shoulders, limbs, extremities, torso, and back—nearly the entire body. She had difficulty standing, sitting, or lying down, and the difficulties worsen as she attempts to carry out voluntary actions. At one point she could not prevent her head from banging against nearby furniture. She could hold a cup to her lips only with great difficulty. Even her respiratory movements are seriously afflicted so that her speech comes out in grunts and gasps amid spasms of her respiratory muscles.

Roberta's current psychotic disorder is most probably also a product of neuroleptic-induced brain disease. Her inappropriate affect—giggling and superficial smiling while in great distress—is typical of brain damage. Roberta may improve somewhat after several months off the neuroleptic drugs, but she will never again have anything remotely resembling a normal life.

Tardive Dyskinesia and Tardive Dementia

Roberta had an unusually severe case of tardive dyskinesia (TD), a disease frequently caused by the neuroleptics. The term "tardive" means late-developing or delayed; "dyskinesia" means abnormal movement. Tardive dyskinesia is a movement disorder that can afflict any of the voluntary muscles, from the eyelids, tongue, larynx, and diaphragm to the neck, arms, legs, and torso.* On rare occasions it can occur after a few weeks or months, but usually it strikes the individual after six months to two years of treatment.

Any of the neuroleptics can cause tardive dyskinesia.† The total dosage probably affects the likelihood of this happening, but the dose relationship is not easily demonstrated, and any amount must be considered dangerous. While some symptoms improve or even disappear after removal from the offending medications, most cases are permanent. There is no known treatment for tardive dyskinesia.

Often the start of disease goes unnoticed, because the drugs that cause it also tend to suppress the overt symptoms. Thus the disease percolates out of sight, finally breaking through with uncontrollable twitches, spasms, or writhing movements. Whenever possible, patients should try to stop the drugs periodically to check for abnormal movements.

Roberta also had tardive dementia, a global deterioration of her mind and mental faculties caused by the drugs. While tardive dyskinesia is a firmly established disease, tardive dementia remains more controversial within the profession, although evidence for its existence seems incontrovertible.

Had She Seen a Different Doctor . . .

Roberta was a college student getting good grades, mostly A's, when she first became depressed and sought psychiatric help at the recommendation

---

*The description of tardive dyskinesia may seem familiar to people who have seen the recent movie *Awakenings*. When the main character, Leonard, deteriorates while taking large doses of L-Dopa, his extreme and disabling involuntary movements are identical to a very severe case of tardive dyskinesia.

†Clozapine is a possible exception (see discussion later in this chapter).

of her university health service. She was eighteen at the time, bright and well-motivated, and a very good candidate for psychotherapy. She was going through a sophomore-year identity crisis about dating men, succeeding in school, and planning a future. She could have thrived with a sensitive therapist who had an awareness of women's issues.

Instead of moral support and insight, her doctor gave her Haldol. Over the next four years, six different physicians watched her deteriorate neurologically without warning her or her family about tardive dyskinesia and without making the diagnosis, even when she was overtly twitching in her arms and legs. Instead they switched her from one neuroleptic to another, including Navane, Stelazine, and Thorazine. Eventually a rehabilitation psychologist became concerned enough to send her to a general physician, who made the diagnosis. By then she was permanently physically disabled, with a loss of 30 percent of her IQ.*

More "Mild" Cases of Tardive Dyskinesia

Most cases of tardive dyskinesia are labeled "minimal" or "mild," compared to "moderate" or "severe." But imagine how you would feel if your mild case of tardive dyskinesia made you stick out your tongue periodically in front of other people, or if you had to blink your eyes spasmodically or crane your neck oddly, or if your voice screeched a little out of control, while others were watching or listening.

An older woman came up to me after one of my lectures at a university. She was warm, friendly, and articulate; but what she was saying seemed undermined by the strange way she kept shrugging her right shoulder. Afterward, a friend of mine, perplexed, asked me, "What's up with her? She sounds rational, but she acts so strangely." I explained that the woman had been treated for years with neuroleptics. The hunching of her one shoulder was a mild case of tardive dyskinesia; but it was disfiguring enough to discredit and distract attention from what she was saying. That she was a former mental patient only made others more certain that her symptom was an expression of "mental illness."

You may recall passing someone on the street, perhaps an old and

---

*I've seen several cases where multiple physicians have continued medication and failed to make the proper diagnosis. It appears as if the second and third doctors too often simply go along with the treatment, or else actually try to cover for the earlier doctor's mistakes. In some cases the denial of the iatrogenic disease becomes grossly negligent. Patients have been seen in emergency rooms and have been psychiatrically hospitalized for days or weeks without anyone on the medical or nursing staff noting the existence of gross tremors, twitches, and other abnormal movements. Even physicians doing physical examinations may somehow neglect to notice or record the telltale signs of drug-induced neurological disease.

disheveled man, who seemed to be chewing a wad of gum. It looked ridiculous, the way he was chewing back and forth, and somehow you knew it wasn't normal, it wasn't just gum chewing. You figured it was a sign of craziness. The odds are that he had another mild case of tardive dyskinesia.

Or perhaps you saw a homeless man standing on a corner bouncing up and down from one foot to another like he had, as the old expression goes, "ants in his pants." That, too, was probably tardive dyskinesia, or a variant called tardive akathisia, which forces a person to move all the time, against his or her own will. It also can induce unbearable tension and anxiety.

The Lessons of Lethargic Encephalitis

Rather than treating a disease, the neuroleptics create a disease.

Delay and Deniker (chapter 3) were the first psychiatrists to experiment with the original neuroleptic, Thorazine, for psychiatric purposes in Paris in the early 1950s. They immediately noticed that small doses produced a neurological disease very similar to a special type of virulent flu virus that killed tens of thousands during and shortly after the First World War.

The type of flu mimicked by the drugs was called lethargic encephalitis (*encephalitis lethargica*), or von Economo's disease. "Lethargic" refers to a typical symptom of the disease, a sluggish or apathetic mental state. "Encephalitis" designates inflammation of the brain.

The similarity between the neuroleptic effect and lethargic encephalitis should have been a colossal warning against using the neuroleptics on human beings. Indeed, the viral disease and the drug-induced effects are so similar that to learn about lethargic encephalitis is to learn about the routine effects of the psychiatric medications. Yet the psychiatric literature has expurgated this important information so that most young psychiatrists are wholly unaware of it.

An esteemed text on the disease, *Lethargic Encephalitis*, was written by New York University professor of neurology Isador Abrahamson and published posthumously in 1935. Abrahamson's description of the effects of viral encephalitis are almost identical to the lobotomizing drug effect as described by Delay and Deniker and other neuroleptic pioneers:

Irritability both to internal and external stimuli diminishes, and the vital tone of the afflicted host lessens. . . . He may display neither conscious nor unconscious initiative . . . There is a complete lack of emotional expression . . . The face, waxen and corpselike, remains an impassive and inscrutable mask . . . In other words, sensory stimuli stream into the brain and the brain ignores them . . . [A]nd volition is practically suspended.*

Abrahamson uses a phrase to sum up the encephalitis victim's robotic condition—"psychomotor inertia." It, too, is almost identical to the phrase commonly used by psychiatrists to sum up the impact of the neuroleptics—"psychomotor retardation."

Similar Neurological Effects

After the mental lethargy that often heralded the onset of viral encephalitis, a variety of severe neurological symptoms manifested themselves as the disease progressed into its acute phase. These so closely parallel the various neurological reactions produced by neuroleptic medications that they can be discussed together.

The encephalitic patients would develop extremely painful, debilitating spasms of their muscles. This "dystonia" occasionally occurs early in the treatment of patients taking neuroleptic drugs.

The encephalitic patients developed bizarre forms of hyperactivity with an inner irritability that drives the person to move about. Sometimes it can reach extreme proportions of anxiety and anguish, with constant motion. This disorder, "akathisia," typically is found in up to half of the patients taking neuroleptics. A recent study by Joseph Lipinksi in the September 1989 *Journal of Clinical Psychiatry* found a rate of 71 percent for akathisia among a sample of 110 patients at Boston's McLean Hospital.

The victims of the virus often developed a variant of parkinsonism, including a tremor of the extremities, rigidity of movement and facial expression, a shuffling gait, and emotional flattening. Parkinsonlike signs occur in most patients treated with neuroleptics and in all patients given high doses. Many psychiatrists used to argue that the drugs could not have their maximum effect without producing some degree of parkinsonism. The muscles can become so rigid that the patient is unable to carry out aggressive actions or any other vigorous, spontaneous activity. This has been called the chemical straitjacket.[1]

Neuroleptic Malignant Syndrome

Psychiatry has focused increasing attention on an especially dramatic toxic reaction to the neuroleptics occurring in a small percentage of patients treated with the drugs. Like the meltdown of a nuclear power

---

*These quotes are taken from chapter 2, "Mental Disturbances in Lethargic Encephalitis," which is reprinted from the May 20, 1920, *Journal of Nervous and Mental Disease*.

plant, the drug reaction can get completely out of hand. The result, neuroleptic malignant syndrome, is largely indistinguishable from an acute, fulminating case of lethargic encephalitis.

If the viral encephalitis were to suddenly reappear, a trained clinician most likely would be unable to distinguish it from an attack of drug-induced neuroleptic malignant syndrome. Both are marked by lobotomylike indifference and then progress to fever and sweating, unstable cardiovascular signs, bizarre dyskinesias, and, in severe cases, delirium, coma, and death.

Similar Permanent Neurological Effects

The most tragic similarity between lethargic encephalitis and the neuroleptics is their frequent production of *permanent* neurological disorders. After lethargic encephalitis, many patients seemed to recover fully. Then months or even many years afterward, many would unexpectedly begin to deteriorate neurologically. They might develop abnormal bodily movements, such as twitches, spasms, or snakelike movements. Most often they developed permanent parkinsonism. Some would deteriorate mentally into psychotic states or dementia.

The profession of psychiatry now agrees that the drug-induced neurological disorders do become permanent in a large percentage of patients. In addition, there is growing incontrovertible evidence that permanent psychosis and dementia also are frequent outcomes. Neuroleptics impact on the patient by *causing a disease rather than by curing one.*

They Knew from the Beginning

We don't have to speculate about whether Delay and Deniker anticipated the potential tragedy they were creating. In a reminiscence published in 1970[2] Deniker says that he knew from the beginning that the drugs could cause a worldwide epidemic of brain disease similar to lethargic encephalitis:

It was found that neuroleptics could experimentally reproduce almost all the symptoms of lethargic encephalitis. In fact, *it would be possible to cause true encephalitis epidemics with the new drugs.* Symptoms progressed from reversible somnolence to all types of dyskinesia and hyperkinesia, and finally to parkinsonism. The symptoms *seemed reversible* on interruption of the medication. (Italics added)

Deniker also pointed out that the permanency of the damage could have been anticipated from the beginning:

Furthermore, it might have been feared that these drugs, whose actions compare with that of encephalitis and parkinsonism, might eventually induce *irreversible* secondary neurological syndromes. Such effects cannot be denied: it has been known for some years that *permanent* dyskinesias may occur. . . . (Italics added)

The Degree of Risk

In 1980, eight years after the first definitive reviews and twenty-five years after the drugs first had been used, the American Psychiatric Association finally completed and published an official task force report on tardive dyskinesia. Its official summary for the rates of tardive dyskinesia in routine drug use over six months to two years are staggering: at least 10 to 20 percent of neuroleptic-treated patients would get more than minimal disease. In older people and longer-term use the rates escalated to at least 40 percent in hospitals and in clinics.

Data in the task force report show that the percentages of affected patients are in fact much higher than reported in their summary estimate. The task force examined one group of 506 patients with special care and tabulated the rates according to age. The rates surpassed 54 percent in men and 59 percent in women age sixty and over. Among more elderly women treated with the drugs, 66 percent suffered from tardive dyskinesia.

The task force cited some well-conducted studies showing tardive dyskinesia rates of 40 to 60 percent in clinics and in state hospitals.

Half or More of Long-Term Patients

As the APA figures suggest, half or more of long-term patients, as well as older patients, are likely to develop tardive dyskinesia. A few drug advocates have acknowledged this openly. In their 1986 *Manual of Clinical Psychopharmacology*, published by the American Psychiatric Press, Alan Schatzberg and Jonathan Cole note that tardive dyskinesia tends to develop at the rate of 3 to 4 percent per year and that "in chronically institutionalized psychotic patients, dyskinesia prevalence rates are often on the order of 50–60 percent" (p. 99). A 1981 pamphlet written by psychiatrist Robert Sovner and produced by the drug company Sandoz, observes that "up to 56%" of "chronically hospitalized patients" will develop tardive dyskinesia.

An Almost Certain Risk?

Some experts have begun to admit that nearly all long-term patients are likely to succumb to tardive dyskinesia. Guy Chouinard of Canada is one of the most experienced and best known researchers in the field. The June 1990 *Clinical Psychiatry News* reports on Chouinard's recent findings: "It appears that drug exposure of 15 years and more would lead to almost certain risk for tardive dyskinesia." Unfortunately, many patients are told they must remain on neuroleptics for the rest of their lives, without being told about the huge and "almost certain" risk of developing a serious neurological disease.

A Court Verifies the Rates

While much of the psychiatric leadership continues to minimize and to misrepresent the risks of psychiatric drugs, the courts have become more convinced of the menace. In a supreme court case in Indiana in 1981, Judge Evan Goodman gave the following opinion:

At the heart of this case is the virtually undisputed allegation that a person medicated with anti-psychotic drugs has a 50% risk of contracting tardive dyskinesia, a disease exemplified by twisting tongue movements, puffing cheeks, smacking of lips, sucking movements of the mouth, and face and body movements characterized by continuous rocking motions, tremors and bizarre postures, and other symptoms, and which at this time is incurable.[3] (Italics added)

What the Public Hears

Generally the profession tells the public and patients very little about tardive dyskinesia and greatly minimizes the risk. A fortunate exception is psychiatrist Jack Gorman in his book *The Essential Guide to Psychiatric Drugs* (1990). He warns the potential patient, "The risk of developing severe TD from antipsychotic drugs probably lies between 20% and 40%, but mild signs may appear in up to 70% of patients. Patients should be examined carefully by the doctor, at least every six months, for signs of TD" (p. 221).

If patients are taking these drugs, it is indeed imperative that the doctor carefully examine them frequently for signs of abnormal movements and that the patient and the family stay alert for them as well.

Confirming High Rates Among Older Patients

Recent investigations have confirmed the high rate of tardive dyskinesia in all age groups and have ruled out spontaneous dyskinesias of unknown origin as a major complicating factor. In *Tardive Dyskinesia* (1988), edited by Marion Wolf and Aron Mosnaim, a team led by Ramzy Yassa from

McGill University found a rate of 41 percent among patients over age sixty-three after only twenty-four months of exposure to neuroleptics.

None of the nondrug controls in Yassa's study developed movement disorders during the test period of two years. Since the aged are the only group thought to be susceptible to an appreciable number of spontaneous motor disorders, this should lay to rest the argument that tardive dyskinesia rates are falsely inflated by nondrug movement disorders. As the September 1983 headline in *Clinical Psychiatry News* had already indicated, DYSKINESIA INCIDENCE HELD VERY LOW IN HEALTHY AGED POPULATION.

Confirming High Rates Among Children

Children frequently are given these medications in hospitals, facilities for delinquents, and, especially, institutions for the retarded. Typically they are used for the control of unwanted behaviors. This well-known fact was confirmed in a 1987 survey of practices in a children's state hospital by Benedetto Vitiello and others in the *Journal of Clinical Psychiatry*.

For a decade after the recognition of tardive dyskinesia, psychiatric experts supported the myth that children are less affected by tardive dyskinesia and that it is safer to give them the medications. Yet the review in my 1983 book *Psychiatric Drugs: Hazards to the Brain* made clear for probably the first time that rates among children are high and that children tend to suffer from especially incapacitating cases of the disease, often involving control of the torso, making it hard for them to sit, stand, or walk.

Fortunately, the myth about children being resistant to tardive dyskinesia seems to be dying. A study of drug-treated retarded children by C. Thomas Gualtieri and his colleagues, published in the April 1986 *Archives of General Psychiatry*, showed that 34 percent of the children developed tardive dyskinesia, the *majority* displaying moderate to severe symptoms. They stated, "One may conclude that TD, including severe and persistent TD, represents a substantial hazard to young retarded people treated with neuroleptic drugs." The risk, of course, is not limited to the retarded, but equally includes every child treated with these drugs. The study also showed that the children went through an especially agonizing period of withdrawal from the drugs, during which their mental anguish increased substantially.

Tardive Akathisia in Children and the Developmentally Disabled

Tardive akathisia—anxiety or nervousness and an uncontrollable drive to move the body—is a particularly insidious problem among children treated with neuroleptics. Especially in institutions for children and among people with mental retardation, the neuroleptics are given in order to control restlessness. It's easier to drug these persons than to provide more interesting and stimulating environments to occupy their energy. But when the drugs are administered for several months or more, there is increasing danger that they will produce tardive akathisia—a permanent need to move about, accompanied by sometimes dreadful anxiety. Thus the drugs create the very symptoms they are supposed to control, and the child ends up in a vicious circle, being given larger and larger doses in order to control the now-drug-induced disorder.

Akathisia, as already noted, is very common during neuroleptic drug treatment. How often it becomes permanent is more difficult to tell, but Gualtieri, one of the world's experts, estimates that tardive akathisia occurs in 13 percent or more of institutionalized developmentally disabled persons who are treated with neuroleptics.[4] It is an irony of tragic proportions that we literally are *creating* hyperactive children and adults, saddled for the rest of their lives with sometimes excruciating inner turmoil and a drive to keep their bodies in motion all the time.

The Professional Reaction to Tardive Dyskinesia

For twenty years the profession simply failed to notice that a large percentage of its patients was twitching and writhing from the drugs. When the first highly visible reports came out in 1973 by George Crane in *Science* and by a joint committee of the American College of Neuropsychopharmacology and the Food and Drug Administration (FDA) in the *Archives of General Psychiatry*, the professional reaction was largely one of denial and rejection. The editor of the *Archives*, Daniel X. Freedman, appended an editorial to the report on tardive dyskinesia in which he warned the reader not to exaggerate the problem because it might impede congressional funding for beleaguered psychiatry. The late Nathan Kline, once the nation's most quoted drug specialist, said he'd never seen a case in his life, even though he conducted research in state mental hospitals where half or more of the patients are afflicted. Nor was Kline alone. Nearly every hospital and clinic psychiatrist in the world was at that time guilty of the same oversight.

The story of psychiatry's failure to take responsibility for injuring its patients is recounted in detail by Phil Brown and Steven Funk in "Tardive Dyskinesia: Barriers to the Professional Recognition of an Iatrogenic Disease" in the June 1986 *Journal of Health and Social Behavior.** Brown and Funk cite George Crane's confirmation that "the majority of psychiatrists either ignored the existence of the problem or made futile attempts to prove that these motor abnormalities were clinically insignificant or unrelated to drug therapy." In a frightening revelation, Crane discloses that psychiatrists tended to increase their use of neuroleptics after he lectured them on their dangers.

Psychiatrists continue to be largely remiss about informing patients and their families about the dangers of tardive dyskinesia. As Brown and Funk observed in 1986, "psychiatrists do not, by and large, inform patients and their families adequately about the risks of TD." As we saw in Roberta's case, they can persistently fail even to recognize the disease they themselves have induced. †

Psychiatry's Special Concern

As the data on tardive dyskinesia piled up, psychiatry became more and more concerned—not for its patients, but for itself. On October 7, 1983, the official APA newspaper, *Psychiatric News*, declared in a headline: TD COURT CASES UNDERSCORE IMPORTANCE OF APA REPORT. It gave the bad news: two precedent-setting cases had been settled for $760,000 and $1 million. Another headline in the January 1984 issue of *Clinical Psychiatry News* shouts out the dreaded words: EXPECT A FLOOD OF TARDIVE DYSKINESIA MALPRACTICE SUITS. I know of no corresponding headline, such as BEWARE A FLOOD OF TARDIVE DYSKINESIA PATIENTS. It's the legal cases that worry psychiatrists.

---

*Brown and Funk point out that at the time of Thorazine's introduction in the United States, its toxic effects and potential for causing damage were almost wholly ignored in the rush to use it as an agent of control in the state mental hospitals. Although it had been tested on only 104 patients in this country, Smith Kline and French promoted Thorazine so successfully that within eight months in 1954 the astounding number of two million Americans had been placed on the medication, nearly all of them involuntary inmates in state mental hospitals.

† In 1987 Peter Weiden and his colleagues from the Cornell Medical Center published a study in the *American Journal of Psychiatry* aptly entitled "Clinical Nonrecognition of Neuroleptic-Induced Movement Disorders: A Cautionary Study." A July 1988 report in *Clinical Psychiatry News* confirms that psychiatrists continue to underdiagnose the disease. Using the standard of mild but definite symptoms, independent researchers in one study found a 48-percent rate of tardive dyskinesia; but the treating psychiatrists had noted signs of the disease in only 12 percent of the same group of patients. The treating doctors were especially prone to miss more subtle signs, such as difficulties in breathing and swallowing. The latter can be life-threatening. But they also missed more obvious signs, such as movements of the arms and legs.

In July 1985 the American Psychiatric Association followed up its task force report of five years earlier with an unprecedented letter to its nearly forty thousand members, which included nearly every psychiatrist in America. It repeated its warning that "at least 10–20% of patients in mental hospitals" and at least 40 percent of longer-term patients would get more than minimal signs of tardive dyskinesia. It also confirmed that children are at risk.

Why the unusual letter? One reason, at least, was self-serving: "We are further concerned about the apparent increase in litigation over tardive dyskinesia."

Since then, malpractice suits have escalated. TARDIVE DYSKINESIA LAW-SUITS ON INCREASE warns a May 1989 headline in *The Psychiatric Times*. Expert Theodore van Putten estimated 400,000 to a million cases of the disease in the United States alone. Out-of-court settlements, the article says, were averaging $300,000, while jury awards were averaging $1 million.

NIMH Waters Down the Rates

As the tragedy of tardive dyskinesia unfolded, some doctors devoted themselves to making light of it. Dilip Jeste and Richard Jed Wyatt of NIMH and St. Elizabeths Hospital estimate a tardive dyskinesia rate of only 13 percent in their 1982 book *Understanding and Treating Tardive Dyskinesia*. While even a rate this high would be a medical catastrophe, the real figures are much higher. Jeste and Wyatt achieve their relatively low figures, first by assuming that one-quarter of reported cases are due to nondrug movement disorders (p. 32) and second by arbitrarily dropping out all cases in the literature except those labeled "moderate" and "severe" (p. 22). Without these manipulations of the data, which are buried in the text, their rate would be more than double the 13 percent.[5]

In reality, the most careful studies have generated the highest rates. Stewart Tepper and Joanna Haas, in a December 1979 review in the *Journal of Clinical Psychiatry*, specifically focused on the better studies and found rates for tardive dyskinesia in the range of 24 to 56 percent for patients undergoing chronic neuroleptic treatment. Studies with low rates were typically very flawed. Tepper and Haas estimated that "close to 200,000 patients may develop tardive dyskinesia as a result of neuroleptics prescribed in 1978." As an example of a well-conducted study, psychiatrist Gregory Asnis and his colleagues, in 1977 in the *American Journal of Psychiatry*, reported using objective rating scales, more than one rater, and videotapes. They found that *among outpatients* in a New York City clinic, 43.4 percent suffered from tardive dyskinesia. Worse still, many had received the drugs for a year or less. One had been treated for only eight months.

The President of APA Tries to Deny the Rates

On the Oprah Winfrey TV talk show on August 17, 1987, I debated the president-elect of the American Psychiatric Association, psychiatrist Paul Fink. Shortly before I was introduced, psychiatric survivor Judi Chamberlin had warned the viewing audience about tardive dyskinesia. Now I further explained, "If individual people want to take drugs, that's their privilege. But they should know that long-term therapy in 50 percent of the cases is producing the neurological disease Judi mentioned."

Fink interrupted adamantly, "Fifty percent of the cases is an outrageous overstatement. Absolutely an outrageous overstatement."

I corrected him, "The Psychiatric Association's Task Force on Tardive Dyskinesia said—"

Fink began shouting and interrupting again, "Never said 50 percent."

"It says 40 percent get *more than minimal* disease," I said, completing my sentence.

"Never said!" he shouted again. "Never says 40 percent."

There it was. The president-elect of the American Psychiatric Association could not possibly be ignorant of the data from the APA report, especially since the 40 percent figure had been published repeatedly in the association's books, journals, newspapers, and even an official letter to the membership two years earlier.

At the next break for advertising, I retrieved from my briefcase my copy of the official APA task force report, *Tardive Dyskinesia*. When the show resumed, I read aloud the statement, quoted earlier in this chapter, that at least 40 percent of long-term patients will be afflicted with tardive dyskinesia.

Newly Recognized Manifestations of Permanent Neurological Damage

There's increasing recognition of variations on tardive dyskinesia, including tardive dystonia, with recurrent muscle spasms that are agonizing to the patient, and tardive akathisia, described earlier in this chapter. As with the other tardive disorders, there are no known treatments for them.

Cases are appearing of patients permanently unable to control their water intake, leading to water intoxication, as well as cases of the chronic disability of temperature control mechanisms, leading to heat stroke. The growing array of problems stimulated a story in the November 1987 issue of *Clinical Psychiatry News* with the headline DYSKINESIA 'TIP OF ICEBERG' OF NEUROLEPTIC SYNDROMES.

Beneath the "tip of the iceberg" of neuroleptic syndromes lurks something far more threatening.

Deterioration of the Mind from Neuroleptic Treatment

When I first began to review the extensive literature about tardive dyskinesia, all of the psychiatric textbooks assumed that it was a disease affecting muscular control without imperiling the mind. Intuitively, and from what I knew scientifically of the integration of brain and mind, it seemed implausible to ruin the motor control systems without harming the mind as well. My research resulted in a lengthy overview on permanent mental dysfunction from the neuroleptics, published as a chapter entitled "Lobotomy, Dementia, and Psychosis Produced by the Major Tranquilizers" in my 1983 medical book *Psychiatric Drugs: Hazards to the Brain*. Seven years later I followed this with an updated, still more detailed review, "Brain Damage, Dementia and Persistent Cognitive Dysfunction Associated with Neuroleptic Drugs: Evidence, Etiology, and Implications," in the *Journal of Mind and Behavior*.[6]

Briefly, the basal ganglia are most clearly damaged during the production of tardive dyskinesia by the neuroleptics. Pathological findings in Parkinson's disease and Huntington's chorea indicate that they influence control and coordination of the muscles. But the basal ganglia also are intimately connected to the higher mental centers, and diseases affecting the region ultimately impair the mind. Tardive dyskinesia is caused by permanent hyperreactivity in the dopamine neurotransmitter system in this area. But dopamine is also the main neurotransmitter ascending into the emotion-regulating limbic system and frontal lobes. The lobotomy effect results from the action of the drugs on these nerve pathways. When this region also becomes permanently hyperreactive in response to the neuroleptics, as we know it does, it would make damage to the higher brain and mind inevitable.

The clinical literature confirmed my initial suspicions and my surmise that permanent damage to the highest mental centers was inevitable. The initial studies of tardive dyskinesia showed that many and sometimes all patients also were suffering from serious mental dysfunction, including dementia. These threatening revelations were literally in small print and in charts, and seldom were commented on.

The Cover-Up of Vital Information on Drug-Induced Dementia

The federal government sponsored a highly publicized nationwide study of the effects on the brain of taking multiple street drugs, such as narcotics and hallucinogens. A serendipitous finding came up in the mental patient control group: *the consumption of neuroleptic drugs was directly associated with a permanent loss of overall mental function.*

If the drug had been marijuana, or even tobacco or alcohol, the results of this authoritative study would have been instantly flashed across the nation by the media. Not so when the brains of mental patients are balanced against the reputations of psychiatrists. The reputations nearly always carry the day.

A complete but unpublished version of the paper was presented at professional conferences. It was authored by Igor Grant, Kenneth Adams, Albert Carlin, Phillip Rennick, Lewis Judd, and others. Senior author Grant was assistant professor and Judd was professor and chairman of the Department of Psychiatry of the University of California in San Diego. Until recently Judd was the director of NIMH, pushing it in the direction of becoming exclusively a biopsychiatric institute.

I was able to obtain the unpublished version that was presented in 1978 at the International Neuropsychological Association in Minneapolis. The unpublished copy reports that the mental dysfunction was found in more than 25 percent of the neuroleptic-treated patients using the Halstead-Reitan Neuropsychological Battery, considered by many to be the best test available for detecting mental dysfunction caused by brain damage. A statistical correlation was found between lifetime ingestion of neuroleptic drugs and persistent mental dysfunction. None of the patients had received psychiatric medications for more than five years.

In the unpublished version the authors declared, "We were struck that the deficit frequently occurred in psychiatric patients" and "that this deficit was correlated with extent of antipsychotic drug use." The final sentence warned, "It is also clear that the antipsychotic drugs must continue to be scrutinized for the possibility that their extensive consumption might cause general cerebral dysfunction."

Gerald H. Dubin, at the time a research psychiatrist at the National Institute on Drug Abuse, was a project officer for the Grant studies. In an interview with me on February 26, 1991, Dubin confirmed the importance of their findings that neuroleptics "might cause" neuropsychological impairment of a lasting nature. He said the studies indicated the need for "extensive research" on the subject by individuals and organizations who do not have a "vested interest" in drugs.

What happened to the published versions of this study?

In February of 1978, the same year that the unpublished version was presented at the Minneapolis conference, a slightly different version appeared in the *American Journal of Psychiatry*, an official journal of the American Psychiatric Association. It covered all of the same material, except for the all-important correlation between neuroleptics and chronic brain dysfunction. That is buried in the statistical analysis, without a single mention in the synopsis, introduction, discussion, or conclusion of the article. Only by reading the article with a mental magnifying glass focused on the statistical analysis would anyone find it.

Even worse, the statistical data in the discussion section of the article points to a correlation between schizophrenia and brain dysfunction, making it seem as if schizophrenia causes the problem. Shockingly, the further correlation with total lifetime consumption of neuroleptics is not mentioned. Moreover, there's no hint in the discussion sections of the published paper that brain dysfunction was primarily correlated with taking neuroleptics.

The study resulted in another major journal article by the same senior authors, Grant and Adams, as well as Judd, in the September 1978 *Archives of General Psychiatry*, published by the AMA. This version does mention the correlation between psychiatric drug ingestion and mental dysfunction, but without stressing that it is permanent dysfunction and without the warnings given in the original, unpublished paper.

In 1986 Grant and Adams published *Neuropsychological Assessment of Neuropsychiatric Disorders.*[7] Unhappily, while they briefly admit to their original findings, they quickly dismiss them in a sentence: "Grant and associates found a relationship between cumulative exposure to antipsychotics and impairment in a small group of younger schizophrenics. It was not clear whether the drugs were causal, or merely reflected a more refractory form of schizophrenia which was characterized by pre-existing deficit" (p. 155). In fact, there was no evidence that their patients were refractory or gravely disabled. Their unpublished paper argues *against* schizophrenia as a cause, in part because the patients were not "chronic," and stresses the correlation between brain dysfunction and lifetime neuroleptic drug intake.

An earlier book with Grant as the sole author, *Behavior Disorders: Understanding Clinical Psychopathology* (1979), dramatically displays his bias against his own findings. Grant fails even to *mention* or to *cite* his own research on drug-induced brain dysfunction. Instead, he declares that "the antipsychotic drugs represent a true milestone in the humane treatment of schizophrenics" (p. 97). Tardive dykinesia is given a mere paragraph and, most incredibly, is called "rare" (p. 105). Thus Grant not only leaves out his own work on irreversible mental dysfunction, he denies the epidemic rates of tardive dyskinesia.

Growing Confirmation and the Continuing Cover-Up

Dozens of studies have since come out indicating that neuroleptic-treated patients have such severe brain damage that it can be detected as shrinkage of the brain on the newer radiology techniques, such as the CT scan, which utilizes computerized analysis of X rays of the brain taken at multiple levels. Often the shrinkage is associated with degrees of mental deterioration. My 1990 review in the *Journal of Mind and Behavior* provides the dozens of citations on which the following analysis is based.

Many—but not all—of my psychiatric colleagues view these findings as the long-sought proof that schizophrenia is a brain disease. But the brain shrinkage cannot be due to schizophrenia. For decades schizophrenia has been called a "functional disorder" precisely because it typically occurs in the absence of any signs of organic brain disease. The recent finding that these individuals have gross organic brain disease flies in the face of this long-standing clinical experience. Confirming this clinical knowledge, autopsy studies in the predrug era failed to find any consistent gross pathology in the brains of schizophrenics. Furthermore, we have animal autopsy studies confirming that the neuroleptic drugs do indeed damage the brain, even in small, short-term doses. And finally, we have studies of additional groups, such as adult patients with other diagnoses and mentally retarded children, who are developing mental deterioration on the same drugs.*

In criticism of the burgeoning brain-shrinkage studies involving schizophrenic patients, psychiatrist Theodore Lidz declared in a 1981 letter to the *American Journal of Psychiatry*: "For hundreds of years investigators have reported a neuropathological or physiopathological cause of schizophrenia. The trouble is that no such findings have been replicated. If the patient suffers from dementia, the diagnosis is not schizophrenia"

---

*Before the neuroleptic drugs came into use in 1954, hundreds of autopsy studies attempted to prove that schizophrenics have brain disease. Then, as now, it was an obsession in psychiatry, every researcher's hope for a Nobel Prize. The methods used were far more sensitive than CT scans. The heads of thousands of recently deceased patients were opened on autopsy and their brains examined under microscopes with special staining techniques. They were, of course, inspected, weighed, and measured most carefully. In Nazi Germany the search for a brain disease in schizophrenics was carried to the ultimate with made-to-order dead patients—hapless individuals specifically and officially murdered so that their "fresh" brains could be studied by avid biopsychiatrists. In the 1959 *American Handbook of Psychiatry*, Sylvano Arieti states under "Neuropathology of Schizophrenia" that, despite an intensive search, no consistent abnormalities of the brain have been found and all such hopes "have remained unfulfilled."

(p. 854). Lidz went on to link brain scan studies to earlier, equally fervent attempts to find a physical basis for schizophrenia, many by the very same investigators. Lidz suggested taking into account the impact on the brain of shock treatment and medications.*

In the next chapter we shall examine compelling evidence from twin studies for the damaging effect of neuroleptics on the brain.

The various brain scan studies of damage and dysfunction suggest that somewhere between 10 and 40 percent of neuroleptic-treated patients are afflicted. Age and total lifetime intake of medication probably influence the rate. The rates are thus substantial but somewhat lower than those for tardive dyskinesia. When both threats to the brain are considered, it is clear that all, or almost all, long-term neuroleptic-treated patients will suffer some sort of permanent brain damage and dysfunction.

The Newest Miracle Drug

A relatively new drug in this country, clozapine (trade name Clozaril), is said to have the neuroleptic impact without as many neurological side effects. It apparently does not suppress dopamine neurotransmission in the motor-regulating areas of the brain, thus reducing the risk of tardive dyskinesia. However, this does not mean that it won't cause tardive dementia, tardive psychosis, and other central nervous system disorders when it blocks neurotransmission in the higher centers of the brain. If long-term studies show that the drug does not cause tardive dyskinesia, psychiatrists will be lulled into believing that it is relatively harmless to the brain. They will have an even greater tendency to forget the more subtle and yet devastating possibility of persistent mental deficits and dementia.

Clinicians I have spoken to in Europe feel that clozapine produces a particularly profound lobotomy effect, adding to concern about long-term dangers of tardive psychosis and dementia. As early as 1977, when the drug was already being used in Europe, U. Ungerstedt and T. Ljungberg warned in *Advances in Biochemical Psychopharmacology* that since the drug seemed more effective in blocking neurotransmission in the frontal lobes, it might also end up producing especially severe reactive psychoses. In an extensive letter to the editor in the 1982 *Journal of Clinical Psychopharmacology*, Guy Chouinard and Barry Jones revived this theme,

---

* Few current textbooks mention the importance of these CT scan studies for the dangerousness of psychiatric treatment. The 1988 American Psychiatric Press's *Textbook of Psychiatry* points out that recent findings of abnormalities "could be a simple direct consequence of neuroleptic treatment" (p. 383), but the devastating implications of such a possibility go unmentioned.

pointing to Swedish observations on reactive psychoses following withdrawal from clozapine.* This means that once patients are put on the drug, it can be very difficult to withdraw them; yet, due to the drug's toxicity, their higher mental functions may be deteriorating the longer they stay on it.

Clozapine also is known to cause an unusually high rate of agranulocytosis, a life-threatening blood disorder that reduces the white blood cell count, rendering the individual less able to respond to infection. It has been found to occur in 2 percent or more of patients. As a result, it was taken off the market in Europe for many years before being approved recently in America.

Sandoz, the manufacturer, has constructed an elaborate plan for distributing the drug, including required weekly blood tests by its own designated laboratory. The total cost will be in the range of $9,000 or more a year per patient.† In addition to its concerns about lawsuits, critics have wondered whether Sandoz isn't motivated by a desire to make as much money as possible before its patent runs out in about four years. Meanwhile, those in favor of the drug are outraged at the price, pointing out that the cost of its anticipated usage would exceed the entire mental health budget of some states and reach a grand total of $2 billion per year in the United States. A Veterans Administration (VA) representative called it "a rich man's drug for a poor man's disease."[8] To those of us afraid of the damage that this drug will do, its price is a blessing.

Sandoz has become very cozy with the parents organization NAMI in promoting this dangerous agent. It has given NAMI five hundred "scholarships" for free clozapine.[9]

Despite all the hoopla surrounding clozapine, there's very little evidence of its efficacy, even by traditional psychiatric standards. It is being slated for only those patients resistant to other drugs, or about 25 percent of those people diagnosed as schizophrenic. Of these, drug advocates estimate that about one-third will be helped.[10] We are talking about a relatively small number of very difficult patients who may or may not have any added effect from the new drug, but who will surely be subjected to a greater risk of brain damage and other serious and potentially lethal side effects.

---

*Chouinard and Jones observed: "This convincing evidence of clozapine's ability to induce supersensitivity psychosis might be related to both the short half-life of the drug and its greater affinity for mesolimbic dopamine receptors" (p. 144).
† Under pressure, Sandoz recently dropped the required testing program.

The Gravest Danger in the Future of Neuroleptic Treatment

We have seen that during the first two decades (1954 to 1973) of wide-spread neuroleptic use, psychiatry in general failed to notice that half or more of chronic state hospital patients were trembling, twitching, and displaying other bizarre drug-induced symptoms. Some psychiatrists then tried to blame the neurological disorder on schizophrenia rather than on the drugs, and some continue to do so.[11] It is even easier to ignore the symptoms of dementia or to blame the patient's innate mental illness rather than the drugs. I am very concerned that clozapine will swell the size of the epidemic of drug-induced dementia while psychiatry continues to find it convenient to ignore the tragedy of destroying the brains and minds of the very people it is supposed to be helping.

Other Side Effects of the Neuroleptics

Not even the experienced psychiatrist can keep in mind all of the potential dangers of using these highly toxic drugs that impair the function of many organs of the body. Without wholly relying on them, patients and their families should read a few textbooks in combination with yearly updated sources, like the *Physician's Desk Reference (PDR)* and *Drug Information for the Health Care Provider* (see appendix B). The readily available American Psychiatric Press's *Textbook of Psychiatry* also has a fairly extensive list. No single source will cover all of the side effects, and some will leave out very important ones. These references can be supplemented with my 1983 medical book and with Dr. Caligari's *Psychiatric Drugs* (see appendix B).

If you believe you must take neuroleptic drugs, be alert for *any* danger signals that your body isn't responding normally. Almost any organ can be adversely affected by the neuroleptics: eyes, nose, and throat; internal organs, such as the liver, stomach, intestines, cardiovascular system, and sexual organs; the skin; and of course, the brain. Be aware that a small percentage of patients suffer disastrous consequences, such as neuroleptic malignant syndrome, sudden unexplained death, cardiovascular crises, seizures, and heat stroke in overheated institutions. These are among the most dangerous medications ever used in medicine.

Of special concern to women, there are a number of reasons to fear an increase in breast cancer. The tendency to demean both women and mental patients and to exalt psychiatric treatments has led to serious underemphasis on this problem. Research suggestive of increased rates of cancer in women have not been followed up adequately, and the profession has not taken the danger seriously.[12]

Above all, don't be fooled into believing that these drugs are actually treating a disease. They are suppressing overall brain function and creating diseases.

Withdrawing from Psychiatric Drugs

While neuroleptic drugs are dangerous to take, they also are dangerous to stop taking too quickly. Disturbing muscular control problems can develop during the withdrawal period. Withdrawal can cause a temporary or permanent worsening of psychotic symptoms, with anxiety and even anguish, as a result of central nervous system rebound from the drugs. This can take weeks or longer to clear or may not clear at all. Insomnia is common. Withdrawal commonly produces a very distressing flulike syndrome, including runny nose, headache, fever, muscle and joint aches, and gastrointestinal upset.*

Because of the withdrawal problems, patients should try to come off the medications while receiving emotional and social support from others and with supervision by someone familiar with the process. It should be understood that withdrawal symptoms may encourage the doctor and patient alike to resume the drug prematurely, when what the patient really needs is time to recover from the drug.

Helping patients come off these drugs can be very difficult. I try to involve people who deal with the patient regularly, such as members of the family, friends, ministers, teachers, and family doctors. Nearly everyone personally associated with the patient is likely to believe that he or she must take the drugs for a lifetime. Symptoms of possible dementia —such as silliness or shallowness, erratic moods, difficulty focusing attention, wandering speech, disconnected thoughts, talking too directly in the listener's face—will be seen as evidence of an innate mental illness. Any withdrawal symptoms, from insomnia and hyperactivity to hallucinations and delusions—also will be attributed to the patient's psychiatric problem. In addition, as the patient recovers from some of the lobotomy effect, old resentments and conflicts may surface between the patient and others. Eventually the drug-free individual may have to deal with his or

---

*The consequences of withdrawal can be so serious that the *American Journal of Psychiatry* in 1989 published two of my letters explaining why we should label these agents addictive. Interestingly, it was a psychiatric survivor I met in Germany who asked me to give more consideration to the addictive qualities of the neuroleptics; but the *American Journal of Psychiatry* felt it would reduce the impact of my letter if I mentioned the source of my inspiration, and it was edited out before publication.

her originally overwhelming passions. People who must deal with the patient on a daily basis may find themselves minimizing the dangers of the drugs in favor of restoring the relative peace and calm enforced by the drugs.

Anyone helping the patient withdraw from the drugs may need to spend time communicating with people other than the patient, encouraging them, too, to support the gradual and sometimes treacherous process. Perhaps the drug-free person won't ever again be as easy to live with, but he or she will be physically healthier and have vastly increased opportunity to get more out of life.

I've known many people in the psychiatric survivor movement who successfully have come off these drugs cold turkey; but I never recommend it in my psychiatric practice, unless the patient has been using the medication for only a brief period of time.

Patients, I believe, should try not to get started on neuroleptics and, once taking them, should do so for the shortest time possible. Whenever possible, patients should periodically attempt to carefully withdraw from them. In contrast to the biopsychiatric viewpoint, I advocate psychosocial approaches as the first choice whenever possible.

The Right to Drug-Free Care

In Sweden, physician Lars Martensson is advocating the right to drug-free care. As long as the government supports, promotes, and even enforces involuntary drug treatment, it's appropriate to require the government to provide drug-free alternatives as well. Martensson's views are gaining political support.

I doubt if the neuroleptics would be legal except for the fact that they are given to mental patients. We tend to hold the health and well-being of psychiatric patients in low regard, a prejudice that has resulted in drastic harm to millions of people.

The Size of the Epidemic

There has been no official attempt to estimate the numbers of patients suffering from tardive dyskinesia. That no such body as NIMH, APA, or FDA has taken this task upon itself is further testimony to psychiatry's desire to turn away from the problem. Organized psychiatry is fond of producing half-cocked statistics on how many so-called schizophrenics or depressives there are in the country, because it helps business. But it is loathe to estimate how many patients it is permanently damaging.

Occasional estimates do pop up in the literature. As we saw, Tepper and Haas suggested that 200,000 new cases were generated in one year, 1978. Van Putten estimated a total of 400,000 to 1,000,000 cases in the United States in 1989, a figure that is accepted by the Tardive Dyskinesia/ Tardive Dystonia National Association, which cites "400,000 to *over* 1,000,000" afflicted Americans. In Seymour Fisher and Roger Greenberg's *The Limits of Biological Treatments for Psychological Distress,* also in 1989, Mantosh Dewan and Marvin Koss estimate at least 360,000 cases in the United States.

I believe that the upper estimate suggested by van Putten is closest to the mark and that *more than one million Americans suffer from tardive dyskinesia.* If we add tardive dementia without signs of tardive dyskinesia, the figures continue to swell. The total number of victims worldwide since 1954 must be astronomical, probably running into the tens of millions.

Where do I derive such frightening estimates? The lower estimates usually are based on the presumed numbers of schizophrenics being treated with the neuroleptics, but the drugs are in fact used for a wide variety of people, from prisoners and children to retarded people and the elderly in nursing homes. Remember that even the American Psychiatric Association, the national trade union of psychiatrists, admits that at least 10 to 20 percent of routinely treated patients will develop more than minimal signs of tardive dyskinesia, and that the figure goes up to at least 40 percent in long-term treatment cases and older patients. Therefore, it is conservative to use an overall rate of approximately 20 percent for all patients under all conditions; it probably is higher. Now all we have to do is obtain some estimates of total numbers of drug-treated patients and multiply it by 20 percent. My own estimate in chapter 3 of five to ten million neuroleptic patients a year would then suggest at least one million tardive dyskinesia patients. Combine that with perhaps double that number accumulating over the years for a total of two million cases in the United States alone.

Informal estimates have been made that at least 250 to 300 million persons have been treated with neuroleptics worldwide since the inception of neuroleptic treatment in 1953–54. According to material described to me and cited by British psychologist David Hill, the drug company Roche Laboratories estimated in 1980 that 150 million people worldwide were receiving neuroleptics *at that time.* In 1985 Hill used that figure to estimate that "38.5 million people are currently suffering from tardive dyskinesia."[13] It seems conservative to say that in 1991, tens of millions of tardive dyskinesia victims are alive around the world, with many more having been afflicted over the years since the mid-1950s.

The point of these estimates is not to come up with an incontrovertible figure, but to communicate that we are indeed talking about millions of victims—a plague of brain damage of huge proportions. It seems fitting to conclude as I did following my discussion of tardive dyskinesia in my 1983 medical book *Psychiatric Drugs: Hazards to the Brain*: "Psychiatry has unleashed an epidemic of neurological disease on the world. Even if tardive dyskinesia were the only permanent disability produced by these drugs, by itself, this would be among the worst medically-induced disasters in history."

Despite the best efforts, we can never fully anticipate all of the damaging effects inflicted on the individual by the neuroleptics and other toxic drugs. We must assume that numerous harmful effects go unnoticed. There is an analogy here to environmental pollution, where likewise we can notice, measure, and anticipate only the most obviously damaging effects. By the time we do become aware of new dangers, we've already done an unconscionable amount of harm, and for the health of many people, it's too late. We need to be extremely cautious in our use of toxic agents in psychiatry. The human body is not the place to dispose of toxic chemicals put out by any industry, including the psychopharmaceutical and psychiatric industries.

Chapter 5

The Biology and Genetics of "Schizophrenic" Overwhelm

In schizophrenia, for example, despite intensive investigations, no alterations in the brain have been found. It seems to me that to reduce other people to the status of depersonalized objects is of no help to them whatsoever.

—*Benno Muller-Hill*, Murderous Science *(1988)*

The dogma that "mental diseases are diseases of the brain" is a hangover from . . . materialism. . . . It has become a prejudice which hinders all progress, with nothing to justify it.
—*Carl Jung (1948)*

. . . even if schizophrenia were largely genetic in origin, it would in no way follow that drugs—or any biological, as opposed to social, treatment —would necessarily be the most effective therapy.
—*R.C. Lewontin, Steven Rose, and Leon Kamin*, Not in Our Genes *(1984)*

I was getting ready to appear on a Canadian television talk show, "The Shirley Show," and I'd brought my son Ben along on the trip. At the time, he was twelve. As I got ready for the cameras to roll, my mind was still on the green room, where Ben was getting ready to watch me on the TV monitor. Why was I distracted when my mind should be on the show? In the green room with Ben were several members of a Canadian organization of parents of schizophrenic offspring. To my dismay, in front of my son, they were trying to rattle me before I went on the air; and now I was concerned about leaving him alone with them.

One parent had been acting very sweetly toward me. Then, as I was leaving to face the cameras, she said, "Now that you've seen how nice I am, won't you feel guilty saying that mothers cause their children to go crazy?" She had written that her own son, a schizophrenic, saw devil's horns growing out of her head. Another member of the parent group, a father, had been bluntly ridiculing me, with knowing glances toward my son. As I left for the studio down the hallway, the man was shouting at me.

The show started and my attention did become galvanized, if only because the audience was packed with parent group members who hooted and hissed whenever I spoke. When I talked about children becoming disturbed in part, at least, due to stresses and conflicts in the family, they tried to drown me out. The parent representative on the panel glowed as she announced that of course science had exonerated her of any role in the breakdowns of her several children. It was all genetic.*

Afterward I asked Ben how it had gone in the green room. Yes, the parent group members had continued to ridicule me while I was on the TV, specifically directing some of their remarks toward him. Fortunately, even at age twelve, Ben was undaunted by their tactics.

I was not surprised by the Canadian group. It was the counterpart of the American parents group, NAMI.

Wanting to Believe in Genetics and Biochemistry

Why would parents so passionately desire to believe that their children suffer from genetic and biochemical defects? Frustrated in trying to influence their children, and perhaps overwhelmed with guilt and shame, they turn to modern biopsychiatric theory to exonerate them. They also turn to psychiatric drugs and electroshock to control their desperately rebellious offspring.

Seeing the hurt and anger in these parents, they, too, must have been damaged by their own parents. Nothing in life is more difficult than holding our parents responsible for the ways in which they have mistreated us. Again, biopsychiatry protects them from having to face the painful realization that they are passing family problems from generation to generation.

So there are many motives for parents to combine with biopsychiatry in blaming their problems with their children on genetics and biochemistry. But the price of these gains is enormous—the abdication of self-

---

*The parents group members in the audience also shouted in outrage when I spoke about the brain-damaging effects of psychiatric drugs. Their felt need to drug their children does not allow them to entertain the possibility that they are damaging them. The Canadian psychiatrist on the show, Barry Jones, at first denied that the drugs cause brain damage; but when I threatened to display several of his own articles on drug-induced irreversible tardive dyskinesia and permanent reactive psychoses—which I had in my coat pocket—he admitted, on the air, that the psychiatric drugs do indeed cause brain damage. Still, the hostess of the show had to pull the admission out of him.

determination, self-esteem, and love for their children. Rejecting all responsibility for the condition of their sons and daughters robs parents of the opportunity to help them by improving the environment in which they all live.*

It's understandable that parents would prefer to think of their children as genetically defective rather than as resentful, rebellious, misunderstood, or even abused. But it's harder to see why people in despair would want to see *themselves* as innately defective, as some patients do. One reason is that they typically feel helpless. Genetic and biochemical theories confirm that helplessness and alleviate the need to overcome it. Often they feel frightened by the seemingly primitive impulses stirring within them, and genetic or biochemical theories help to explain those impulses away. Frequently they feel guilty about their passions and their problems—and especially about their resentment toward their parents—and biopsychiatry relieves them of facing these personal conflicts.

More and more frequently, psychotherapists find that biopsychiatric propaganda discourages their clients from learning about themselves and taking charge of their lives. Typically these clients have been reading the science column in their local newspaper, which tells them, day after day, that genetics and biochemistry lie at the root of their problems. Nothing more thoroughly strips a person of his or her psychospiritual verve than biopsychiatric ideology.

Why psychiatrists themselves would favor biochemical and genetic theories is no secret. Their entire professional identity depends on this ideology, and in the case of researchers, their funding can be totally dependent on it (see chapter 15).

What the Public Hears

What the profession communicates to the public through the media is summed up in a recent newspaper headline: GENETIC BASIS OF SCHIZO-PHRENIA SAID TO BE FOUND.

Books written for laypeople also make the claim that the hereditary basis of madness is a fact rather than a bias or a conjecture. In the 1985 mass-market book *The New Psychiatry*, psychiatrist Jerrold S. Maxmen cites adoption studies and concludes, "These findings provided overwhelming evidence that genes were the principal source of schizophrenia" (p. 149). Assertions of this kind are so frequent that even sophisticated scientists in other fields assume that schizophrenia must have a proven genetic link.

---

*Chapters 2 and 16 discuss how families can help their members deal with or overcome severe states of psychospiritual overwhelm.

Similarly, a constant stream of propaganda from psychiatry tells the public that all forms of human distress are due to biochemical imbalances or even gross brain damage. A recent twin study that we'll examine was highly publicized as demonstrating shrinkage in the brains of people labeled schizophrenic.

We begin by looking at genetic theories and then turn to biochemical explanations.

What the Experts Tell the Profession About Genetics

Within the confines of professional books and reviews, the claims are considerably more muted, if still badly exaggerated. In *Biological Psychiatry* (1986), in a chapter entitled "The Genetics of Psychiatric Disorders," Steven Matthysse and Seymour Kety acknowledge "the absence of a consistent and generally accepted mode of genetic transmission of schizophrenia." They repeat a constant theme in the professional literature: "The task is a daunting one, but it must eventually be carried out. . . ." Notice the use of "eventually." Kety himself jointly authored the key study cited by Maxmen in *The New Psychiatry*, and even Kety doesn't think it proves the case for a genetic origin.

In Armand Nicholi, Jr.'s *The New Harvard Guide to Psychiatry* (1988), the chapter on "Genetic and Biochemical Aspects of Schizophrenia" is again written by Kety and Matthysse. Their opening statement is hardly the stuff to run to newspapers with: "Psychiatric genetics, in its relatively short history, has encountered unusual difficulties in understanding and interpretation." One problem is that schizophrenia is still difficult to define, so much that "there is little reason to insist that it represents a single disease." Needless to say, that makes it difficult to discover schizophrenia's presumed genetic origin.

"In the Family" Does Not Mean Genetic

Schizophrenia does tend to run in families. About one in ten families with a schizophrenic parent will have a schizophrenic offspring. To their credit, Kety and Matthysse concede the fact that this "does not necessarily constitute strong evidence for the operation of genetic factors." Families share both a genetic and an environmental influence. "Pellagra, which also shows a strong familial tendency, was at one time erroneously regarded by some on that basis as a simple genetic disease," these researchers point out. It turned out to be due to niacin deficiency. Similarly, families share political outlooks, national feelings, cultural values and prejudices, and language; but nowadays scientists do not consider these traits to be genetic in origin.

The Meaning of Twin Studies

Identical twins have shown a tendency toward concordance for schizophrenia; that is, if one of the identical twins displays symptoms of schizophrenia, so does the other, but usually much less than half the time.

Can we think of any good reasons, other than genetics, why madness might sometimes afflict both members of a pair of identical twins? Indeed, wouldn't we *expect* it to happen sometimes as a result of the similarity of their environments as children? Especially in the decades in which these studies were done, parents typically tried to rear twins with a rigorous sameness, right down to their clothing. Compounding this trend, twins themselves often go through periods where they try to look and act alike, and where they feel themselves drawn together and dependent on each other as a unit.

Since their sex is always the same, identical twins are especially likely to face more nearly identical environmental stresses than do fraternal twins or other siblings. Any sexual or physical abuse probably would be aimed at both of them at the same time.

While twin studies may seem straightforward, in fact they are not. In the best book about genetics and psychiatry, *Not in Our Genes* (1984), R. C. Lewontin, Steven Rose, and Leon Kamin question the methodology of the twin studies, including whether the twins were really identical and whether their diagnoses were reliable. The authors confirm that in most instances, when one identical twin becomes schizophrenic, the other does not. They conclude that the twin data is more compatible with an environmental influence than a genetic one.

In "Biological Theories, Drug Treatments, and Schizophrenia: A Critical Assessment," in the Winter 1986 *Journal of Mind and Behavior*, David and Henri Cohen similarly conclude that "the only unquestionable result of twin genetic studies is that they demonstrate the extensive contribution of 'environmental' factors to the etiology of the disorder." This is so seemingly out of step with what the public is told, it bears repeating: identical twin studies support an environmental theory of schizophrenia rather than a genetic one.

What about the more definitive study of identical twins raised apart from their families? When laypersons think of twin studies proving the genetic basis of schizophrenia, they naturally assume that the studies are of twins raised apart. But no such studies of psychiatric disorders exist. The numbers of identical twins raised apart are simply too small to study a problem that affects a tiny fraction of the population. It's a case of the public filling in the blanks with information that isn't there.

The Most Relied-On Genetic Study

When the twin studies failed to produce the hoped-for data, genetic researchers turned to studies of children raised more or less apart from their parents. In an NIMH-sponsored Danish-American study, adopted children in Denmark who developed schizophrenia were located. Then their biological families were located and evaluated to see if they, too, had schizophrenic members. If so, it was reasoned, then a genetic factor might be at work, since the adopted children presumably had been raised in a "normal" environment separate from their parents.

These studies are by far the most often cited in support of the genetic theory of schizophrenia, and the investigators came with the highest possible credentials. Seymour Kety was a psychiatry professor at Harvard, and psychologist David Rosenthal and psychiatrist Paul Wender were at the National Institute of Mental Health. Fini Schulsinger was the chief psychiatrist in Copenhagen.

When I located the original 1975 summary report on the Danish study by Kety and his colleagues in the book *Genetic Research in Psychiatry*, I was shocked by what I found. There was no increase in so-called schizophrenia among the close biological relatives, including the mothers, fathers, full brothers, and full sisters. Thus the studies actually tended to *disprove* the genetic origin of the presumed illness.

So what data were they using to prove a genetic tendency? They had made a most strange finding: *the half-brothers and half-sisters on the father's side did have an increased rate of "schizophrenia."* * In other words, we have a miracle gene that skips the biological mothers, fathers, brothers, and sisters—and even the biological half-brothers and sisters on the mother's side—and strikes only the half-siblings on the father's side.

Obviously this finding is so ridiculous, so clearly an error or a chance

---

* I referred to the half-siblings on the father's side as supposedly schizophreniclike. The coding system indicates that four out of six were in reality diagnosed as "latent schizophrenia." In the then-current APA *Diagnostic and Statistical Manual of Mental Disorders* (*DSM-II*, 1968), which the study used, latent schizophrenia is a hodgepodge, catchall diagnostic group, including patients who have "symptoms" of schizophrenia but no actual episode of schizophrenia and including "borderline" cases and "prepsychotic" cases whom the investigators judge to be potential schizophrenics who have never fully manifested their "illness." In more recent versions of the diagnostic manual (*DSM-III* and *DSM-III-R*) the diagnosis is dropped entirely. Indeed, examining the chart in the Danish study, we find that the total number of paternal half-siblings with schizophrenia was eighteen, fourteen of whom were "latent." What extreme efforts these investigators went to in order to give the impression of a familial genetic influence.

finding, that Kety, Rosenthal, Wender, and the other investigators are reluctant to describe their full data to their colleagues. Therefore, the actual nature of the alleged genetic tendency goes unmentioned in their reviews and requires deep digging into the original data itself.

Furthermore, the NIMH study involved so few families that this peculiar finding of increased diagnoses of schizophrenia among the half-siblings on the father's side depended on one large family with six offspring who supposedly were suffering from schizophreniclike disorders. One must wonder if there was incest or some other abusive practice occurring on the paternal side of this family. (See the chapter on women for further discussion.)

In April 1990 I had the opportunity to debate one of the authors of the study, Fini Schulsinger, in a public forum at the University of Copenhagen. I repeated the point about the unaccountable loading of his study with a group of distant relatives made up of half-brothers and -sisters on the father's side. Did he produce some statistics to prove me wrong? To the contrary, he conceded the point. Yet the whole genetics of schizophrenia rests on this house of cards. What hocus-pocus!

This is only the beginning of the flaws in this study, but I think it is sufficient to make the point.

As the authors of *Not in Our Genes* observed, the weaknesses of the Danish study are so obvious that it's hard to understand how "distinguished scientists" could have promoted them as valid. In the March 16, 1990, *Psychiatric News,* Yale psychiatrist Theodore Lidz reminded readers of his own earlier criticisms. "Our published reexamination of the Danish-American adoption studies show that the researchers' interpretations of their data are untenable, distorted to support their hypothesis."

There is simply no evidence in the most highly touted studies for a genetic factor for schizophrenia. Instead, their failure to detect *any* genetic influence tends to confirm an environmental origin for schizophrenic overwhelm. It discredits psychiatry that these studies have been used to prove the opposite of what they really show and that the public has been consciously propagandized with misleading information.

A more recent study by the Finnish psychiatrist Pekka Tienari and several other investigators, including the American Lyman Wynne, was published in 1987 in *Schizophrenia Bulletin* (vol. 13, no. 3). Like the Danish study, it studied children who became schizophrenic after being adopted away from their original families. Tienari finds some evidence for a genetic influence, but hidden in the fine print is the fact that the children had lived with their original parents until up to the age of four years and eleven months. Whatever apparent genetic influence Tienari found could easily be due to early environmental exposure to the biological parents.

A much more striking finding was generated by Tienari's careful psychological examination of the adoptive parents. In every case that a child became diagnosed as schizophrenic there was serious diagnosed mental disorder in one of the adoptive parents. Tienari states flatly, "There were no borderline or psychotic offspring who were reared in healthy or mildly disturbed families." He concludes that *environment must play a role in the development of schizophrenia.*

If there is any pattern here, it is that the genetic hypothesis remains unproven, while the environmental hypothesis has been confirmed repeatedly by the very studies aimed at proving a genetic component.

The Diminishing Evidence

Because of psychiatry's influence in the media, most people think that there is a growing body of studies supporting the genetic origin of psychiatric disorders, such as so-called schizophrenia.

In reality, literature supporting a genetic cause for "schizophrenia" has grown sparser over the years. We have fewer and fewer studies claiming a genetic basis. Old ones have become discredited by the hundreds, while new ones are rare indeed. If anything, the evidence seemed much more convincing in the 1930s and 1940s, when genetic researchers inspired Hitler's eugenic legislation and the enforced sterilization of tens of thousands of people in the United States and then in Germany. At that time, dozens of progenetic studies typically were cited in reviews. If there has since been a scientific revolution in genetic psychiatry, it has been in the opposite direction—toward discrediting the old studies and casting skepticism on the few new ones. But that's not what the public is told.

A Specific Gene for Schizophrenia Has Been Located!

Recently the public has been encountering another kind of genetic study—those claiming to have located specific genes for specific psychiatric problems, such as schizophrenia, depression, and alcoholism.

In the British journal *Nature*, in November 1988, a team headed by Robin Sherrington of the Molecular Psychiatry Laboratory of the University of London reports locating a gene for schizophrenia on "the long arm of human chromosome 5" in seven families from England and Iceland. The exact gene could not be identified, but it was thought to be dominant. Those carrying it would supposedly become schizophrenic or have a related disorder. "This report," they claim, "provides the first strong evidence for the involvement of a single gene in the causation of schizophrenia."

An editorial in the same issue of *Nature* proclaimed a breakthrough in psychiatry: "New research has shown some schizophrenia to be, in part, genetically determined." The president-elect of the American Psychiatric Association, Herb Pardes, leaped on the promotional opportunity and proclaimed the study to be a "tremendous advance." Newspapers all over the world carried the story without a hint of skepticism.

Apart from the hazard of making too much of a single study, there was a logical fallacy in this one that rendered it highly suspect from the start. When scientists succeed in locating a single dominant gene for a physical disease, such as Huntington's chorea, their finding makes sense because the disease is already known to be transmitted by a dominant gene as a result of studying the medical family tree of the patients. If one parent has Huntington's, for example, the odds are exactly fifty-fifty that each of the offspring also will have it. But this is not the case with so-called schizophrenia. Every family study—including the ones we have looked at—shows that a single dominant gene does not exist for people diagnosed as schizophrenic. This has been known for decades. So anyone familiar with the field could have dismissed the discovery of a dominant gene even before looking at the study. Yet the study was heralded by psychiatry as a powerful confirmation of its genetic bias.

An actual examination of the study brought out more absurdities. Drawing on seven families, it contained 104 individuals. From the family tree reproduced in the study we find the following examples of extraordinary prevalence for schizophrenia and other disorders among these families: one set of parents had five of seven children with psychiatric disorders, including three who were said to be schizophrenic or otherwise psychotic; another had four out of seven with diagnosed schizophrenia or other psychoses; another had seven out of ten with psychiatric disorders. The typical rate for children diagnosed as schizophrenic in families with a schizophrenic parent usually is estimated to be less than 10 percent. These families could vie to be in the *Guinness Book of World Records* for being the most crazy family.

What can be learned from such a group of families in terms of schizophrenia? Probably nothing. It would be far more interesting to check out the patterns of child abuse and neglect required to produce such rampant misery.*

Curiously, the same issue of *Nature* contains a study in which James

---

*Even the title of the study, "Localization of a Susceptibility Locus for Schizophrenia on Chromosome 5," is specious. The statistical correlations were not between the alleged gene and schizophrenia, but between the alleged gene and a hodgepodge of schizophrenic and schizophreniclike disorders, other psychoses, and something called "fringe" diagnoses. Again, few in the field believe that one gene could account for such a wastebasket of diagnoses. The investigators obviously were hard-pressed to massage the data to come up with a statistical correlation.

Kennedy and his colleagues find, as the title states, "Evidence Against Linkage of Schizophrenia to Markers on Chromosome 5 in a Northern Swedish Pedigree." The Swedish study specifically and precisely refutes the English study.*

Now, the English study has gone the way of all such studies, lost in the shifting sands of science; yet the public has never heard the refutations.

Despite the single-minded promotion of genetic explanations in both the psychiatric and the popular press, occasionally a more realistic appraisal crops up. The March 1987 issue of *Psychiatric Times* carried an article headlined CONFIDENCE WANES IN SEARCH FOR GENETIC ORIGINS OF MENTAL ILLNESS. It declares, "The reason: Researchers are finding it difficult or impossible to replicate earlier reports claiming to trace various psychiatric illness to particular chromosomal locations." Genetic advocate Elliot Gershon of NIMH is quoted as admitting, "The major problem is all the nonreplications." It concludes, "But so far the evidence is so equivocal that some competent observers deny that there is any convincing evidence for the genetic basis of any major psychiatric illness."

Investigator Bias—or Worse?

Suppose a team of modern biopsychiatrists at last publishes a genetic study in which the data, if true, strongly confirm the genetic theory. Do we believe it? Do we take for granted that nothing has been fudged?

There's always good reason to be circumspect, considering the number of reports that have made the news recently concerning cheating in scientific research. But we have more direct confirmation of the need for skepticism. In psychiatry, biological research is guided, indeed driven, by the profession's need to justify its existence as a medical specialty. In this light it is useful to look at what motivates some of the most important researchers in the field.

---

*But Kennedy and his colleagues didn't want to overturn the genetic apple cart by dismissing their colleagues, even though they had proved them wrong. So they wrote that their study did not invalidate the British one. They rationalized that there must be different genes causing schizophrenia in different cases. But this makes no sense, because the English study located the alleged gene in *several different families* over a *wide variety of psychiatric diagnoses* in *two different countries*. It had to be a very common gene for schizophrenia, if not *the* gene for schizophrenia. Therefore, the failure to find the same gene in a separate study was a refutation of the English study. To top it off, a couple of days later in the *New Scientist*, still another research team failed to find a link between chromosome 5 and schizophrenia.

Ernst Rudin, Hero of Nazi Genetics

Ernst Rudin was the single most important psychiatric researcher in the field of genetics during the highly active period of the 1930s. He was a professor of psychiatry and director of the Department of Heredity at the Kaiser Wilhelm Institute in Munich. The Kaiser Wilhelm was perhaps the most honored psychiatric research center in the world, and when it suffered financial problems during the German prewar inflation it was bailed out by the Rockefeller Foundation. Rudin himself came as a visiting dignitary to America in 1930 with the support of the Carnegie Foundation. He wrote dozens of papers proving the genetic origin of schizophrenia and was the most respected genetic scientist in the field of psychiatry until the outbreak of World War II isolated him from the remainder of the Western scientific community.

How objective was this scientist? How unbiased were his motivations? When Hitler came to power, Rudin was ready for him. It was Rudin who influenced Hitler, not Hitler who influenced Rudin. The psychiatrist became the architect and official interpreter of the first legislation establishing the Nazi eugenics program that lead to the castration and sterilization of tens of thousands of individuals accused of being schizophrenic, retarded, epileptic, or in some other way physically or mentally "defective."

On his sixty-fifth birthday Rudin was praised by Wilhelm Frick, Hitler's minister of the interior, as "the indefatigable champion of racial hygiene and meritorious pioneer of the racial-hygiene measures of the Third Reich." He was awarded the Iron Cross by Hitler; but at the end of the war he had to flee for his life from the outraged families of murdered mental patients. Rudin's mountainous publications on genetics, pivotal in justifying the mass murder of "genetically defective" mental patients under German rule during World War II, stimulated acceptance of the eventual slaughter of the Jews as well.

Franz Kallmann, Hero of American Genetics

The second great influence in genetic psychiatry of that era was Franz Kallmann, chief of psychiatric research at the New York State Psychiatric Institute and professor of psychiatry at Columbia. He was, in more ways than one, Rudin's American counterpart, and probably his chief competitor for dominant influence in the field. As late as 1959 he authored the key chapter on "The Genetics of Schizophrenia" in the widely read *American Handbook of Psychiatry*. The reader may find that Kallmann's name has a ring of familiarity; his work was widely read in college courses in the 1950s and 1960s.

Kallmann had been trained in Germany, and he strongly supported Hitler and Rudin's eugenics programs. Indeed, he stayed in Germany under Hitler until the last minute, when he was forced to flee because he was half Jewish. Geneticist Benno Muller-Hill has written in *Murderous Science* (1988) how Kallmann, while still living in Germany, called for more radical sterilization measures than the Nazis were willing to implement. He wanted to sterilize every possible member of any family tainted with schizophrenia and any person showing signs of eccentricity or minor anomalies that might suggest a latent gene for the supposed disease. Muller-Hill also points out that Kallmann became a witness for Rudin at the latter's denazification tribunal (p. 176). In *Not in Our Genes*, Lewontin, Rose, and Kamin also cite Kallmann's pronouncements in Germany and describe how two Nazi geneticists rose to reject his schemes to sterilize relatives of so-called schizophrenics as unfeasible and unwarranted. In addition to documenting and condemning Kallmann's "totalitarian passion for eugenic sterilization," the authors of *Not in Our Genes* offer a scathing scientific analysis of the eugenicist's research.

Writing in *Eugenical News* in 1938, Kallmann persists in his totalitarian aims. He laments that the most extreme eugenic measures suggested in the United States—enforced sterilization of all psychiatric hospital inmates—would hardly begin to dent the problem of eradicating the bad genes from our society because, as already noted, the supposed genes had to be recessive and infrequent in the population. He believed that it required two of them to make a crazy person; therefore, even latent carriers of the gene had to be sterilized against their will. That, he determined, would mean sterilizing relatives of these patients and preventing the marriages of eccentric people and borderline cases. More specifically, Kallmann argued, "compulsory sterilization of all hospitalized schizophrenics would not prevent more than 1 percent to 3 percent of schizophrenic individuals" from being born. Again going beyond the Nazi sterilization program, he called for "legal power" to sterilize "tainted children and siblings of schizophrenics" and to prevent marriages involving "schizoid eccentrics and borderline cases." Kallmann had to be aware of the unfolding events in Nazi Germany, the country he had so recently been forced to leave; his article in *Eugenical News* was followed by another describing and praising Hitler's mass sterilization program for dealing with "these useless, hopeless, and harmful people" called the mentally ill.

The Final Solution

The ideology of men like Rudin and Kallmann eventually led to the mass murder of several hundred thousand mental patients in Europe, followed by the extermination of Jews and others deemed unfit in Germany. In the words of Muller-Hill,

When Hitler came to power, psychiatrists and anthropologists were enthusiastic, since they saw in him someone who would realize and give due prominence to their ideas. . . . The laws which were passed or planned, and which required the sterilization of "schizophrenics", "psychopaths", and "social misfits", which forbade "Jews" and "schizophrenics" to choose their lovers freely, which required the killing of "schizophrenics", all had their origins in the proposals and demands made by these learned specialists.[1]

Even in America the "learned professionals" sought to bring about a psychiatric holocaust. An official editorial in the *American Journal of Psychiatry* in July 1942, entitled "Euthanasia," calls for the killing of people incurably genetically defective with mental retardation. An article by psychiatrist and neurologist Foster Kennedy in the same issue advocates the murder scheme, and now the journal officially adds its approval. It quotes Kennedy's assertion that "with no good brains there can be no good mind" and, like him, calls for the extermination of the "completely hopeless defective—nature's mistake." It directed its lethal intentions broadly toward those with "mental disability," "the feebleminded," the "low-grade defective," and the "helpless, inarticulate idiot." It used euphemistic language such as "a lethal finis to the painful chapter," "merciful passage from life," and "a method of disposal which . . . would bring relief to all concerned." It concluded by positioning psychiatrists as the ones to help parents overcome their "unhappy obsession of obligation or guilt" about killing their children (pp. 141–43).

Rudin and Kallmann Today

Rudin and Kallmann were the international bulwark of psychiatric genetics prior to World War II, and Kallmann maintained his influence long after. What's the status of their work today? If you check the reviews I've mentioned in *Biological Psychiatry* (1986), for example, you won't find them listed among the 349 references. But biopsychiatrists of late are becoming more bold. Kallmann, and even the Nazi Rudin, are being cited again as legitimate scientists, as in the 1988 American Psychiatric Press's *Textbook of Psychiatry*.

The Genain Quadruplets: A Study in Child Abuse

Modern biopsychiatrists are mostly too young to have been identified with the events in Nazi Germany. We must look to other contexts to understand the nature and intensity of their prejudices. In recent time, Paul Wender and David Rosenthal have been among the most influential geneticists. They are joint authors of the Danish study mentioned earlier. Wender's ideology, especially his radical biological bias, will become apparent when we review his impact on child psychiatry in chapter 12.

NIMH psychologist David Rosenthal is the editor of a book entitled *The Genain Quadruplets: A Study in Heredity and Environment in Schizophrenia* (1963).[2] The book examines in detail the lives of four young women, identical quadruplets, all of whom apparently became mad. Various investigators look at the lives of these children from every possible perspective. Rosenthal himself assumed that schizophrenia in four genetically identical females was prima facie evidence of a genetic cause, and he tells the reader he named the family "Genain" by deriving it from the Greek words meaning "dire birth" or "dreadful gene." Nonetheless, he assures the reader that "my position is one which considers both genetic and environmental factors important in such disorders."

So, could something other than their genes have driven all four girls crazy?

The father of these four twins is an alcoholic, subject to fits of paranoia. He impregnates at least two women other than his wife during the time when the twins are young children and is notorious for his affairs. He beats his children and his wife, restricts them to the home, and allows them no outside contacts and no deviation from robotic regimentation. When his wife threatens to leave, he tells her he will follow her anywhere and murder her.

Obsessed with his family's sexuality, he "plays sexual games" with at least one of the girls, and "if his wife or daughter ate a piece of darkly toasted bread, he accused them of 'trying to get sexually stimulated.' " When his preteen daughters are found masturbating, he puts acid on one of their genitals. That failing to stop them, he sends two of them off to a sadistic surgeon who mutilates their genitals, severing nerves and cutting out substantial flesh. So notorious is the surgeon that he is driven out of private practice and goes on to work in a state mental hospital.

The father, in the mother's words, is "always so angry and hateful and mean." During sex, he frequently bites her face so badly that it bleeds and swells up. On one occasion the mother has had to knock down her husband in self-defense in front of her brood of four young girls. Once he banged two of the girls' heads together to stop their crying.

The mother herself, as one can readily imagine, has her own problems.

When the children are young and in their formative years, she is despondent and suicidal. She, too, has bizarre ideas, participating in the use of acid and mutilating surgery on her children's genitals and probably communicating her own fear that masturbation breeds madness. When one of the girls develops the first hints of breasts, she explains that they are bruises and treats them with salve. She takes one of the children to a psychiatric clinic to stop her from masturbating, and the psychiatrist describes her as "very inflexible, a very controlling kind of person." She doesn't return when he cannot "magically" stop her daughter from touching herself. When three of the girls are later sexually assaulted, she tells them to forget it and offers no sympathy.

The mother participates in the creation of a home that "most" outsiders consider " 'fear ridden,' devoid of fun and humor, and very restrictive." There is a "coldness" in the house and the children "needed more warmth," according to outside observers. Indeed, their teachers feel sorry for them because of their restricted life. The four girls are not allowed to participate in normal school activities and come to school "marching" like an army squad doing double time. It's no wonder that people describe the quadruplets as "passive, timid, and unusually quiet children who showed little spontaneity or initiative." They show no curiosity in school and do not have a "good childish laugh."

This is a heart-rending tale of extreme child abuse—the emotional, physical, and sexual abuse of four female children who happen to be quadruplets. Yet this is not how Rosenthal presents the "cases." He presents them as a scientific study of genetic and environmental influences on the development of the "disease" of schizophrenia, with heavy emphasis upon genetics, including elaborate reviews of presumably relevant genetic studies.

The book presents one of the most tragic chronicles of child abuse recorded anywhere. Yet at no time is the abuse discussed as such. In no place in the book is it summarized. The data is strewn throughout the six hundred pages in the reports of the various professionals. Much of it is contained in footnotes. The synopsis I have provided was put together from these scattered observations.

Reading and retelling the story leaves one overcome with pity. Imagine what it was like to have lived such lives. For Rosenthal to suggest that the study supports a genetic theory of schizophrenia itself constitutes a form of child abuse. To fail to underscore or to summarize the outrages perpetrated against the children constitutes intellectual complicity with the child abuser. To leave the reader to dig the abuse out of hundreds of pages is to invite the question, Why wouldn't this renowned NIMH geneticist face the facts directly? It's no surprise that Rosenthal's most famous and influential accomplishment—the Danish adoption study of schizophrenia—also was grossly oversold to the profession and to the public.

A Theoretical Impossibility

Psychiatrists suffer from the repression of painful memories as much as anyone else does. Genetic psychiatrists not only must repress the lessons of Nazi Germany, they have to forget about the lessons of their own research, which ultimately has undermined their position. As a result, the history of genetics is largely expurgated from reviews on the subject. In *The Schizophrenic Disorders* (1978), Manfred Bleuler, who himself keeps hoping for a genetic breakthrough, offers a glimpse of how futile the search has been:

Today it is possible to declare simply and briefly that the old method of familial research did not succeed in discovering for schizophrenia a mendelian hereditary process by which to trace it back to a mutation in the biological heritage. Certainly ample attempts to accomplish just that have not been lacking. (P. 460)

Bleuler recounts how disappointed biopsychiatrists in the 1930s sought to discover a way around their own conclusion that their hundreds of studies had failed to disclose a genetic factor. They explored complex mathematical formulas seeking a combination of multiple individual genes with varying degrees of influence over the outcome. This "monumental mathematical effort," Bleuler tells us, "actually came to naught, except, perhaps, to prove that a mendelian hereditary process for schizophrenia could not be proved."

Bleuler raises another issue that is no longer discussed in public by psychiatric geneticists—the *theoretical impossibility* of an ordinary genetic transmission for schizophrenia.

People diagnosed as schizophrenic have a very low reproductive rate. This results in part from their social isolation and psychological helplessness as well as from their frequency of long-term incarceration in mental hospitals. Physically abusive biopsychiatric treatments, stigma, and social handicaps also reduce their tendency or ability to have children. Why, then, don't we see a great decline in their numbers over the centuries and decades? Why hasn't the "disease" been eradicated entirely, as Hitler and his psychiatrists attempted to do in Germany? Bleuler argues that the mathematics of epidemiology prove that "schizophrenia" would have been wiped out early in human history if it were an ordinary inherited disease.

Three Centuries of "Bad Blood"

Much as the alleged genetic basis of schizophrenia, the alleged biochemical basis of schizophrenia is touted constantly by the experts to the media and to the public. Most biopsychiatric reviews boast about the rich and varied number of hypotheses about the cause of schizophrenia. We have more and more suppositions and conjectures, rather than fewer and fewer. The public is told that this plethora of hypotheses indicates progress. To the contrary, in science the number of conjectures and hypotheses is inversely proportional to nearness to the truth. The truth, in scientific terms, is established as *one* hypothesis gains acceptance over others.

Before examining current theories, a medicinal dose of history is needed to put these conjectures into perspective. Leaders in psychiatry, nearly one and all, have long declared that mental disorders are physical in origin. The claim has been made loudly and with determination since psychiatrists first appeared on the world stage. After all, we psychiatrists are physicians. Why would we want to make any other claim, when any other claim would make irrelevant all our years of medical studies, invalidate our basic philosophies of life, undermine our authority in the field, and threaten our power to treat mental patients against their will?

Claims for a biological defect in mad people have focused recurrently on the blood and blood vessels, providing us the opportunity to glance at changing claims over the centuries. In 1668 the British publication *Philosophic Transactions* presented "an extract from a letter written by J. Denis, Doctor of Physick and Professor of Philosophy and Mathematics at Paris." A madman with a long history of bizarre behavior was bled and then transfused with calf blood in the hope that "its mildness and freshness might possibly allay the heat and ebullition of his blood." He was improved with the first transfusion and, after going into shock with the second, became "perfectly recovered" from his madness. The scientific breakthrough was witnessed by several physicians and surgeons certified by author Denis as too intelligent to be swayed by anything but reasonable proof.

Benjamin Rush, author of *Medical Inquiries and Observations upon the Diseases of the Mind* (1812), stood in the long tradition of bleeding the mentally and physically ill. His own pet theory, allegedly proved by autopsy, was that the source of madness resides in the blood vessels of the brain; and perhaps that conjecture led him to utilize bleeding after other medical practitioners had abandoned it as outmoded.

In addition to being revered as a signer of the Declaration of Independence, Rush's head is enshrined on the seal of the American Psychiatric Association. He also invented a tortuous restraining device called the tranquilizer chair, which rendered the victim immobile for hours at a time. One wonders if he used it on his son, whom he had committed to his mental institution.

Rush also is notorious for having bled George Washington to death. Does it mean something that the Father of Psychiatry killed the Father of the Country?

Rush killed a lot of other people, too. We may conjecture that he did so within his psychiatric institution, but we know he did so en masse by applying his psychiatric techniques to the treatment of plague victims in 1793 in Philadelphia. In *Bring Out Your Dead*,[3] first published in 1949, J. H. Powell describes how Rush bled and purged people who already were debilitated to the point of death by loss of fluids. He administered toxic mercury in amounts described by others at the time as "a murderous dose," "a devil of a dose," and "a dose for a horse." Powell himself observes that "the mercury purge and copious blood letting were erroneous, surely fatal, treatments."

Powell is careful to document that Rush was not following flawed traditions, he was inventing his own approaches. Indeed, many other plague victims were being treated successfully in the contemporary French tradition with supportive, nonintrusive methods, including nursing care, good food, rest, and the administration of fluids. The French doctor Jean DeVèze viewed Rush's toxic therapy as "very fatal" and sought instead to assist nature as gently as possible. He was critical of Rush, declaring —in what might be a critique of modern psychiatry—that "any one who, seduced by the brilliancy of a system, will force nature by the rules of the method he has adopted, he, I say, is a scourge more fatal to the human kind than the plague itself would be" (p. 172).

Powell wonders how "the brilliant Benjamin Rush could have come to believe as he did," but misses the point that Rush simply was applying his psychiatric theory and know-how to the plague. Forcing radical treatments on the patient, bleeding and purging people near to death, and wholly ignoring the patient's need for nurturing care are all time-honored psychiatric traditions.

Ironically, Powell describes Rush himself as deluded by his medical prowess: "Rush was expansive and jubilant. Now he entered that state of self-delusion which was to shape, first with praise, then with blame, his permanent reputation in the history of medicine" (p. 121). In what remains today a description of the modern psychiatrist and his toxic treatments, Powell says this of Rush: "Yet as he watched death a thousand times that fall, he continued to believe himself right, his cure successful, his patients helped. He grew ever more courageous, ever more determined, ever more convinced" (pp. 130–31).

Leaping ahead in our historical survey of bad blood in biopsychiatry, on November 2, 1951, the *Long Island Press* declared in a headline

CREEDMOOR DEVELOPS INSANITY BLOOD TEST. Three doctors at the venerable state hospital announced the development of a blood test that supposedly was 83 percent accurate when tried out on seventy-three psychotics and nonpsychotic controls. The method sounded highly sophisticated, using ultrasound to induce clotting, followed by electronic analysis of the clot. Naturally, the state commissioner of mental hygiene, Newton Bigelow, was thrilled. He declared to the media that the test was able to "discriminate with a high degree of statistical accuracy" between the blood of psychotic and nonpsychotic patients.

Throughout the 1950s and 1960s investigators continued to report the discovery of causative substances in the blood of schizophrenics. Psychosurgeon Robert Heath, director of psychiatry at Tulane University, found a "blood protein factor" he called "taraxein." (Heath also was known for putting hundreds of electrodes into the brains of individual patients as a prelude to melting brain tissue.[4]) Adrenochrome, a breakdown product of adrenaline, was thought by others to be a hallucinogenic factor in the blood of schizophrenics. The 1959 *American Handbook of Psychiatry* held out much hope for these and other blood factors, noting that they were "being explored intensively in schizophrenia, and [that] the next few years should give decisive answers concerning their relevance." Nowadays, taraxein, adrenochrome, and the like don't get passing mention in textbooks.

More recently, kidney dialysis has been used to cure schizophrenia, again to cleanse the blood of the elusive toxin. John Cade, who first used lithium to subdue mental patients, has been a strong advocate of the toxic blood theory and kidney dialysis, which he personally showed to be effective as a treatment. In the June 19, 1982, *Lancet*, Petr Skrabanek responded by ridiculing the concept and placing it squarely in the same old "bad blood" tradition. Once a darling of the psychiatric newspapers, kidney dialysis for schizophrenia is now a professional embarrassment.

The Dopamine Hypothesis of Schizophrenia

The most frequently cited possible cause of schizophrenia is an abnormal hyperactivity of the dopamine neurotransmitter system in the brain. The 1988 American Psychiatric Press's *Textbook of Psychiatry* calls it "the most widely accepted pathophysiological explanation for the symptoms of schizophrenia" (p. 382) and *The New Harvard Guide to Psychiatry*, also published in 1988, discusses no other hypothesis in detail. The 1989 *Comprehensive Textbook of Psychiatry* says, "The notion that a fundamental excess of dopaminergic activity is related to the development of schizophrenia has been the most promising and widely accepted hypothesis of schizophrenia" (p. 718).

What is the theory? In a nutshell, since the neuroleptics probably achieve their effect on schizophrenic patients primarily by suppressing dopamine nerve transmission, we may speculate that dopamine neurotransmitters are abnormally hyperactive in schizophrenics.

The neuroleptics do suppress dopamine activity in various parts of the higher brain, including the main nerve pathways to the frontal lobes and emotion-regulating limbic system. As we saw in chapter 3, the circuits they suppress are closely related to the ones that are cut in psychosurgery. Surgical lobotomy cuts the fibers *to and from* the frontal lobes; the neuroleptics suppress the fibers mostly *to* the frontal lobes from the deeper brain because they are mediated by dopamine.

Because the neuroleptics inhibit dopamine nerve transmission in the frontal lobes, should we suppose there's something wrong with these areas of the brain? Not at all. We've seen that these drugs have the same effect on all people, regardless of their diagnosis or mental condition. They always inhibit passion and willpower. They even have this effect on animals.

Consider surgical mutilation of the frontal lobes. Does its effectiveness in controlling psychiatric inmates and patients prove that the surgery corrects an abnormality of the frontal lobes? The lobotomy effect is nonspecific; it blunts humans and animals regardless of the state of their minds or brains. Why, then, should the effectiveness of neuroleptic-induced chemical lobotomy be used as evidence for an abnormality in the frontal lobe neurotransmitters? It's not scientific thinking, it's wishful thinking.

Consider alcohol and its impact on us. For many people, alcohol provides at least a brief sense of relaxation, and maybe even euphoria. Alcohol accomplishes this by impeding brain function, and, with chronic use, it disables brain cells and can kill them. Does this mean there is something wrong with these brain cells because people "feel better" when the cells are disabled or even dead? The same question may be asked in regard to the tranquilizing effects of nicotine in tobacco or the energizing effects of caffeine in coffee. Must we assume the prior existence of a defect in the brain in order to explain our "need" for nicotine or caffeine?

Studies have been done to try to determine whether so-called schizophrenics do have abnormally active dopamine pathways, and some of the studies confirm that they do. The trouble is that in nearly all of these studies the patients have been treated with neuroleptics, and chronic exposure to these drugs causes these nerve pathways to compensate by becoming hyperactive. As the American Psychiatric Press *Textbook of*

Psychiatry admits, there's no way to prove the hyperactive dopamine hypothesis at present, because the studies are almost always done on patients who have taken neuroleptic drugs. The *Comprehensive Textbook of Psychiatry* similarly indicates that the most frequently cited biochemical theory of schizophrenia is speculative at best, resting largely on the mechanism of action of the neuroleptics.

So there's no significant evidence for a biology of schizophrenia. Psychiatrists admit this in their books and journals and then hope and pray that maybe the dopamine hypothesis will prove true. But what do they say in public? Typical is Jerrold S. Maxmen in *The New Psychiatry* (1985). On one page he tells us that "many psychiatrists believe that schizophrenia involves excessive activity in the dopamine-receptor system," and a few pages later he slides into the conclusion, almost as an aside, that "mental illness clearly involves abnormal receptors and neurotransmitters." He does not add, as he should, "but not until toxic psychiatric drugs start pouring into the brain."

The Chicken and the Egg

Suppose future studies of schizophrenic patients do document a relative degree of dopamine hyperactivity in some or all of them. Would this prove that these people's brains are abnormal or that dopamine causes the schizophrenia? Common sense and experimental evidence indicates that certain passionate states are associated with corresponding changes in brain function. Prolonged mental stresses of almost any kind, as well as physical trauma or stress, cause the brain to stimulate increased production of certain hormones, such as steroids. Conversely, if you are relaxing right now, your steroid output may decline. In each of these instances the mental state influenced the brain, rather than vice versa.

We find the same results examining brain waves. If you are excited, with intense focus of your attention, your brain is likely to generate fast, low-amplitude electrical waves on the electroencephalogram (EEG). If you then relax, the EEG will show alpha waves—slower, with a higher amplitude. In each case, the mental state influenced how the brain reacted, not vice versa.

Indeed, a whole new field is developing, psychoneuroimmunology, based on the theory that our state of mind affects our brain, which in turn affects our immunological system.

Clearly, proving an association between a particular state of mind and a particular reaction in the brain doesn't indicate which came first. Yet the biopsychiatrists, without discussing it, usually assume that the brain is the egg from which the chicken—mental disorder—is born. They search for signs of hyperactivity in the dopamine system of schizophrenics without acknowledging that if they find it, it could be the *normal* response of a *normal brain* to the prolonged expression of an intense emotional state.

Do Schizophrenics Have Shrunken Brains?

In recent years, brain imaging techniques have been demonstrating shrunken brain tissue and brain size in a significant number of schizophrenic patients, nearly all of whom have been treated with neuroleptic drugs. Biopsychiatrists presume that the cause is schizophrenia, but as we found in the previous chapter, the drugs are the cause.

On March 22, 1990, the *New England Journal of Medicine* published a much-promoted report on the biology of schizophrenia by an NIMH team led by Richard Suddath and including biological extremists E. Fuller Torrey and Daniel Weinberger, men who have devoted their professional lives to proving the genetic and biological basis of madness. Long before this particular research project, Weinberger frequently had declared schizophrenia to be a proven biological disease. He would cite brain-scan studies of patients without mentioning that they already had been treated with electroshock and with years of toxic drugs. Torrey, the chief investigator for the NIMH-funded study, is a spokesman and the patron psychiatrist of NAMI. He has supported NAMI's attacks on psychiatrists who disagree with NAMI and with him. None of these obvious biases was mentioned in the press that lavished attention on the study.

NIMH director Lewis Judd quickly publicized the results. He told Daniel Goleman in the March 22, 1990, *New York Times* that the new study provided "irrefutable evidence that schizophrenia is a brain disorder."

The study of fifteen sets of identical twins, using brain-imaging techniques (MRI), found that in almost every case, the diagnosed schizophrenic twin had shrinkage of brain tissue while the normal twin did not. The report, and an accompanying editorial, claims to have proven the biological basis of schizophrenia. The investigators assume that the cause of the brain shrinkage is the presumed disease of schizophrenia and mention no other possibility in their lengthy abstract and introduction. Tucked toward the end of the article was the admission that the results "cannot rule out" treatment as the primary cause of the damage.

The facts favor neuroleptic treatment, plus electroshock, as the cause of the brain shrinkage. Two of the patients had shock treatment yet, unaccountably, were not dropped from the study. All but two of the patients were receiving neuroleptics at the time of the study, and all of them had been given massive drug treatment, averaging a decade or more.

That the patients were recruited through NAMI, the parents organization that pushes psychiatric drugs, suggests they were given unusually heavy drug therapy over the years. And indeed, we are told that their total lifetime medication ranged from 10,000 to 103,000 mg. fluphenazine (Prolixin) equivalents. Even the lowest lifetime dose, the equivalent of 10,000 mg. fluphenazine, is a significant one. The *Physician's Desk Reference* (1990), for example, says that less than 20 mg. daily usually controls patients during the acute stage and that 1 to 5 mg. generally is sufficient for maintenance. Thus the patient with the *least* drug exposure had the equivalent of two thousand to ten thousand days—five and a half to twenty-seven years!—of maintenance dose. Clearly, each of these patients had substantial exposure to toxic medication.

More shocking in some ways, the authors don't deal with the probability that most of the patients already had a known drug-induced brain disease, tardive dyskinesia. The median length of illness for these patients was over ten years, indicating that many or most had been exposed to neuroleptics for a decade. Given that tardive dyskinesia strikes more than 40 percent of long-term neuroleptic-treated patients, many or even most of the patients in this study must have been suffering from the neurological disorder already. But the authors fail to tell us how many of the patients had tardive dyskinesia. In fact, they don't even *mention* tardive dyskinesia. Given that other studies already have shown correlations between tardive dyskinesia and brain shrinkage,[5] the failure to discuss the issue in this study is inexplicable.

I asked psychologist Bertram Karon, a professor of psychology at Michigan State University and an expert on schizophrenia research, to evaluate the study. On June 6, 1990, he wrote me that the published data was insufficient to fully check their statistics but it appeared that the strongest correlation was between the drugs and the brain damage. *"The conclusion most consistent with the presented data is that the authors have found strong evidence that neuroleptic medication is brain-damaging,"* he summarized.

How did the psychiatric press respond to the study? *Psychiatric News* (April 6, 1990), the *Psychiatric Times* (May 1990), and *Clinical Psychiatry News* (April 1990) each touted the study as providing new evidence for a biological basis for schizophrenia. None discussed the misinterpretation of the statistics noted by Karon, gave serious consideration to drugs as the cause of damage, or noted the glaring omission of any discussion of tardive dyskinesia. Nearly every American psychiatrist reads one or more of these newspapers, and many went to bed resting more easily in their convictions about the presumed biology of schizophrenia.

We have found consistently that biopsychiatrists view their data and their reports as proving the biological and genetic basis of schizophrenia, although instead they end up inadvertently confirming the brain-damaging effects of psychiatric drugs. They also end up undermining their pet genetic and biological theories. This most recent study yields one of the strongest confirmations to date for the brain-damaging effects of the neuroleptics. Since identical twins clearly did not share the diagnosis of schizophrenia, it also undermines genetic theories of schizophrenia. Yet the profession uses it falsely to prove the biological basis of schizophrenia. Clearly, psychiatry is not easily swayed by scientific evidence.

Implications for Peer Review

That the twin study appeared in its distorted form in the *New England Journal of Medicine,** perhaps the world's most respected medical publication, is unsettling. It indicates how thoroughly medicine has closed ranks with psychiatry against openmindedness and fairness in psychiatric research. The peer review system in medical journals is supposed to guarantee a high standard by requiring each manuscript to pass through a panel of experts in the field before acceptance and publication. In the field of psychiatry and, I suspect, elsewhere in medicine, peer review has become one more old-buddy network guaranteeing that critical viewpoints never see the light of day while badly flawed studies supporting the establishment are rushed into print. †

Recently I was interviewed by a newspaper reporter who was writing an article obviously slanted in favor of neuroleptics. In the course of our interview she challenged, "If you've seen so many cases of brain damage from drugs, why don't you publish your data in the *New England Journal of Medicine?*" To those unsophisticated about how the old-buddy system works, it's not an outrageous question. But any such submission to that journal on brain damage from any psychiatric treatment will be sent for

---

*See chapter 12 for a similar oversight in an article in the same journal dealing with brain atrophy in autistic patients.
†I have not found that medical research or practice in general suffers from as much bias and outright corruption as in psychiatry. For example, in medical school at Case Western Reserve University (1958–62) our professors urged us to question and challenge contemporary beliefs—except in psychiatry, where we were asked to accept all of the prevailing dogma, from psychoanalysis to electroshock. Where the foundation is most flimsy, dogma is most firm.

"peer review" to the same "experts" who have been denying this damage for years, the very experts who make their living promoting the drugs, shock treatment, or lobotomy. And as we'll see in the chapter on the psycho-pharmaceutical complex, the drug experts often benefit directly from the largess of the drug companies.

Implications for Contemporary Values

Genetic and biochemical theories of human problems are becoming a part of our culture. Recently a psychiatric patient returned from her hospitalization looking "completely blitzed" to her coworkers, who explained it away as her "biochemical imbalance." The source of her biochemical imbalance was the drugs that were stupefying her.

The notion of biochemical imbalance has become so commonplace now that it appears as a jest in modern stand-up comedy routines and in plays and movies. Instead of "You're neurotic," we hear "You've got a chemical imbalance."

On a more serious level, what will it mean as increasing numbers of people view psychospiritual crises, personal conflict, behavioral deviance, rebellion, and other human phenomena as biochemical in origin? We are creating a new way of dismissing people and their problems, especially people in direct conflict with us. From so-called hyperactive children and rebellious adolescents to despairing middle-aged women and abandoned street people, we shall be able to dismiss troubled or troubling individuals as physical aberrations hardly worthy of human sympathy or consideration. This may turn out to be the worst legacy of biological psychiatry.

In summary, we do not fully understand the human experience that gets labeled schizophrenia, but we have some good ideas about its environmental origin and psychospiritual meaning. As a later chapter on psychosocial interventions will further show, we also know a lot about helping people get through the experience in a creative, valuable manner when they ask for and desire our help. What begins as disintegration or breakdown, a psychospiritual overwhelm, can become a journey of renewal and growth. It often involves facing meaningful conflicts about the nature of life, love, relationships, and responsibility. It gains its particular flavor, which has been called madness, from its often flamboyant psychospirituality, combined with its typically overwhelming feelings of fragmented identity, humiliation, and helplessness.

Instead of offering human understanding to these overwhelmed people, psychiatry has fabricated biological and genetic explanations. It has used these explanations to justify a massive drug assault that has taken a profound toll in terms of damaged brains and shattered lives.

Although many of us can find hints of the experience within ourselves, the extremes of passion, irrationality, and overwhelm that often characterize "schizophrenia" may seem foreign to us. In part II we will examine something that seems less foreign to most people: depression. Sadness and depression, in moderate degrees at least, are a familiar and even expected part of living. But we shall find that contemporary psychiatry deals with it much as it deals with schizophrenia—as a disease to be suppressed or eliminated.

"Depressive" and "Manic-Depressive" Overwhelm, Antidepressants, Lithium, and Electroshock

Chapter 6

Understanding the Passion of "Depressive" and "Manic-Depressive" (Bipolar) Overwhelm

Sadness and Gladness succeed each other.
—*Thomas Fuller (1732)*

[Winston Churchill] is a mass of contradictions. He is either on the crest of a wave, or in the trough. . . . When he isn't fast asleep, he's a volcano. There are no measures in his make-up. He is a child of nature with moods as variable as an April day.
—*British minister of defense Hastings Lionel Ismay in John Connell,* Auchinleck *(1959)*

In my opinion the manic-depressive cycle represents, primarily, a physical and metabolic disturbance of the nervous system. The great quantity of research in brain function over the past fifteen years has shown that chemical changes and abnormal brain metabolism combine to interfere with neural circuits, thus slowing down or speeding up nervous activity.
—*Psychiatrist Leo Cammer,* Up From Depression *(1972)*

Depression and elation are among the most common human experiences. They are familiar in our own lives and in those of our friends and family, and we tend to think of these ups and downs as natural responses to being alive. Even when someone we know becomes extremely depressed, we often are able to attribute the reaction to something specific, such as a death in the family, the loss of a job, a failure in love, passing a landmark in aging, feeling trapped or unproductive in one's life, or coping with a life-threatening or debilitating physical illness. If the response seems excessive to us, we may find additional explanations, such as "He was too dependent on her" or "She needs to handle setbacks better" or "It's hard to start over again at her age." When the causes do not seem so obvious, we often can identify basic attitudes or personality traits that help to explain the depressed reaction. We might decide, "He had a tough childhood and he's never gotten over it" or "She's had a string of bad things happen to her" or "She gets scared and depressed whenever things are going too well."

Despite its familiarity with depression as a natural response to living, the public has been bombarded recently with medical explanations for depression and elation. The media have been filled with claims for the discovery of a gene for manic-depression. A whole new type of depression has been defined—seasonal affective disorder (SAD)—a presumed light deficiency to be cured with special lamp technology. And, of course, there's the biochemical imbalance theory, a veritable psychiatric gospel. Antidepressants have become nearly a religious mania, with *Newsweek* adoringly featuring a Prozac capsule on one of its 1990 covers. Even electroshock for depression is being promoted with renewed vigor, a phenomenon to which a whole separate chapter will be devoted.

Depression and the Business of Psychiatry

Psychiatry and the pharmaceutical industry have been marketing depression as a "real disease" in need of medical treatment. Accordingly, the *Diagnostic and Statistical Manual of Mental Disorders, Revised (DSM-III-R*, 1987) of the American Psychiatric Association has determined that severe or major depression occurs in up to 26 percent of women and 12 percent of men during their lifetimes. That's enough business in itself to sustain all of the psychiatrists in the country.

In *The Good News About Depression: Cures and Treatment in the New Age of Psychiatry* (1987), psychiatrist Mark Gold tells us in no uncertain terms that "depression *is* a brain disease." He begins one of his chapters with: "Depression literally flows out of the brain and into the body. The endocrine system provides the channel" (p. 223).

Genetic and biological theories of depression also dominate neurologist Richard Restak's popular book *The Brain* (1984). I have a hardcover edition that I bought at a used bookstore. It is stamped "Compliments of CIBA-GEIGY, Corporate Underwriter of *The Brain*, A Public Television Series." Enclosed in the book is an expensive color brochure by Ciba-Geigy advertising the TV series. The drug company manufactures many psychiatric medications, including the widely used antidepressant Ludiomil as well as Ritalin and a lithium product, Lithobid.

Despite all of this biopsychiatric propaganda—which we'll scrutinize in the next chapter—depression is a readily understandable expression of human despair that is frequently responsive to psychosocial help.

A Promise to God

The causes of depression can be buried so deeply in the past that the individual seems to have a physical disease that unaccountably strikes him or her down.

Phil was in his thirties when he came to therapy in part because of recurrent depressions. Periodically he would fall into "a black hole." His suicidal mood, lasting for a few days to a few weeks, was so despairing that it would cast a feeling of gloom over his wife and children. Even during good times he frequently suffered from a sense of impending doom.

In therapy we noticed on two occasions that the depressions struck when the rest of his family were catching colds. Alert to the latest scientific fads, Phil decided he might suffer from a variant of depression caused by a mild viral inflammation of the brain. But there was one serious flaw in the theory: in his entire adult life, Phil had never shown any other symptoms of a cold. He had never gotten a runny nose, sore throat, stiff neck, headache, or achy muscles.

During the second bout of depression Phil realized he'd gotten a fever and become dehydrated, still without getting any classic cold symptoms. He wanted me to write him up in a journal as a new kind of viral depression.

Instead I urged him to search his memory for something in his past connecting cold symptoms to a powerful loss. Then one night when his family was away, he experienced a dreadful sense of isolation. Prepared by his therapy sessions, he didn't run away from the feelings by watching violence on TV or by taking a drink or a drug. Instead he urged his feelings to come on full force, seeking their underlying meaning. And then the crucial memory came back to him.

Phil had been twelve when his closest friend, Roy, died of an acute, fulminating polio only two days after wrestling with him. Phil was overcome, first by the loss of his best friend, and then by the dread that he must have caught the disease while wrestling with him. Phil's mother called the family doctor, who told her, "There's nothing we can do but wait and hope. If little Phil gets any symptoms, bring him in right away." The symptoms, which Phil's mom warned him about, were a runny nose, sore throat, stiff neck, headache, and sore, aching muscles.

That night Phil went to bed in a mixed state of terror and loss, and he made a secret pact with God. If God would make sure he never got any of those symptoms, he would try to be the best little boy who ever lived. Then he repressed the entire event, including all memory of the death of his friend and the anguish surrounding it. No longer in his conscious awareness, the pact with God and the events surrounding it dominated much of his psychospiritual life.

Now, years afterward, Phil continued to feel an overwhelming compulsion to be "very, very good." Much of the time, that compulsion kept him from succumbing to depression. But when a cold began to strike, with the dread signs of polio, he would collapse into depression again.

The night that Phil recalled the death of his friend and his pact with God, his nose began to run, his throat got sore, his neck got stiff, his head throbbed, and his muscles ached. His body, so long suppressed in its natural reactions to the cold virus, let it all burst out at once. Amid the rampaging cold symptoms, he laughed and cried with relief.

The sources of depression are usually too subtle and too complex to be explained by one traumatic event in the past, and even in Phil's unusually focused story there were other contributing factors. For example, Phil's parents rarely paid any attention to the boy's feelings, and despite his anguish at the time of his friend's death, they never discussed it with him.

Over a period of two years Phil was able to overcome his recurrent depressions and to ameliorate his compulsion to be good. He never again lapsed into anything so dismal as his "black hole," and with time he was able to replace his childlike compulsions with a more adult perspective on how to live his life.

Intern on the Surgical Ward

Sometimes the causes of depression seem obviously rooted in the immediate present and require no in-depth analysis of the past. During my medical internship, when I was doing a rotation on surgery, one of the patients on the ward, a middle-age woman named Mrs. Wright, had terminal cancer.

Mrs. Wright's cancer had proven to be largely inoperable, but enough of the tumor had been removed to enable her to eat and drink during her remaining days. Yet she had stopped taking food or drink and therefore was destined to die even sooner than otherwise expected, and she was in a state of despondency. She began rejecting visits from her husband and children and spiraled downward on a despairing course of death.

I could see that Mrs. Wright's family loved her and wanted to be close to her in her last days; and so I felt confident in talking with her about the possibility of facing death by creating something good in the face of something so apparently dreadful.

Dressed in my white intern's jacket, stethoscope dangling from my pocket, I must have looked out of place perched on her bedside with a tray of food in my lap; but gradually she accepted my encouragement to eat and to drink. This required an hour or two, feeding her much as one would a child, until eventually she took over feeding herself. Meanwhile I talked openly with her about her fear of death and the pain she was enduring, as well as about her family, their love for her, and their wanting to share her experience and ease her loneliness.

She told me that everyone would be better off if she died without seeing them again.

I told her, "Your family doesn't want you to live your last days all alone. It's not good for you or for them. There's plenty of time for all of you to be together in a loving way."

The following morning even her physical pain had diminished or lost its grip on her, as she felt moved by a purpose—to share love in her last days.

Her family welcomed the change and drew closer to her for the remainder of her days.

What, most likely, would happen to Mrs. Wright today? When Mrs. Wright stopped eating, the surgeon would ask for a psychiatric consultation, with or without the patient's consent. The psychiatrist, probably arriving unannounced and perhaps without identifying himself, would spend half an hour or less with the patient to confirm the obvious "diagnosis"—major depression. Very possibly he would order an antidepressant drug, perhaps Triavil, which combines the antidepressant drug Elavil with a potent neuroleptic to suppress her anxiety over dying. In a sufficient dose this combination would blunt her mind, causing her to die in a state of drug-induced fogginess.

The busy psychiatric consultant almost surely would not have the inclination or the time to help Mrs. Wright create a loving reunion with her family. Unschooled in matters of love—but heavily indoctrinated in biochemical theories, drugs, and shock—he probably would not give consideration to a psychospiritual alternative. Since she was dying, he would not consider her as a candidate for even short-term psychotherapy. And if her nurses couldn't get her to eat, it wouldn't occur to him to try. He'd probably find spoon-feeding a patient demeaning, as well as a poor use of his time.

Even worse, the psychiatrist might prescribe a course of electroshock for Mrs. Wright. To the layperson this might seem preposterous; but it is a distinct possibility. Not long ago a patient of mine had to resist a psychiatrist's attempt to give her father shock treatment a scant few hours before he died. Recently there was a report in a psychiatric newspaper alerting psychiatrists to look for "major depression" in medical patients much like Mrs. Wright. Major depression, it said, is best treated with drugs or electroshock.

Understanding Depressive Overwhelm

Patients labeled schizophrenic, we found in chapter 2, often express a combination of intense passion and psychological helplessness. This is true as well in depression, although the component of passion may be more covert. In Phil's case, bouts of passionate despair were obvious. Mrs. Wright was more withdrawn and her passion was more hidden; but as she opened up, she expressed profound feelings of loneliness, guilt, and despondency. In both people, feelings of guilt and even self-hate were lurking beneath the surface. Depression often is comparable to a smoldering volcano. Beneath the distant rumbling and the dark wisps of smoke, there's molten emotion—under pressure and ready to explode.

Feelings of overwhelm or psychological helplessness were apparent in both Phil and Mrs. Wright. When depressed, both stopped taking good care of themselves and both stopped responding to the needs of others. Both were ready to give up—Phil by imagining he had a biochemical imbalance or viral disease, Mrs. Wright by deciding her remaining life wasn't worth living.

When It's Hard to Understand Depression

When we cannot readily identify with the depressed person's plight, more often it is due to our own lack of understanding than to the obscurity of the causes.

A young woman, Vivian, came to me for psychotherapy following the death of her cat. She had been careless in leaving the door to her home ajar, and her cat had escaped and been killed by a car. After weeks of bitter self-recrimination she began to feel that she no longer deserved to live. She also started to experience obsessive fears. Certain she had run over an animal on the road, she would pull over on dangerous thruways to see if there was bloody fur smeared on her car.

Isn't it an inexplicable "mental illness" for someone to have such a strong reaction to the death of a pet?

Although she had wholly pushed it out of her mind, it turned out that Vivian had once loved another cat. Given to her by a neighbor, the pet had been her only solace throughout a lonely childhood punctuated by sexual abuse at the hands of her father. When Vivian reached her early teens and began to take an interest in people outside the home, including boys, her resentful father drowned the cat. Why? He told Vivian, "You weren't around enough to take care of it anymore."

The recent death of Vivian's cat re-created the anguish over the murder of her childhood pet, restimulated the guilt feelings provoked by her father's accusation, and reevoked her stifled rage at her father's abuse of her and his murder of the cat. It was too much to handle head-on until she came for psychotherapy.

In therapy recently with a young man named Mike, we uncovered a repeated pattern of depression during the fall holiday season each year. Mike then decided that he probably had SAD, a much-promoted but highly controversial diagnosis within the profession. People with SAD supposedly become depressed with the coming of winter because of a biochemical need for sunshine. When I asked him if anything traumatic had happened to him in the past during the fall holiday season, he did remember that a grandparent had died during the fall in his childhood; but that revelation seemed to have little impact on him.

So we continued to search for significant past events. Abruptly, Mike got a startled expression on his face and then he began to sob. His closest boyhood friend had died unexpectedly five years earlier in a swimming accident. The event had been so painful and guilt-provoking that he had pushed it out of his memory. I asked him to recall the exact date of his friend's death and it turned out to be the holiday weekend that had passed less than a week before our session. This was a powerful revelation and he continued to cry as he recalled the tragic loss, remembered his own feelings of guilt at the time, and talked about his love for the person whom he had pushed out of his memory. Mike left the office free of depression and convinced that he now had the psychospiritual tools to combat it in the future. He wasn't over his problems, of course, but he'd taken a giant stride in improving his emotional life.

Depression, Guilt, and Mental Paralysis

Depression often seems rooted in profound conflicts that no choice can resolve. A man wants to leave his wife, but his religion and upbringing have taught him that such a wish is forbidden. Besides, he cannot bear to bring so much anguish upon his young children. Yet he feels as if he is dying in the marriage. He becomes paralyzed and sinks into quiet despair. A forty-five-year-old woman wants to break free of old fears and constraints and go to college; but her aspirations conflict with how she was raised and with her husband's demands for her time. She becomes afraid she cannot be a "good wife" and a "successful person" at the same time, and this leaves her unable to act. She, too, becomes depressed.

Beneath depression we often find feelings so painful that the person cannot handle them and, especially, cannot take meaningful action. The mind, as if acting on a signal from a frustrated will, shuts down. The therapist's job is to help unlock the trap—to help the individual deal with otherwise unacceptable feelings and impossible conflicts—and in the process to encourage hope for a better way of life.

Guilt often fuels the mental paralysis. Psychotherapist Larry Tirnauer has reminded me how guilt blocks our awareness of angry feelings, encourages our mental paralysis, and hence cuts off our understanding and our options. Vivian, for example, repressed her memories of her cat partly because of her guilt feelings over his death and her outrage at her father. Phil and Mike both felt guilty about the death of boyhood friends. Mrs. Wright felt guilty about being a burden to her family. These people lapsed into psychological helplessness in part because they couldn't face their feelings of guilt and in part because the losses or issues in their lives seemed too overwhelming.

Comparing "Schizophrenic" and "Depressive" Overwhelm

In the psychospiritual overwhelm that becomes labeled schizophrenia, the helplessness usually is expressed by a futile and often self-destructive blaming of others. The person's fantasies overflow with how other people are to blame for his or her problems. Typical of humiliation, the anger is directed outward, and in the extreme the person tries to hurt someone.

In depression and guilt, blame is directed toward oneself as evil, bad, harmful to others, and deserving of punishment. Typically, the individual rejects his or her own right to happiness and, especially, to be loved. Anger is directed inward, and in an extreme case the individual may attempt suicide.

In schizophrenic madness, the focus is on threats from outside the individual. A man may believe people are menacing him, plotting against him, snickering about him behind his back, influencing him through radio waves or covert hypnosis.

In the typical depressed madness, the scenario is reversed. A woman believes that she is bad or dangerous to others. She harms people by her very existence. She is a burden of such proportions that people would be better off if she were dead. She may believe that she is physically rotting from the inside out. Her evil is so great she can smell it—a stench emanating from her own body. She is not threatened by external poisons or pollutants; she is the polluter.

In contrast, the person overwhelmed with humiliation—and frequently diagnosed as schizophrenic—feels worthless and impotent, literally of no account whatsoever. The guilt-ridden, depressed person feels bad and able to do harm. The distinction between worthless and bad may not be apparent immediately, but it is critical. The shame experience is that of lacking any significance, meaning, power, control, or influence in relation to other people or of having a very low status and value in their eyes. The shame experience is connected to abandonment, utter rejection, and invisibility. One's whole identity or selfhood can seem near extinction.

The guilty depressed person feels that he or she has impacted on the world, but in a noxious way. The guilt-ridden person may believe that others are actually profoundly interested in his or her evil and will confess openly in the hope of appeasing them. He or she has a more solid identity, albeit a negative, guilt-ridden one.

Guilt-provoking parents often take more notice of their children than do shaming parents. They make them feel as if they have a significant but negative impact on the family. Typically the parents blame their own suffering on the child. Their classic axioms include "Children aren't worth the pain they cause" and "Wait until you have children and see the pain they cause you." The children may be called "bad" or "burdensome" and be taught that they caused pain and travail from the pregnancy throughout their teenage years and even into adulthood. As they grow up, these children become dominated by duty and obligations—often felt as guilt—in their relations with others.

Depression and Cultural Influences

Many of the men and women who seek professional help for depression are caught between the pursuit of their own chosen adult values and those taught to them as children by their religious, educational, and family institutions. In separation and divorce, in particular, people frequently are paralyzed by the conflict between a growing desire for a more loving mate and the moral imperatives taught to them before they could reason. For example, the macho imperatives of our culture can keep a man from reaching for the love he needs, encouraging him to live amid an unrecognized, continuous sense of gloom.

Women, as we've already noted, are far more often diagnosed as depressed than are men. In the past psychiatry blamed this on their wombs or their hormones. In recent times biopsychiatry has brought us full circle back to these oppressive biological explanations. As we'll elaborate in chapter 14 on women, there are cultural reasons why women so often lapse into despair.

Depression in Two African Communities

Sometimes, if we look at communities that seem somewhat unfamiliar or alien to our own, we are more readily able to see common human principles at work. Outside the usual psychiatric literature, I did locate two books about "primitive" jungle cultures in which the authors approach depression as a psychosocial and even spiritual phenomenon pertaining to loss of companionship and love.

The famous doctor who authored the first book describes the roles of "friendship," "love," and "altruism" in the community, citing, for example, how relatives and friends risked their lives for each other against frightening attacks from wild animals. Males cooperate in the hunt and females share in the raising of any orphaned offspring.

Little Flint, the subject of a touching vignette, was eight and a half years old at the time of the death of his mother, Flo. Flo was the matriarch of the family, but little Flint was born when Flo was seemingly too old to bear children. She was becoming ill as well, and in her infirm state she had "insufficient strength to enforce the independence" of little Flint. For example, "she continued to give in to his demands to sleep with her at night" and, despite her infirmity, she also acceded to carrying him about on her back "like an infant" when he was old enough to walk by himself.

The study includes photographs of Flint and his family. They show a surprisingly aged-looking mother with a heavily lined face, a sagging countenance lacking in animation, and a body that has lost its strength of carriage. The older siblings are full of sparkle in these pictures, and so is the small child Flint, who looks bright eyed, endearing, and eager for attention.

The unexpected death of a sibling when Flint was only five frightened and disturbed him and, combined with his mother being increasingly "unable to cope," made Flint more excessively dependent on her. He indulged in "very little play" and became especially "nervous" around bigger, older boys. Meanwhile, Flint's father paid little or no attention to him; but this was a routine phenomenon in their culture, and perhaps not that different from ours.

The doctor—whose name I will withhold for the moment—said of Flint, "He was unusually dependent upon his very old mother" and "when she died in 1972, Flint was unable to cope with his state of depression." Flint "showed gradually increasing signs of lethargy." He suffered a "loss of appetite" and had "sunken eyes." Finally he died of an inflammation of the gastrointestinal tract. His doctor concluded, "It seems likely that the psychological and physical disturbances associated with loss made him more vulnerable to disease."

Other members of the community had recognized Flint's need and reached out to him, but because of his immaturity and history of losses, he had been unable to respond to their love.

By any standard, Flint died of a major depression. Indeed, he perfectly fits the official criteria of the APA's *DSM-III-R.* Major depression is frequently considered genetic and biochemical, and the usual treatment is drugs. In Flint's depressed state he might have been given shock treatment, even as a child.

But the doctor who told the story of Flint did not see him as having a genetic or biological vulnerability to depression; he had a family vulnerability based on the death of a sibling, his ailing mother's incapacity to raise him properly, and her premature death.

The great irony about this analysis of Flint's all-too-human response to a difficult childhood is that he's not a human being. The doctor was not a physician or psychiatrist. Not even a psychologist. She was the world-renowned ethologist Jane Goodall. Her marvelous 1983 book is *The Chimpanzees of the Gombe.* Yes, Flo and Flint were chimps. And it's true that, unlike any modern psychiatric textbook, Goodall's book has subchapters on themes like "Helping and Altruism" and "Love and Compassion."

While Goodall acknowledges the role of genetics in influencing broad behavior patterns, such as aggressivity in males, even in this arena she points out the importance of environment. But with no psychiatric ax to grind, she recognized that obvious psychosocial experiences, such as depression, are not genetically based.

Ethologists studying primates have discovered their many fundamentally psychospiritual qualities, including the capacity for altruism and love, and their corresponding darker side of "depression" and even madness. At the same moment, psychiatrists studying human beings are discarding psychospiritual concepts as outmoded. In short, the ethologists see their animals in human terms, while psychiatrists see their patients in what we used to think of as animal terms.

Jane Goodall's loving approach to primates, including her psychospiritual understanding of depression, is echoed among other ethologists. In *Gorillas in the Mist* (1983) Dian Fossey tells a very similar story about a depressed young ape, Simba, who was abandoned by her mother. An uncle did his best to help Simba recover, but after her mother finally died, she lapsed into a lifetime of withdrawal and depression. Fossey and her biographer Farley Mowat (*Woman in the Mists,* 1987) described how Fossey herself nursed an orphaned ape out of depression and near death through love, physical intimacy, and constant attention. Again, these animals met the technical criteria for major depression.

Before she became involved with gorillas, Fossey worked in human rehabilitation, and she apparently learned some of her more gentle and cautious approaches to the animals from helping autistic children. But human kids rarely are given this kind of attention by professionals in the field of autism. Increasingly there is little place for loving approaches in conventional psychiatric practice because they are being ruled out by biopsychiatric dogma.

Flint and Simba Meet the Psychiatrist

In addition to their meeting the diagnostic criteria for major depression, modern psychiatry would find other compelling reasons for treating Flint and Simba with drugs and even electroshock. First, they had many physical signs associated with their depressions, including loss of appetite and cosmetic and physical deterioration. Often these are assumed to indicate a physical origin. More important, they had *recurrent* depressions. Flint's problems seemed to start or to worsen with the death of a sibling, and then to worsen again with the death of his mother. Similarly, Simba had two distinct depressive episodes, one on the disappearance of her mother and another on her death. In modern psychiatry, as Ronald Fieve argues in *Moodswing* (1989), the fact that Flint and Simba suffered recurrent depression would be taken as further proof that each suffered from a physical illness. That Flint died and Simba never recovered would be used as additional evidence that these were not "normal" or "natural" responses but rather the product of disease, thus strengthening the psychiatric argument that individuals like them need drastic physical interventions.

Imagine the outcry if a captive Flint or Simba became depressed after the loss of a parent and was scheduled for shock treatment at the local city zoo? There would be picket lines. Outraged citizens would offer to adopt the animals to give them proper foster care. Animal protection advocates would chain themselves to the cages. There are many local "zoos" filled with human children and adults being subjected to precisely that sort of abuse, and very few people are protesting.

Every time I have gotten to know someone suffering from so-called major depression I have found a story similar to that of the primates and human beings described in this chapter. There has been no need to resort to genetic or biological theories. Without elaborate explanations, their life stories tend to explain their desperate feelings. The deepest depressions, if anything, are often the most easy to understand. People who suffer severely from emotional problems usually have been exposed to very destructive life experiences, often starting early in childhood.

That depression is typically precipitated by losses and other stresses was confirmed by all three psychiatric experts at the April 6, 1991, "U.S. Depressive Disorders Update" conference in New York City sponsored by Eli Lilly. Nonetheless, all three promoted the use of drugs along with psychotherapy. That all three included psychotherapy in the treatment program may signal changing policy within psychiatry as the profession loses increasing numbers of patients to psychologists, social workers, counselors, and other nonmedical talking therapists. The continued insistence that drugs are important serves the purpose of convincing people to go to medically trained psychiatrists for both talk and drugs (see chapter 15 for a further discussion of psychiatric economics).

Meanwhile, a whole new body of research based on direct observation is confirming the negative effects on children of poor maternal nurturing. Not surprisingly, depressed parents produce depressed or withdrawn children. Recent studies are presented in D. Cicchetti and V. Carlson, eds., *The Effects of Maltreatment on the Development of Young Children* (1989).

Helping Severely Depressed People

But can severely depressed humans be helped by psychosocial interventions? Psychotherapists do it routinely. Here are two stories from my own experience as a young psychiatrist working in mental hospitals.

One night when I was alone on duty as the psychiatrist in charge of the hospital, I received word that a Mrs. Merr would be coming in for emergency evaluation in a state of psychotic depression. She had had several earlier hospitalizations, spanning a number of years. Each time, she showed up in a state of physical collapse from failing to eat and drink, and each time, she "exhibited bizarre delusions and hallucinations." Each time she had received shock treatment.

Mrs. Merr had no family and was brought by the police, who had been notified by her landlady. She was disheveled and filthy, half-starved and very dehydrated. She was practically mute, and when she did speak, she muttered about "things crawling." She offered no resistance but didn't actively cooperate.

The night nurses helped her shower and then, at my request, agreed to share part of their bag lunches to see her through the night. There were lots of drugs available for late-arriving patients, but no food.

Mrs. Merr at first refused to eat. She said her food at home had been poisoned and that it might be poisoned in the hospital as well.

"I'll be your official taster," I declared, taking some sips of milk and a mouthful of food.

Reassured somewhat, she began the process of eating.

Then I noticed her picking at her skin.

"What's the matter?" I asked.

"Can't you see them?" she retorted with irritation.

"Them?"

"The worms."

Mrs. Merr cringed when I reached out to touch her where she saw the creepy crawly things on her skin. Then I patted her, communicating that I neither saw nor felt anything awful coming out of her body. I also talked with her about how bad she must feel about herself that she imagined such awful things coming from inside her. She listened, nodded, but gave no direct assent as she continued to eat and to drink.

In the morning I presented her case for evaluation by a senior psychiatrist, who happened to recall her from her previous admission.

"She won't need shock this time," he announced after interviewing her. "She's got no hallucinations or delusions, and she's eating and drinking fluids. She's not nearly as sick on this admission as she was two years ago."

I tried to explain that she had arrived in at least as bad a condition as the previous time and had responded well to several hours of attention, but the senior psychiatrist couldn't believe it. After all, no one in the hospital had ever tried to help people like Mrs. Merr by "just talking to them," and it made no sense to him.

Of course, I didn't "cure" Mrs. Merr. I'm sure I hardly dented her vast problems. But I was able to get her through her crisis without further damaging her brain.

Mrs. Pulsky, whom I had been unable to reach with a few weeks of psychotherapy, remained extremely depressed, plagued by the belief that various organs in her body were rotting. She was diagnosed as having involutional or endogenous depression, implying that her organs were indeed defective. It was another case in which psychiatric theory paralleled and reinforced the helpless person's worst view of herself—that bodily defects beyond her control were responsible for her anguish.

When no progress was made, my supervisor ordered shock treatment for her, despite my protests. When they didn't help either, he told me she'd soon be shipped to the state hospital—in those days a place of no return. I confronted Mrs. Pulsky with this dreadful alternative and urged her to talk with me about what was troubling her; but she went on muttering about her putrefying body parts.

In desperation I decided to call together everyone in Mrs. Pulsky's family who was willing to come in for a conference. Her husband, her mother and father, and a sister showed up.

After a gloomy silence, Mrs. Pulsky's mother broke into tears and begged her daughter to talk about what was bothering her. Her sister also pleaded with her.

Then the patient's husband burst out, "I want you home, damn it!"

Mrs. Pulsky, as if shocked from a stupor, snarled back at him, "Never with you! Not when you make me do those filthy things in bed."

In the tumult that followed, Mrs. Pulsky haltingly explained that certain sexual acts revolted her and that her husband was using force to make her perform them. She'd rather go to the state mental hospital than return to being sexually abused.

Her family, including her outraged father, rallied to her side, and her husband slunk from the room. She needed only to make sure she would never again have to submit sexually to her husband. The family agreed, and as a start she was to move in with her sister.

Within minutes Mrs. Pulsky no longer looked depressed. She looked frightened and angry. With still more support from her family and from me, she began to look determined.

Everyone was now ready for her to go home, but Mrs. Pulsky was an involuntary patient, and I knew I could never convince my supervisor to let her go so abruptly. Just a few minutes earlier she'd been considered a hopeless case suffering from an intractable psychotic depression of biological origin.

As I was preparing to discharge Mrs. Pulsky about a week later, her husband came barging into the hospital. He caught up with me in the corridor and threatened to attack me physically. Then he abruptly whirled around and stalked from the hospital. Soon afterward he packed his things and left home, much to the relief of Mrs. Pulsky and her family. Mrs. Pulsky went home to her own house.

I continued with my psychiatric training, wondering more than ever if there wasn't something fundamentally wrong with the whole process of diagnosing people and treating them with drugs and shock. I wondered as well how many of my so-called mental patients actually were victims being victimized one more time, this time by psychiatry. I don't think I thought sufficiently about how many of my female patients were being sexually or physically brutalized; my full awareness of that took many more years to come.

In chapter 16, we'll look further into the psychotherapy of depression, including controlled studies of its efficacy.

Getting High on Oneself

Mania is an extremely exaggerated and irrational high or euphoria, which in psychiatry is considered a psychosis or severe mental illness. Often people who experience mania will also experience depression, either flip-flopping from one to the other or passing in and out of each condition at different times in their lives. When both tendencies are demonstrated in one person it is called a bipolar disorder or a manic-depressive disorder. The two are synonymous.

The experience of going from low to high, or vice versa, is not unusual among human beings. Watch any football game or soccer match around the world, and if the stands are evenly divided, at any one moment half of the people may be displaying "depression" and the other half "elation." Should the course of the game take an abrupt turn, a "bipolar" reversal might occur, with dramatic changes in the mood on each side of the field.

The man jumping up and down, his eyes bulging, adrenaline pumping through his veins, screaming and shouting as if by sheer vocal force he could change the fate of the world, looks perfectly adjusted to life—in the stands at an exciting football game. So does the vastly dejected fan whose team has just lost the championship. But suppose there were no real-life football game going on. Suppose a woman is getting high or low about her own life. Suppose she's just desperate enough to be wildly rooting for—or against—herself.

There's no biochemical test to distinguish the so-called manic-depressive person from the elated or despondent football fan. Nor is there any reason to assume that the manic-depressive's inner experience is driven by twisted molecules while the football fan's is driven, at worst, by twisted values.

We don't call the behavior of football fans a "mental illness" or a "disease," because we understand and accept the context in which it takes place and because it seems harmless and short-lived. When we don't understand and accept the context of a human experience, and especially when it seems harmful or bad and lasts a long time, we tend to label it mental illness.

The remarkable thing about manic-depressives is that they can generate such dizzying heights of conflicting energy wholly from within themselves without benefit of external support from a football team, a crowd of boisterous companions, or alcoholic intoxication. Yet is this so surprising? Human beings always have shown a remarkable capacity to generate all sorts of miraculous and calamitous responses wholly from within their own imaginations.

Why People Become Manic

What drives people into mania? Why would someone find himself or herself taking such a bizarre psychospiritual route? Often mania seems like nothing more than the flip side of depression.

In mania the individual feels like the most wonderful person in the world. The businessman who was disappointed in himself now gets high on himself and all his projects and feels invulnerable to failure. He's filled with ideas and projects and spills them out in a rush of words.

Mania is a great escape, a shortcut to psychospiritual heaven on earth. As already noted, it often attempts to deny and overcome grave feelings of guilt and depression. It declares, "I'm not feeling low, I'm feeling high!" But it also can be driven by extreme humiliation or worthlessness, emotions more commonly seen in people who get diagnosed as schizophrenic. As such, mania declares, "I'm not a nobody; I'm the greatest, most successful guy in the whole world!" In his struggle to overcome feelings of humiliation he may become blaming and hostile. Thus the person labeled bipolar may end up at other times with a diagnosis of schizophrenia, or a mixed diagnosis such as "schizoaffective disorder." Again we find that psychiatric labels refer to human conditions that cannot be pigeonholed, because they are not diseases, but subjective experiences that exist along a complex continuum.

Alfred Adler has given one of the better analyses of how and why people become so falsely elated:

Mania, in common with melancholia and severer neuroses, is a barricade erected by the patient to block his own approach to the real business of life, and it is sometimes preliminary to the establishment of psychosis in the form of manic-depressive insanity. The most formidable phase of the mental disorder, as we have seen, occurs invariably when some urgent problem presses for solution and the patient has lost courage. In mania there is an effort to overcome this cowardice, and the patient pushes himself forward, exaggerates his actions, and talks and laughs with needless excitement. He is high-spirited and irritable, has great projects, is very superior and boastful of his power, and displays strong sexual inclinations.[1]

For Adler, mania is, like all psychospiritual crises, a moral and social phenomenon to be understood in the context of basic human needs and strivings.

Most frustrating to those of us who are psychotherapists, people who can become manic almost invariably have a tendency to avoid the work of learning about themselves and their self-defeating patterns, even at their most rational moments between their bouts of elation or depression. If they've been hospitalized or thrown into jail in the past, they typically try to deny that their own conduct got them into trouble. They rarely think that they are in danger of ever getting out of control again. In retrospect they think others have exaggerated their manic state and are too worried about future outbursts. They don't have any problems; everything is fine in their lives. In other words, they have a "manic life-style."

Their episodes of mania are but very gross exaggerations of their basic approach to living.

Anyone willing to escape from guilt or humiliation into wild euphoria must have a general willingness or penchant for escaping from most serious problems rather than confronting them. It's therefore not surprising that such a person is likely to display a tendency to avoid, escape, or deny difficult personal issues or conflicts on a routine basis.

Since mania, then, is not a disease, but the ultimate expression of an attitude toward life, it is entirely relative. Some people get a little high once in awhile and some people get wildly euphoric on repeated occasions. Some people actually do creative work during their highs, and some people simply waste their resources and their time. Some exceptionally creative people would be diagnosed as manic except for the fact that they are highly productive and can come down from their highs when necessary.

The Challenge of People Who Become High

To offer psychotherapy to people who became manic can be a frustrating experience. Since they often don't admit to having any problems, they don't feel they need any help. And even when they seek or accept help, they have a most difficult time focusing on their inner life, their emotions, and their responsibility for their actions.

Watching people plunge hell-bent into disastrous activities, we feel compelled to enforce what we perceive to be common sense and reality upon the rebellious individual. Nothing strains the ethics of freedom as much as dealing with such persons in one's own family; they can wreak havoc so quickly on everything from the family reputation to its finances.

My own ethical and political opposition to enforced medication or psychiatric incarceration is sorely challenged when dealing with individuals caught up in mania. It is tempting to abort their driven activities with drugs while controlling the individual with enforced hospitalization.

Acutely manic persons rarely submit to treatment voluntarily, although between episodes they sometimes agree to the long-term use of lithium in the hope of controlling their mood swings. Drug therapy may appeal to people with a manic attitude toward life, because they often resent the work of self-insight and want quick, easy solutions. This is one reason they sometimes welcome lithium treatment.

But should doctors encourage psychological helplessness by offering or enforcing physical treatments? While I recognize the right of these patients to find doctors to give them drugs, personally I don't wish to encourage their self-defeating attitudes. Nor do I wish to expose them to the many risks inherent in the long-term use of toxic drugs.

If society decides that manic persons must be locked up temporarily for their own apparent benefit or that of others, it should be seen for what it is—a police activity, not a therapeutic one. Psychiatrists should not have the legal right to lock people up. The power corrupts psychiatrists, encourages brutal and oppressive treatments, and makes psychotherapy, or other attempts to help, nearly impossible.

Fortunately there are very few psychiatric patients who are so obviously self-destructive and yet so adamantly against being helped. The average psychiatrist in private practice will see severely manic patients only on rare occasions. The vast majority of obviously disturbed people are amenable to help that is respectfully offered. For the few self-destructive people who reject help, there are no easy solutions. I wish that we had safe havens available for them, where they would not be forced to submit to drugs or electroshock (see chapter 16). If psychiatry offered caring, respectful, and voluntary alternatives, more people would turn to them. Above all else, the existence of this small minority of self-destructive persons who reject help should not be used to justify the whole oppressive system of involuntary institutional and biological psychiatry. That system injures and drives away people who do need and want help.

Both depression and mania are easy to understand as human phenomena rooted in the individual's experience of life; and depression is often readily overcome with loving, informed help from other human beings. Meanwhile, the public has been exposed to an enormous amount of propaganda about the genetic and biological basis of depression and mania and the efficacy of drugs and electroshock. Let us look at the facts.

Chapter 7

The Biology of "Depressive" and "Manic-Depressive" Overwhelm

It is reassuring for new patients to learn that there is a biochemical basis for an illness they thought for years resulted from unconscious conflicts in their personalities, deeply rooted since childhood, and probably from sexual, aggressive, or guilty feelings toward parents or siblings. . . . Their learning of the biochemical cause of their illness seems to result in a marked diminution of guilt in patients and families about behavior during attacks.

—*Psychiatrist Ronald Fieve,* Moodswing *(1989)*

By three months of age, [Tiffany] Field says, infants of depressed mothers developed their own brand of "depressed" behavior, characterized by lack of smiling and a tendency to turn the head away from the mother and other adults. These babies become more upset when they look at their mother's unresponsive face than when they see her leave the room, Field adds.

—Science News, *report from the 1990 annual meeting of the American Psychological Association*

People who are depressed sometimes feel "defective," as if "my brain is slowed down; it isn't working right." There's a sense of something gumming up the mental works. This feeling makes patients susceptible to psychiatric pronouncements about chemical imbalances in their brains and encourages reliance on psychiatric authority.

Whatever the scientific basis for a biology of depression, it's good for the business of psychiatry. Treatments for physical diseases are reimbursed by insurance companies much more generously than those for "mental illnesses." A report in the March 4, 1988, *Psychiatric News* describes how an Arkansas appeals court ordered Blue Cross/Blue Shield to reimburse a policyholder at the payment rate for coverage of physical disorders, even though the patient was diagnosed as manic-depressive. Four out of five psychiatrists testified that manic-depressive disorder was indeed a "biological" disease. One was quoted as stating under oath that "overwhelming research" proves its "biochemical basis."

Organized psychiatry welcomed the ruling. Paul Fink, president-elect of APA at the time, declared that "all major illnesses are physical, mental and medical." Only in psychiatry is the existence of physical disease determined by APA presidential proclamations, by committee decisions, and even, at times, by a vote of the members of APA, not to mention the courts.

The very sound of the term *bipolar disorder* smacks of hard science. A synonym for the older term *manic-depressive disorder*, it has become associated in the public's mind with biological disease and lithium therapy. That was psychiatry's purpose in promoting the term.

What the Public Is Told

In the introduction to his 1989 edition of *Moodswing*, Fieve presents a seemingly proven scientific truth: "The outlook for the patient suffering from depression is bright, for he or she is experiencing a treatable biochemical imbalance." Similarly, the chapter headings in psychiatrist Mark Gold's 1986 book *The Good News About Depression* are ablaze with biopsychiatric conviction: "Depression Is a Brain Disease" and "Depression Is Too Many Hormones and a Mistimed Bio-Clock."

The Biological Theory of Depression

For years the dominant biological theory of depression, like the dopamine neurotransmitter theory of schizophrenia, was derived from speculations on how and why medications sometimes seem to alleviate depression. One of the earlier groups of antidepressants, the monoamine oxidase inhibitors (MAOIs)—such as Parnate, Marplan, and Nardil—tends to increase the levels of available norepinephrine in the central nervous system. So it was hypothesized that depression might result from the opposite—too little norepinephrine. Later studies showed that some so-called antidepressants also cause an increase in the availability of another neurotransmitter, serotonin. So the theory was enlarged: some forms of depression may be due to too little serotonin as well. This is the theory that Demitri and Janet Papolos aptly criticized in *Overcoming Depression* (1987) as too "simplistic."

Eventually the theory was punched full of holes by contradictory evidence. For example, some drugs that mimicked these biochemical effects did not seem to alleviate depression, and others that are thought to sometimes relieve depression have a wholly different biochemical mechanism. Furthermore, the supposed efficacy of the antidepressants, as we'll see, is much in doubt.

Suicide, Murder, and Serotonergic Sluggishness

Despite the failure to construct an overall biochemical theory of depression, evidence has been accumulating over two decades that *some* expressions of depression—especially suicide—may in some instances be correlated with low levels of serotonergic neurotransmission (see chapter 8). Personally, I have grave doubts whether this research will hold up any better than similar efforts we have examined. However, in the April 1990 *Journal of Clinical Psychiatry*, Gerald Brown and Markku Linnoila review correlations between reduced serotonergic activity and "impulsive, destructive behaviors, particularly where aggression and violence are involved." In an interview with me, Linnoila stated that this association, while not wholly consistent, is considered probably the best established in biopsychiatry. Similar conclusions are reached by Ronald Winchel and his colleagues in a chapter on "Biochemical Aspects of Suicide" in *Suicide Over the Life Cycle* (1990), edited by Susan Blumenthal and David Kupfer.

Meanwhile, no causal relationship has ever been established between a specific biochemical state of the brain and any specific behavior, and it is simplistic to assume it is possible. What we do know is that some changes can increase the *likelihood* of one kind of activity or another, but only in the most general fashion, usually based on the individual's preexisting attitudes. Thus alcohol is sometimes associated with violent behavior, but it is more often associated with passive, relaxed responses. It's the person, and to some extent the situation, much more than the drug, that determines human conduct. Similarly, uppers such as amphetamine, PCP, and cocaine do tend to cause a "high" or euphoria that can deteriorate into paranoid, aggressive behavior, and after "crashing" from these drugs, depression and despair can follow. Yet considering the widespread use of these agents, sometimes under provocative or upsetting circumstances, it is relatively rare for individuals to become violent or severely depressed in response to using them.

Some drugs are used to treat depression on the theory that they enhance serotonergic neurotransmission; but in reality they cause extreme imbalances in the system, including a relative compensatory *shutdown* of serotonergic neurotransmission. As we'll see in chapter 8, this is especially true of the most widely used antidepressant, Prozac, which has recently been implicated as a potential *cause* of murderous and suicidal acts. Thus, even if we eventually substantiate an association between some harmful behaviors and abnormal brain function, we are in no position to safely tamper with the extraordinarily complex activities of the brain. Since the brain typically tries to compensate for any artificially induced biochemical imbalance, drugs are too likely to achieve the opposite of what we intend.

Current Status of the Biochemistry of Depression

We cannot at present scientifically confirm the suggested relationship between sluggish serotonergic neurotransmission and some destructive or self-destructive behaviors. Meanwhile, there is even less evidence that people routinely diagnosed as depressed by psychiatrists have biochemical imbalances. Scientific reviews of the biochemistry of depression have failed to identify a consistent biochemical basis.[1] The most recent psychiatric textbooks review the biochemistry of depression, sometimes in detail, as if a great deal must be known about the subject; but they end up admitting that the theories are conflicting and remain speculative. The summary concerning the biology of depression in *The New Harvard Guide to Psychiatry* (1988) is pockmarked with phrases like "important clues," "intriguing clues," and "still preliminary" (p. 136). The American Psychiatric Press's *Textbook of Psychiatry* (1988) ends up referring to "ultimate, as yet unknown, factors that cause the illness" and hopes that "unraveling the causal connections awaits a better understanding of the genetic vulnerability" (p. 423). Somewhat buried amid all the scientific reflections in the text is the blanket admission, "As it is true for most other major disorders in psychiatry, the etiology of affective illness is still unknown" (p. 417).

That last sentence bears rereading, as it confirms much of the substance of this and several other chapters in this book.

Similarly, the *Comprehensive Textbook of Psychiatry* (1989) recognizes that the twenty-year-old biological hypotheses that have been relied on are no longer viable, that the field is now in a "new phase of development," that the data cannot be "nicely fitted into any one theoretical framework," and that the very latest research remains "still preliminary" (pp. 877–78).

As yet there is no biology of depression. But can there ever be? Or is it a theoretical impossibility?

The new edition of the *Comprehensive Textbook of Psychiatry* further observes, "It seems highly unlikely, however, that there will be a truly comprehensive understanding of the etiology and pathophysiology of depressive disorders until a parallel description of the functional neurochemistry and neurophysiology of the normal brain becomes available"

(p. 878). Put simply, we can't begin to understand the biology of depression until we understand the normal brain, and we don't understand the normal brain. Seen from a *scientific viewpoint*, most biopsychiatric research is misleading and futile, since it attempts to locate an *abnormality* in the brain when depression usually develops in people with normal brain function who have been subjected to psychosocial stress and conflict.

Again, the Chicken and Egg Problem

The fact that biochemical changes take place in the brain in association with intense moods proves nothing about which comes first. This confusion has led to misguided conclusions about the much-investigated and much-ballyhooed response of the pituitary gland during some cases of chronic depression. Some people who are depressed display what has been labeled an "abnormal" hormonal response.

Cortisol is secreted into the bloodstream by the adrenal glands during prolonged stress of any kind. The increased cortisol in the bloodstream then acts as a hormonal feedback to the pituitary, causing it to stop stimulating the further production of cortisol by the adrenals. This is a self-regulatory feedback mechanism.

It was found in some chronically depressed patients that the feedback mechanism failed. This could be demonstrated by what is called the dexamethasone suppression test (DST). Ingesting the steroid dexamethasone did not seem to suppress the pituitary as expected.

Hundreds of papers have been written about the DST in the hope that at long last a psychiatric diagnostic laboratory test for depression had been discovered. Some of these papers used the "abnormality" to show that depression is physical in origin. The news media flashed the story as evidence of proof of the biology of depression.

The effort was largely a waste of time from the beginning. It has long been known that all kinds of stress, including head injury and chronic fatigue, can cause exactly the same effects. Cortisol is put out in response to any severe stress, and with time, in some cases at least, the feedback mechanism gets sluggish. The fact that some depressed people respond in the same way is not surprising, says nothing about the biochemical nature of depression, and in no way suggests that the depression itself is biochemical in origin. As it turns out, the test has been useless. Very few psychiatrists bother to order it anymore, and most sophisticated researchers pooh-pooh its usefulness.

In *The New Psychiatry* Jerrold Maxmen remarks, "Psychiatrists have always yearned for a laboratory test that could diagnose mental illness.

It's almost as if by having such a test, psychiatrists could prove they are 'real' doctors" (p 108). He then goes on to observe succinctly, "Unfortunately, the DST isn't what it's cracked up to be. The test is often positive in conditions other than depression, and not all severe depressions yield a positive test" (p. 109).

When Hormones Do Seem to Cause Depression

Some hormonal disorders, such as Cushing's disease, with an excess output of steroids, do produce depression in a significant percentage of patients. Hypothyroidism also is associated with depression. Thus there is a relationship between some hormonal disorders and depression, but we don't know if the depression is actually caused by the hormonal imbalance. The depression could be a psychological response to the fatigue and mental disability that the disorders cause. Many other diseases that cause extreme fatigue, such as chronic viral infections and liver disease, tend to result in depression. Just as children will get irritable when they're tired but don't want to go to bed, many adults get depressed when they become fatigued or mentally impaired and cannot perform as well as they are accustomed to.

Brain tumors will sometimes precipitate depression before any neurological signs turn up. But again, we don't know why. Is it due to toxins released into the brain by the tumor or by dying cells around it? Or is it due to the individual's dim and unformulated awareness that something is desperately the matter in his or her head? It is difficult to know. What's important now, however, is that the depressions routinely seen by psychiatrists almost always have obvious psychosocial causes. And if a psychiatrist is faced by a depression that is genuinely hormonal or biochemical in origin, the worst thing he can do is to give the patient psychiatric medications, all of which worsen the biochemical condition of the brain.

Nor can psychiatrists necessarily be trusted to detect such a real disease when it turns up. I'm aware of a malpractice case against several biologically oriented psychiatrists who failed to diagnose a flagrant case of Cushing's disease over many years and instead gave the patient multiple psychiatric hospitalizations, drugs, and electroshock.

The Genetics of Depression and Bipolar Disorder

There's no more evidence for a genetic role in depression or manic-depressive disorder than there is for one in schizophrenia, but the informed reader is likely to have heard about an Amish family study of manic-depressive disorders.

The full promotional potential of psychiatry came out to tout the Amish study. It was everything psychiatry had been hoping and waiting for; a PR miracle! On the basis of this one study, NIMH held a press conference and the media hummed with the news.

The study, authored by Janice Egeland and a host of others, was published in *Nature* on February 26, 1987, and entitled "Bipolar Affective Disorders Linked to DNA Markers on Chromosome 11." It claimed to show that in a genetically pure family of Old Order Amish in southeastern Pennsylvania there was a link between "two DNA sequences located on chromosome 11 and a locus conferring a strong predisposition to bipolar affective disorders."

Right away two facts stand out that the press reports do not emphasize. Despite the PR, they didn't find the gene, they found "evidence" for the gene in a particular pattern of DNA combinations. This is important, because the finding is several steps removed from the gene itself, vastly increasing the possibility of errors of one kind or another. In addition, they're not talking about a one-to-one gene-to-disease linkage, but "a predisposition." Having the specific genetic makeup doesn't necessarily mean you'll get the psychological problem. Nor does it mean it's a disease. The gene might be for sensitivity, creativity, or passion—traits likely to run afoul of Amish clannishness and authoritarianism.

There is something else that the PR doesn't tell us: the entire study rests on a very complex and obviously controversial interpretation of statistics. Even though only nineteen patients are involved, the findings are so complex and abstract that they cannot be contained in a chart or table, but only in mathematical formulae. Furthermore, in fine print under a table the authors tell us that they doctored the published family tree to protect the family's privacy, so we have no objective data on which to base our own analysis.

Previously, the authors had written numerous papers on the diagnoses of the patients in the study, but we can't rely on those earlier reports, either. The authors tell us: "Systematic screening methods were used to update changes in psychiatric status on a yearly basis for pedigree 110 [the family being studied]. Consequently, the diagnoses used in these analyses do not correspond completely to those originally published for this family. . . ." In short, they altered the original diagnoses as the study progressed. We have no way of knowing what they did to reach their conclusions, and they aren't going to tell us.

The little they do tell us about the diagnoses is significant, however. The title of the study claims to link a specific genetic defect to bipolar illness. This makes the study look especially significant, because biopsychiatric theory predicts that bipolar disease is a specific entity. But the authors are misleading us with their title. They admit that of the nineteen family members diagnosed with psychiatric disorders and counted as bipolar for the study, only twelve actually fit the diagnostic standards for that disorder. The original intent was to show a relationship with bipolar disorder; it didn't show up on statistical analysis, yet the authors left the unproven connection in the title of their paper, making it look as if they had succeeded. It worked, and the study was widely reported, even in the psychiatric press, as showing a direct link between a gene and manic-depressive or bipolar disorder.

The authors themselves point out a number of mathematical manipulations in their calculations that are controversial. In October 1988, while at a conference in Germany, I asked six geneticists, each from a different university or institute, about the status of the Amish study in the eyes of geneticists around the world, and each said the study was badly flawed. Meanwhile, it continued to be touted to the public.

The authors even fail to review all of the studies that had already contradicted theirs. For example, a report published three weeks later in *Nature*, on March 19, 1987, reviews eight previously published research projects that already had produced conflicting data, including wholly negative results, about presumed genetic sites for depression. None of these is mentioned in the Amish study. This editorial sleight of hand allowed the Amish study to be presented like an unblemished finding to the press, the profession, and the public.

There's still more bad news about the alleged genetics of manic-depression. In one of the world's most highly regarded medical journals, *Lancet*, the well-known geneticist Julien Mendlewicz and his team failed to confirm the Amish study. Their negative finding was published on May 30, 1987, only three months later, but received very little attention in the media or the profession. Furthermore, the *Lancet* report points out something that the PR from NIMH also failed to tell us: three other studies of Icelandic and North American families also had failed to confirm the Amish study.

The Final Word on the Amish Study

After I had written my analysis of the Amish study for this book, confirmation of my viewpoint came more quickly and decisively than I had expected in a report by Harold Schmeck in the November 7, 1989, *New York Times*. The addition of new family members to the statistical analysis of the Amish study completely undid their original report. The authors were forced to conclude that there was no correlation whatsoever between genetics and the mood disorder among the Amish studied. One of the investigators, Arthur Kidd from Yale, declares, "It means we are sort of back to square one." Reporting on Kidd's remarks made at the Eighth World Congress of Psychiatry, the December 1989 *Clinical Psychiatric News* summarizes, "In fact, there is no definitive evidence that such a gene causes manic-depressive disorder even in some Amish families, he [Kidd] said at the congress." Still more recently, a study by Wade Berrettini and a team from NIMH, published in the April 1990 *Archives of General Psychiatry*, undermines another whole series of earlier research projects purporting to show a genetic linkage in manic-depression.

As with the genetic studies in schizophrenia, the main genetic study in manic-depression was more PR than science. Nor was I the only psychiatrist to grasp the shallowness of the much-touted study or to decry the PR psychiatry was generating around it. In an April 1987 letter to the editor of *Psychiatric News*, John Fort takes the newspaper to task for making so much of the Amish study. He points out that genetic linkage studies of this kind were really a "shot into the dark." As Fort said, "There are at least 300,000 human genes and several billion subsets of DNA— most of them uncharted." Fort also takes issue with the psychiatric newspaper's hope that the discovery of a genetic factor somehow will reduce the "stigma" attached to becoming depressed. He already had encountered one family that was planning not to have children as a result of the PR around the Amish study.

When Biology Equals Politics

The biology of depression is based less on science than on politics—the wish of psychiatry to maintain a medical image, to uphold its dictatorial authority, to garner federal funds, and to convince patients to seek psychiatric help. Psychiatry has tried to make depression into a political issue in America, much like poverty, unemployment, or AIDS. Because nearly everyone has some experience with depression as a part of living, it's easy to make claims about the prevalence of the "disease" and to inflate the statistics on prevalence at will.

The lead article in the November 1988 *American Journal of Psychiatry* is entitled "The NIMH Depression Awareness, Recognition, and Treatment Program: Structure, Aims, and Scientific Basis." The program's acronym is DART. DART was conceived at the highest levels of leadership at NIMH and within organized psychiatry. It is a sophisticated political and media sell aimed at getting more Americans to go to psychiatrists when feeling unhappy. For those Americans who aren't willing to shell out the money themselves, it's aimed at getting the federal government to do it for them.

As the summary of the article declares, DART is "a multiphase information and education program designed to alert the health professions and the general public to the fact that depressive disorders are common, serious, and treatable."

NIMH was shocked to discover that most Americans (78 percent) would rather handle depression on their own than go to a health professional. Perhaps in response to the Just Say No to Drugs campaign, only 12 percent said they would take medication for depression. This is bad news for psychiatry, and so DART developed "a wide variety of public education materials, including radio and television public service announcements, posters, flyers, print advertisements, bus cards, bookmarks, and educational brochures at various age and educational levels in English and Spanish."

As a marketing program for biopsychiatry DART promotes genetic and biological theories, specifically citing the Amish study. Every biopsychiatric treatment is touted, from the old standards of antidepressants and shock to light therapy and sleep deprivation, treatment fads hardly worth evaluating. The only treatment that gets no support is placebo—that harmless sugar pill—even though, as we'll find in the next chapter, it's probably the best medicine of all. The NIMH article on the DART promotion says next to nothing about psychological or spiritual origins of being depressed and mentions limited forms of psychotherapy in passing.

If a religion or philosophy were to establish a national campaign to get depressed people to believe in it and to use its services, everyone would know what they were doing: promoting their particular worldview for their own advantage. Whether we agree or disagree with the religion's approach to overcoming depression, we would understand the goal—getting more converts.

When NIMH, APA, and other psychiatric interest groups promote a theory or a treatment for depression, its aim of selling psychiatry is often beclouded by scientific trappings. Average citizens who see DART advertisements are unlikely to protest, "They're trying to sell me shock treatment and drugs on the subway posters" or "They're trying to get me to pay medical doctors to solve my psychological and spiritual problems."

Let us now look at the treatments most frequently prescribed by psychiatrists for depression—medication and electroshock.

Chapter 8

Suppressing "Depressive" and "Manic-Depressive" Overwhelm with Lithium and Antidepressants, Including Elavil and Prozac

Many patients and their families regard lithium as a wonder drug and have great expectations for its curative value. . . . These patients are educated in the concept that lithium is a perpetual preventive much like insulin.

    —*Ronald Fieve*, Moodswing (1989)

The increasing use of lithium carbonate as the treatment of choice for patients with bipolar affective disorder highlights a major concern with respect to memory functioning. . . . Several studies have found cognitive and memory functioning to be impaired in patients receiving lithium therapy.

    —Psychiatric News, *December 5, 1986*

Warnings About a Miracle Drug. A swift and sweeping popularity is often followed by a stinging backlash. This is as true for medical therapies as it is for hit TV series and fashionable restaurants. The latest example: Prozac. . . .

    —Time, *July 30, 1990*

Although it is often possible to help depressed people through caring, enthusiastic psychotherapy (see chapters 6 and 16), biopsychiatrists typically reject psychological approaches and instead make extraordinary claims for the efficacy of drugs.

One antidepressant, Prozac, recently generated a *Newsweek* cover story, leaped to the top of the drug charts, and then ran into a storm of controversy. Sales figures for August, September, and October 1990 show that more than 400,000 *new* prescriptions for Prozac are being written *each month* in the United States. Total sales in 1991 are expected to

150

reach one billion dollars. Meanwhile, a flood of lawsuits is pending against the manufacturer, Eli Lilly.* This chapter will provide an analysis of the actual effects and potential dangers of the drug.

Barely Escaping the Antidepressants

The young man sitting with me in my office had a broad grin on his face as he reminded himself of how much better he now felt. A few months earlier he'd been hospitalized for severe depression with feelings of utter worthlessness and thoughts of suicide; but when antidepressants had been urged on him, he had managed to say no. Probably the doctors would have forced the drugs on him, except that his parents, advocates of more natural cures, had supported his rejection of the drugs. He'd been discharged AMA (against medical advice) and was now virtually free of depression after a relatively short time.

"I was lucky," he said, "because my friends told me the effects they saw on other students who got them. They said, 'Don't take them. They space you out, and they're hard to get off of. They're addictive.' "

The hospital doctor had said the opposite: "Antidepressants don't affect the mental processes at all, and aren't addictive."

The antidepressants also are being pushed by nonpsychiatric physicians. One of my clients, a young man, was going through a period of severe distress when he went to his family doctor for a cold. A shy person, he didn't mention he was seeing a psychiatrist. The family doctor, noticing his emotional distress, gave him a mimeographed handout stating that antidepressants have no serious side effects and that they correct a biochemical imbalance. The handout also said that depression is no longer believed to be psychological in origin. The doctor then prescribed Elavil; but the first dose so "zonked" the young man that he had thrown the bottle away by the time he came to see me again. Eventually he got over his distress without drugs.

A friend of mine whom I hadn't seen in years, a forty-year-old professional woman, stopped by one day recently to say hello. In the course of conversation, she asked me about Prozac. She was a recovering al-

---

*If it turns out that Prozac received especially favorable treatment from the FDA, or that it had an extraordinary boost from certain media leaders, political influence may be at work. Eli Lilly, based in Indianapolis, was a large contributor to the senatorial campaigns of Dan Quayle. In addition, according to the October 2, 1988, *Washington Post*, "Quayle's uncle, William C. Murphy, opened Lilly's government relations office in Washington in 1964 and his 1980 campaign manager, Mark D. Miles, went to work for the company in 1982 as director of communications" (p. A25). Quayle was instrumental in passing legislation described by a Lilly spokesman as the most important drug measure before Congress at that time.

coholic and her psychiatrist had prescribed Prozac as a "substitute" for drinking. After taking the drug for about a year, her doctor wanted her to stay on it indefinitely. She then tried to come off it on her own, and a few days after stopping, she became overwhelmed with exhaustion. It was so debilitating that she started the drug again and was immediately relieved.

Although she's a bright individual, it never dawned on my friend that she had undergone a drug withdrawal reaction. She mistakenly concluded that she must need the drug to fight off depression. How these withdrawal reactions come about is not hard to understand (see ahead), but the danger is not told to patients or even mentioned in current textbooks.

Antidepressants: Widespread and Growing Usage

Antidepressants are very much in vogue, but they have been around for a long time. Elavil (amitriptyline) and Parnate (tranylcypromine), for example, have been in use for three decades. In 1984, thirty-four million prescriptions were written for antidepressants, placing them a distant second behind the minor tranquilizers; but the Prozac craze is narrowing the lead. More than two-thirds of antidepressant prescriptions are for women.

The great majority of antidepressant prescriptions are written by non-psychiatric physicians. Psychiatrists, however, set the tone for the widespread use of these agents. Right now psychiatrists are advocating their use for a variety of disorders, from depression and anxiety to eating problems, premenstrual tension, phobias, and obsessions and compulsions. They have become a jack-of-all-trades drug. This in itself should warn us not to trust the claims being made.

Tricyclic Antidepressants: Some General Principles

The antidepressants represent a varied group of agents, and their effects on the brain and mind are little understood. We can, however, make some generalizations about one group of antidepressants, the tricyclics, which are the best studied among them. With generic names in parentheses, they include Tofranil or Janimine (imipramine), Elavil or Endep (amitriptyline), Adapin or Sinequan (doxepin), Surmontil (trimipramine), Norpramin or Pertofrane (desipramine), Aventyl or Pamelor (nortriptyline), and Vivactil (protriptyline). Another, Anafranil (clomipramine), is advocated for obsessive-compulsive problems and will be discussed in chapter 11.

Closely related to the tricyclics is Asendin (amoxapine), which turns into a neuroleptic in the body and presents all of the hazards of that class of drugs, including tardive dyskinesia and tardive dementia (see chapter 4). Triavil and Etrafon combine a tricyclic and a neuroleptic, entailing the various dangers of both drugs, including tardive dyskinesia and tardive dementia from the neuroleptics, compounded by the unpredictable complexity of their interactions.

Limbitrol is a combination of the tricyclic Elavil and the minor tranquilizer Librium, a sedative or antianxiety drug that is highly addictive (see chapter 11).*

Several generalizations can be made about tricyclic antidepressants. First, evidence for their usefulness is very slim indeed. Research studies generate extremely variable results and indicate that they are hardly much better than placebo.

Second, they have a dulling effect on the mind. In effective doses they can produce lethargy and disinterest, that feeling of being "zonked." They also tend to produce generalized mental dysfunction and, as we shall see, sometimes relieve depression by rendering the brain and mind unable to generate higher psychospiritual responses. But often they are given in smaller doses, which may have a lesser impact or a placebo effect.

As a third general principle, many of the tricyclics have a sedative effect that aids sleep, for a time, much as does any sedative.

Fourth, they can cause severe withdrawal symptoms and can therefore become very difficult to stop taking.

The tricyclics are extremely lethal in overdose and have numerous side effects.

Antidepressant Side Effects

The tricyclic antidepressants originally were tested as neuroleptics because chemically they are very similar to Thorazine (chlorpromazine). They are, in many ways, neuroleptics in disguise. Their side effects stem mainly from suppression of the cholinergic nerves of the autonomic nervous system and the brain, and when the individual tries to stop taking them, the cholinergic system rebounds with great force, making it hard to get off them.

Nearly all of the antidepressants commonly produce the following side effects: various autonomic nervous system signs, such as blurred vision, dry mouth, and suppressed function of gut, bladder, and sexual organs,

---

*In general it is best to avoid combining psychoactive drugs, since their effects when mixed become even more unpredictable and are poorly understood.

as well as low blood pressure on standing, weight gain, sleep disturbances, seizures, and impaired cardiac function. They can bring about anxiety, produce or exacerbate psychotic symptoms, and cause delirium.

They frequently produce sedation, lethargy, and a blunting of emotional responsiveness, although this often goes unacknowledged by psychiatrists.

The antidepressants can cause death when only a few doses are taken at once. In combination with other depressants of the central nervous system—such as alcohol, neuroleptics, lithium, sleeping pills, painkillers, and minor tranquilizers—the antidepressants become increasingly dangerous. They suppress central nervous system function, thereby impairing respiration, and they cause cardiac arrhythmias, leading to heart failure. Caution must be taken in regard to their use by the elderly.

A number of years ago antidepressants replaced sedatives as the prescription medications most frequently involved in successful suicide attempts. Obviously, there is a built-in danger to giving such lethal drugs to depressed patients who have a high and unpredictable suicidal potential.

Withdrawal from Tricyclic Antidepressants

Recently one of my patients, a man in his twenties, was trying to taper off small doses of Elavil prescribed by another physician. Over a period of several weeks we cut back on the medication, until it was stopped. Within a day or two of complete withdrawal he began to feel ill. It seemed exactly like the flu. He felt lethargic and his muscles ached. He lacked appetite, felt sick to his stomach, and vomited in the morning. Despite his tiredness, he had trouble falling asleep and staying asleep. He felt increasing anxiety as well. A complete physical evaluation by an internist produced no evidence of an infection, and I was forced to conclude he had a typical flulike drug withdrawal syndrome. He gradually recovered over a few weeks, vomiting for the last time about a month after ending the medication.

In an article with an extensive bibliography entitled "Antidepressant Withdrawal Symptoms" in the 1987 *International Clinical Psychopharmacology*, DiSalva and his colleagues estimate that 55 percent of adults will undergo withdrawal symptoms when stopping these medications. In addition to the flulike symptoms, withdrawal symptoms from antidepressants often make the person seem irrational and even crazy, with high levels of anxiety and disturbing dreams that awaken the individual in a state of panic or dread. Often there is jitteriness or irritability. There are reports of patients becoming high or manic on withdrawal. Patients also can become depressed, perhaps in response to the fatigue and lethargy associated with withdrawal.

In the May 1981 *American Journal of Psychiatry*, William Law III and his colleagues report on their review of the charts of twenty-two children who had been removed from high doses of a tricyclic antidepressant, Tofranil (imipramine). Each of the children suffered from two or more of the following categories of withdrawal symptoms: (1) gastrointestinal complaints, including epigastric pain, abdominal pain, nausea, vomiting; (2) drowsiness and fatigue; (3) decreased appetite; (4) tearfulness; (5) apathy and withdrawal; (6) headaches; and (7) agitation. Tapering didn't seem to help.

The mental health professionals working with these children often incorrectly attributed their withdrawal symptoms to "mental illness," to specific stresses, such as "changing visits from family, visiting home, dealing with 'loaded issues,' " allergies, or viral illnesses. Unfortunately, antidepressants were reinstituted for some of these children, who were mistakenly diagnosed as relapsing during the withdrawal period.

Anyone being started on an antidepressant should be informed in advance that withdrawal symptoms are very common and that they can be both confusing and distressing. For the same reasons discussed in regard to the neuroleptics, the antidepressants should be considered addictive.

As in withdrawing from the neuroleptics (chapter 4), patients trying to stop taking antidepressants may need emotional support and patience. The patient and the doctor, and members of the patient's inner circle of friends and family, may have to put up with troublesome symptoms and behavior during the withdrawal period.[1]

Permanent Mental and Neurological Damage?

There is an ominous aspect to these withdrawal symptoms, most of which are produced by rebound hyperreactivity of the suppressed cholinergic nerves. Cholinergic nerves of the autonomic nervous system activate the so-called vegetative or digestive processes of the body,* and when they rebound, flulike symptoms develop. However, the cholinergic nerves in the brain play a major role in mental processes, and when they rebound, they cause mental disturbances, such as anxiety, depression, or mania.

---

*The cholinergic (or parasympathetic) nerves of the autonomic nervous system cause the smooth muscles of the stomach, intestine, and bladder to contract. They tend to increase digestive processes, promote salivation, slow the heart, lower the blood pressure, and narrow the pupils. In general, they act in opposition to the energizing adrenergic (sympathetic) nerves.

We have seen how a similar rebound hyperactivity of a different neurotransmitter produces permanent mental and neurological disorders after long-term exposure to the neuroleptics (chapter 4). The questions must be asked, Are we producing permanent symptoms of mental dysfunction, including anxiety, depression, or mania, by giving patients antidepressants? How often do we induce a vicious circle in which patients attempt to come off the medications and then experience withdrawal symptoms that are mistaken for a recurrence of depression or other mental dysfunction—leading to further treatment with the offending medication?

Innumerable animal studies have documented that chronic exposure to antidepressants produces hyperreactivity of the neurotransmitter systems of the brain.[2] It also can produce chronic subsensitivity or reduced reactivity. These findings sound a serious—but almost wholly ignored —warning about the danger of permanent negative effects on the human mind as a result of antidepressant treatment. If the lessons of neurophysiology hold true, the brain frequently does not fully revert to normal functioning after prolonged exposure to toxic medications.

Tardive Dyskinesia and Tardive Dementia from Antidepressants

Many clinicians continue to believe that only the neuroleptics, and not the antidepressants, cause tardive dyskinesia, with its permanent, untreatable tics and spasms of the voluntary muscles. However, some studies suggest that the tricyclic antidepressants also produce tardive dyskinesia, but much less frequently. These findings are not surprising in light of the similarity between the chemical structures of the tricyclics and the phenothiazine neuroleptics. One report found a relatively high incidence of 6 percent.[3]

Since the tricyclic antidepressants closely resemble neuroleptics, and since all antidepressants powerfully affect the brain and mind, I am very concerned about the largely unexplored danger of permanent cognitive dysfunction and brain atrophy similar to that found during prolonged neuroleptic treatment. Patients diagnosed with "affective disorders" (depression, manic-depression, and schizoaffective disorder) are showing up with atrophy on brain scan, suggesting that antidepressants may play a role in causing brain damage. However, the studies done thus far do not rule out electroshock, neuroleptics, and other drugs as possible culprits. Many patients with diagnoses of affective disorders have received a broad spectrum of brain-disabling treatments. Of course, the biopsychiatrists who perform the studies assume that the brain pathology is due to mental illness.[4]

Depression *Caused* by the Antidepressants?

There are reports that administration of the antidepressants can cause depression, especially early in the treatment. Namir Damluji and James Ferguson discuss "Paradoxical Worsening of Depressive Symptomatology Caused by Antidepressants" in the October 1988 *Journal of Clinical Psychopharmacology*. They describe four cases of major depression that were exacerbated to the point of suicidal behavior. Improvement followed immediately on stopping the medication.[5]

Any drug that disrupts mental function can make people feel more helpless and despairing.[6] Drugs that cause mental confusion, sluggishness, and physical fatigue are especially prone to precipitate or worsen depression. Harvey Greenberg and H. Robert Blank report a series of cases who felt dazed, fatigued, and confused in the June 15, 1973, issue of the *New York State Journal of Medicine*; but little attention is paid to these problems in the literature or clinical practice.

Meanwhile, some psychiatrists persist in telling patients and the public that these drugs have no "psychoactive" or mental effects at all.* When uninformed patients then feel numbed or "zonked" from the medication, they are very likely to think their condition is worsening, thereby encouraging suicidal feelings. Dr. Caligari's *Psychiatric Drugs* puts it bluntly:

What psychiatrists call "depression"—lethargy, apathy, nervousness, hopelessness, helplessness and unhappiness—is a serious problem often unrecognized as drug-related (drug-induced). Because of their depressant and debilitating effects, psychiatric drugs can make people feel so bad they want to kill themselves. (P. 18)

Antidepressants and Suicide

In helping seriously depressed people, reducing the suicide rate is one of the first concerns. Do antidepressants have a beneficial impact on suicide? Despite the relative ease of conducting objective studies of suicide rates —the criterion of death is an indisputable one—there is no published evidence that the antidepressants are helpful in reducing suicide. In the *PDR*, the manufacturers of the various antidepressants warn practitioners not to rely on the medications to prevent suicide.

One study, "Mortality in Depressed Patients Treated with Electrocon-

---

* This is so remarkable that I may need to be more specific. When debating psychiatrists about the impact of antidepressants, a few have literally argued that the drugs have no effect on the mind. How they reconcile this with an alleged antidepressant impact is difficult to understand.

vulsive Therapy and Antidepressants," by David Avery and George Winokur in the September 1976 *Archives of General Psychiatry*, shows an *increased* suicide rate among patients receiving antidepressant therapy.

Since antidepressants are now the drugs most commonly implicated in successful suicides, it would seem far more appropriate to designate them as "suicide drugs" rather than antisuicide drugs. Yet psychiatrists persist in giving them to depressed patients who are suicidal.

Do They Work?

The antidepressants have many drawbacks, but do they work? Is there convincing evidence for efficacy to balance against the costs and risks of taking these toxic agents?

It is difficult to evaluate the effectiveness of drugs for depression. Spontaneous improvement of depression (that is, with no psychiatric treatment whatsoever) takes place in at least one-quarter of patients within the first month or so of becoming depressed and in one-half or more over a few months. Even people with severe depression have a high rate of recovery without psychiatric treatment. Since it takes most antidepressants a month or more to have their presumed beneficial effect, it easily overlaps with spontaneous recovery. In addition, placebo has a potent effect on depressed patients; most experts indicate that 40 percent or more will improve during the first month or two of taking a "sugar pill."[7]

The slightly higher rates of improvement for antidepressants over inert placebos, such as a sugar pill, may itself be a special kind of placebo effect. I call this the enhanced placebo effect. Consciously or not, when taking an inert placebo the patient realizes that his mind and body are not being impinged upon strongly by the medication. In sharp contrast, the antidepressants have many obvious physical side effects, so the patient receiving them is likely to believe that he or she is taking a powerful medicine. The concept of the enhanced placebo reflects the wisdom that led hucksters to make patent medicines taste awful.[8]

Ironically, enthusiasm for the use of antidepressants has been skyrocketing among practicing psychiatrists at the same time that research has cast more and more doubt on their efficacy. In *The Limits of Biological Treatments for Psychological Distress* (1989), Seymour Fisher and Roger Greenberg conclude that years of research have failed to provide justification for their use. Here are some highlights from their thoroughly documented review:

- Even the most positive reviews by drug advocates indicate that 30 percent to 40 percent of studies show no difference between the drugs and placebos. Since it is relatively harmless,* placebo may be the best treatment.

- When the standard of "substantial improvement" is used in antidepressant studies, the reported rates of improvement average out to a very meager 25 percent.
- Active placebos that cause side effects are rarely used in controlled studies and would probably perform as well as antidepressants.
- Powerful investigator bias is often at work, since some teams repeatedly find considerable efficacy while others find very little or none. Placebo efficacy, for example, varies from zero to 91 percent in one series of studies (p. 21).
- There are no standard criteria for determining "improvement" and psychiatric standards are often behavioral, such as "sleeps better" or "gaining weight," rather than psychological, such as "feels better about life" or "actively building a better future."
- Controlled studies of the newer, more highly promoted antidepressants provide still less evidence of efficacy: "An overview of all 16 studies indicates that the majority (62%) show no difference in the percentage of patients benefiting from an active drug as opposed to a placebo" (p. 19).
- Controlled studies comparing drugs and psychotherapy tend to favor psychotherapy: "Psychotherapy had its main effect on mood, apathy, suicidal ideation, work, and interest, whereas medication mainly influenced sleep and appetite" (p. 13). They conclude, "Although drugs may help patients with their sleep disturbances, research shows they are often less efficient than psychotherapy in helping patients with depression and apathy and frequently ineffective in aiding patients in their social adjustment, interpersonal relationships, or work performance" (p. 16).

Psychotherapy Versus Antidepressants at NIMH

NIMH coordinated a large-scale, highly publicized study at several medical centers, comparing cognitive behavior therapy, interpersonal psychotherapy, antidepressants, and placebo over a sixteen-week period. A recent publication, by senior author Irene Elkin in the November 1989 *Archives of General Psychiatry*, confirms how difficult it is to find any differences under these conditions between brief psychotherapy, drug

---

*Even placebo is not wholly harmless, since many people taking them believe that they are having side effects and actually develop symptoms. Furthermore, an active or enhanced placebo will of necessity have some side effects.

therapy, and placebo. When the treatments—including placebo—were compared for the entire sample of 250 patients, *no difference* was found among them.

For more severely impaired patients there was a relatively greater benefit from interpersonal psychotherapy and the antidepressant. In these cases the drug performed slightly better than psychotherapy, according to the investigators; but the data show no meaningful difference. To find the drugs slightly superior required fancy statistical footwork based on a limited number of criteria. This did not prevent biopsychiatrists from making much ado about nothing in the press.

Most experienced psychotherapists would probably do far better than those working within the strictures of the NIMH comparative study. First, sixteen weeks for psychotherapy is very short and the time limit is very arbitrary. Depressed patients want to know that their therapist will be much more available than that. Second, the therapy methods used were stilted and routinized to conform to distinctions between cognitive behavioral and relationship models. Most therapists would never limit themselves to one orthodoxy, and they rarely list either one of the NIMH techniques among their repertoire. For example, hardly anyone in the membership directory of the American Academy of Psychotherapists includes either one among the many and varied approaches. Considering such handicaps, psychotherapy performed surprisingly well.

Monoamine Oxidase Inhibitors

The monoamine oxidase inhibitors are among the most dangerous agents used in medicine. They include Marplan (isocarboxazid), Nardil (phenelzine), Parnate (tranylcypromine), and Eutonyl (pargyline). Another, Eldepryl (selegiline), is recommended only for the treatment of parkinsonism and is considered very useful.

Careful adherence to a special diet is required to avoid very severe and life-threatening cardiovascular reactions. The list of foods to avoid is too wide for discussion here (see textbooks and the *PDR*), but includes all those containing tyramine, such as beer and wine, aged cheese, chocolate, fermented foods, yeast, yogurt, chocolate, raisins, and many others. MAOIs also interact dangerously with many other medications, increasing the risk of cardiovascular crises, including hypertension and stroke, as well as brain dysfunction and mental distress. Headaches are frequent and can be a warning sign. They often cause restlessness and insomnia and can produce confusion, disorientation, and a euphoric or manic reaction. They are very lethal in overdose, a special hazard in potentially suicidal depressed patients. Withdrawal from an MAOI can produce depression or its opposite, euphoria.

For many years these drugs were viewed as too dangerous for routine use, and some experts rejected them entirely. With the resurgence of radical biopsychiatry they are becoming more commonly prescribed.

Stimulants

Another group, seldom used as antidepressants today, includes the highly addictive stimulants, such as Ritalin and Dexedrine. They pump up the sympathetic nervous system. We will discuss them in regard to the treatment of children with behavior problems. Until their addictive qualities were fully appreciated they were liberally prescribed for weight reduction. Most physicians no longer recommend them as a treatment for obesity or depression.

Newer Types of Antidepressants

Newer antidepressants of mixed types are sometimes called the atypical antidepressants. They include Asendin (amoxapine; whose extreme hazards are described earlier in this chapter), Ludiomil (maprotiline), Desyrel (trazodone), and Wellbutrin (bupropion). Most textbooks of psychiatry, as well as Fisher and Greenberg's *The Limits of Biological Treatments for Psychological Distress*, confirm that these drugs have not proven themselves more effective than the old standbys, the tricyclics, whose efficacy itself is highly in doubt. We are dealing with a more questionable subclass of a very questionable class of drugs.

Ludiomil carries most of the risks of tricyclics, including sedation, hypotension on standing, skin rashes, and disturbed mental reactions. A special danger is the increased rate of seizures.

Desyrel also carries many of the risks of tricyclics, including heart problems, a special threat among the elderly. All tricyclics can produce sexual dysfunction, but Desyrel carries a particular risk for priapism—uncontrolled, permanent penile erection—sometimes requiring surgical intervention.

Wellbutrin is a very new drug and in a class of its own, which means that anyone taking it in the next several years will be contributing to research on its side effects. It has a fourfold greater tendency to cause seizures than have the tricyclics. Many patients became agitated and unable to sleep while taking it, so sedatives are often required. It also has many other side effects similar to those of the tricyclics.

Prozac: The Most Recent "Miracle Drug"

Prozac (fluoxetine), introduced in January 1988, is one of the latest of a new generation of antidepressants. The March 26, 1990, *Newsweek* sports the picture of a huge Prozac capsule on the cover—a kind of "pill of the year" award. Beneath the giant PROZAC headline, the subhead announces A BREAKTHROUGH DRUG FOR DEPRESSION.

The story sports a photo of a smiling woman, captioned "I'm nowhere near perfect, but it's a big, big improvement." Without embarrassment, *Newsweek* reports how one patient exclaimed to her doctor, "I call myself Ms. Prozac." The story anticipates that "these breakthrough drugs may change the lives of millions."

At a recent picnic I met a woman who had just been prescribed Prozac—by another psychiatrist at the previous party she'd attended. Apparently he wrote out a prescription on the basis of the brief "consultation." Another woman on Prozac explained that her psychiatrist said he himself was taking the drug, even though he wasn't depressed; it just made him feel better.

Surprisingly, recent psychiatric textbooks and many experts take the position that Prozac is no more effective than any other antidepressant, and maybe even less so. The 1988 American Psychiatric Press's *Textbook of Psychiatry* gives it a dubious endorsement: "studies show it to be as efficacious as imipramine in the treatment of depression." Imipramine (Tofranil) is among the oldest antidepressants and is one of those old standbys whose entire credibility is being challenged by researchers like Greenberg and Fisher. Similarly, the 1989 *Comprehensive Textbook of Psychiatry* observes that Prozac is "at least as effective as standard antidepressants."

The most sophisticated analysis, found in the four-volume *Treatments of Psychiatric Disorders*, by the American Psychiatric Association, finds that expectations for the newer generation of antidepressants, specifically including Prozac, have not panned out: ". . . it is apparent that no currently available agent at the time of this writing either offers enhanced efficacy or is free of toxicity limitations." Speaking of Prozac it warns, "Whether this agent's spectrum of efficacy will be more favorable than that of other antidepressants remains to be observed" (p. 1799).

Rarely do psychiatric textbooks display such uniformly conservative evaluations of a new drug. It's a disconcerting contrast to the feverish promotion being generated by the drug industry through the media.

Prozac seems especially exciting to doctors, patients, and the press because it is described as selectively affecting the neurotransmitter serotonin. It is suggested that this selectivity for serotonin somehow makes Prozac more limited in its impact on the brain and mind, and less likely to produce complex or dangerous side effects. These are false conclusions. Serotonin nerves spread throughout most of the brain—including the emotion-regulating limbic system and frontal lobes—and are thus involved in multiple functions that defy our current understanding or imagination. Prozac makes serotonin more available by inhibiting its removal from the synaptic region between nerves.* When this biochemical imbalance is created, many other related neurotransmitter systems, such as dopamine, are forced to undergo changes as well, creating more widespread disruptions. There should be no comfort associated with the idea that Prozac is selective for serotonin. The brain, an integrated organ blessed with harmonies and balances beyond our ken, is thrown out of balance by any such biochemical intrusion.

The relative safety of Prozac is acclaimed by the *Newsweek* cover story; but in reality it's too early to hold out such hopes. Nor does the literature confirm such positive expectations. For example, an August 1989 report in the *Journal of Clinical Psychiatry* compared Prozac with a much more thoroughly tried antidepressant, Desyrel (trazodone). It found no therapeutic advantage to Prozac and no fewer adverse symptoms. Forty-three percent of the Prozac patients complained of two or more side effects, including headache (29 percent), nausea (24 percent), and somnolence (19 percent). It is also well-known that Prozac causes anxiety and agitation, as well as insomnia and bizarre dreams, in a large percentage of patients. It can also result in loss of appetite, diarrhea, dry mouth, sweating, dizziness, impotence, inability to achieve orgasm, seizures, and rash. It can cause hypoglycemia with anxiety, chills, cold sweats, confusion, weakness, and other symptoms of low blood sugar. On rare occasion, a severe rash develops with symptoms of fever, joint pain, and swollen lymph nodes. A "Prozac syndrome" may develop, with hot flashes and flushing, agitation, nausea, muscle tremors, and sweating. Using tryptophan can increase the risk of Prozac syndrome. Convulsions and a few deaths have been reported from massive overdoses. Combination with MAOI antidepressants and other drugs can be dangerous. From the initial studies, it was also apparent that a small percentage of Prozac patients become psychotic. And as we shall see, there are still more ominous problems associated with Prozac, including serious neurological and psychiatric disorders.

The *PDR* warns that Prozac has not been systematically studied for its

---

*This is called blocking re-uptake of serotonin.

potential to cause withdrawal reactions. Earlier in this chapter, I described a patient with such severe withdrawal symptoms that she felt compelled to resume taking the drug. The *PDR* further states, "it is not possible to predict on the basis of this limited experience the extent to which [Prozac] will be misused, diverted, and/or abused once marketed." That is, the drug may yet turn out to be habit-forming or addictive.

Murder and Suicide Associated with Prozac

Newspaper and scientific reports are pointing to an association between Prozac and compulsive self-destructive and murderous activities in a growing number of patients.* In "Murder Trials Introduce Prozac Defense" in the February 7, 1991, *Wall Street Journal,* Amy Dockser Marcus reports, "A spate of murder trials in which defendants claim they became violent when they took the antidepressant Prozac are imposing new problems for the drug's maker, Eli Lilly & Co." An article by Natalie Angier on the same day in the *New York Times* declared in its headline, "Suicidal Behavior Tied Again to Drug: Does Antidepressant Prompt Violence?"[9] On February 28, 1991, a "Donahue" TV talk show put together a group of individuals who had become compulsively self-destructive and murderous after taking Prozac and the clamorous telephone and audience response confirmed the problem.

The clinical literature also displays a growing number of reports of compulsive suicidal behavior in people taking Prozac. An article by Martin Teicher and others in the February 1990 *American Journal of Psychiatry* described six cases of obsessive, violent suicidal thoughts after starting Prozac,[10] and more recently a variety of individual case reports have reinforced these initial observations. I am personally familiar with several cases of compulsive suicidal or violent feelings developing after taking Prozac. Recently I presented a seminar on Prozac and its dangers at the psychiatric grand rounds of a hospital. After I concluded, one of the psychiatrists in the audience summarized a case of his own in which a highly responsible corporate executive had unexpectedly become very violent one week after starting to take Prozac. The patient had no prior history of violence and described the impulse as taking him over. He had to be subdued by several men after he attacked a stranger without provocation during a minor quarrel.

---

*See chapter 7 for my criticism of directly associating particular biochemical alterations with specific behaviors.

How Prozac Could Cause Seemingly Paradoxical Reactions

As noted in chapter 7, some researchers believe they have found an association between diminished or sluggish activity of serotonin and impulsive acts such as suicide and murder.[11] While Prozac is supposed to enhance serotonin neurotransmission, the brain in fact reacts to the first dose by *reducing serotonergic activity*, including that to the emotion-regulating centers. Researchers for the pharmaceutical company itself, Eli Lilly, first described this reaction before the drug was even named. In *Life Sciences* (1974), Ray Fuller and colleagues from the Lilly Research Laboratories reported that one dose of Prozac (then called Lilly 110140) caused a marked *drop* in serotonin nerve activity for more than twenty-four hours. They suggested that this was the result of a "compensatory mechanism" in reaction to initial overstimulation. As further documented by Claude de Montigny and his team in the December 1990 *Journal of Clinical Psychiatry* and by Pierre Blier et al. in the 1988 *Navnyn-Schmiedeberg's Archives of Pharmacology*, Prozac and similar drugs initially cause a *suppression* of serotonergic neurotransmission that gradually returns to normal over a three-week period. In a phone call interview with me in early 1991, Montigny agreed that this compensatory serotonergic shutdown mechanism could possibly account for the out-of-control destructive reactions to initially taking the drug; but he considered the suggestion "speculative." However, it is no less speculative than the drug company's claim that Prozac alleviates depression by enhancing serotonergic neurotransmission.

Prozac can also produce a relative shutdown of serotonergic neurotransmission during long-term use through another mechanism called down-regulation. When neurotransmitter systems are overstimulated, some of them tend to become relatively nonreactive. One way this occurs is through a reduction in the density of the receptors for the neurotransmitter. Prozac-induced down-regulation occurs[12] and is even mentioned in the 1991 USP DI *Drug Information for the Health Care Provider*, but without indicating the potentially disastrous outcomes associated with it.

Prozac as a Stimulant

There are still other ways of understanding how Prozac could produce both murderous and suicidal behavior. Prozac often affects individuals as if they are taking stimulants, such as amphetamine, cocaine, or PCP. When testing a drug for amphetaminelike or stimulant qualities in animal research, the two main criteria are an energizing effect and an appetite suppression effect—and Prozac has both. Indeed, this stimulant quality may be the main reason for Prozac's popularity.

Although Lilly makes no mention of Prozac's stimulant profile in the *PDR* or in its advertising, the response of many Prozac patients is indistinguishable from reactions to the amphetamines or cocaine—"elevation of mood, a sense of increased energy and alertness, and decreased appetite."[13] Like amphetamines or cocaine, Prozac can produce the whole array of stimulant effects, such as sleeplessness, increased energy, jumpiness, anxiety, artificial highs, and mania. Some patients taking Prozac do indeed look "hyper" or "tense," and even aggressive, without realizing it. The 1990 *PDR* states that "abnormal dreams and agitation" are "frequent." Prozac also has other side effects frequently associated with stimulants, including loss of appetite, tremors, various abnormal bodily movements, sweating, and headache. Indeed, the FDA's internal review of Prozac side effects by psychiatrist Richard Kapit twice mentions the drug's "stimulant" effects, but these important observations were not included in the final labeling requirements.

The *PDR* lists the symptoms of Prozac overdose—"agitation, restlessness, hypomania, and other signs of CNS excitation," as well as seizures—and these are similar to stimulant overdose.[14] Consistent with this, there are many published reports of patients becoming "manic" or otherwise psychotic on Prozac. I suspect that violence in individuals taking Prozac may sometimes be associated with amphetaminelike psychoses. And finally, there is already one published report by Mark Pollach and Jerrold Rosenbaum in the January 1991 *Journal of Clinical Psychiatry* that shows that some patients can use Prozac to withdraw from cocaine. We must await further animal and human studies to learn to what degree Prozac can actually substitute for cocaine and other stimulants.

The public has begun to catch on that Prozac is a stimulant. It is being referred to in the popular press as "the Yuppie Upper" and in the January 1991 *Life* (p. 96) as "Prozac, the new Puppie [*sic*] Upper."

Some people react paradoxically to uppers by becoming depressed. More important, in psychopharmacology "what goes up must come down," and we would expect some patients to crash after being high on Prozac, producing still another potential for depressed, suicidal behavior.

Are there precedents for stimulant and other addictive drugs that initially were greeted with unbounded enthusiasm? Yes. Amphetamines for weight reduction and depression were an enormous fad before doctors and the public caught on to the danger of addiction, psychosis, and bizarre behavior. Minor tranquilizers were at first dispensed freely because they were thought to be relatively safe and nonaddictive. They turned out to be very dangerous in combination with other drugs and highly addictive (see chapter 11).

Permanent Depression from Prozac?

Laboratory research in animals shows that subsensitivity can become permanent after exposure to other antidepressant drugs, and while there is as yet no direct evidence for this danger, I fear that Prozac will prove no exception. In some cases the brain may end up needing increasing amounts of Prozac to compensate for the subsensitivity. Are we creating a permanent need for Prozac in some patients—a virtual addiction? Although we do not yet have research confirmation, it seems highly probable to me. If Prozac can indeed alleviate depression by making more serotonin available in the brain, then with time it may produce incurable depression by making the brain relatively unresponsive to any amount of serotonin.* While Prozac does not commonly produce dulling effects on the mind as obviously as the tricyclic antidepressants do, it does disrupt serotonin neurotransmission to the frontal lobes and cerebral cortex. If subsensitivity becomes permanent in that region of the brain, Prozac may also end up causing subtle irreversible lobotomylike effects.

Other Potential Long-Term Risks

Although I've not seen it discussed elsewhere, I also fear there is a potential danger of *permanent* neurological disorders with the long-term use of Prozac. The drug can produce temporary neurological reactions similar to those caused by neuroleptics. In the September 1989 *Journal of Clinical Psychiatry*, Joseph Lipinski, Jr., reports on five cases of akathisia caused by Prozac. The symptoms were objectively and subjectively indistinguishable from those produced by neuroleptics, including "severe anxiety and restlessness," floor pacing and sleeplessness, severe "jerking of extremities," and "bicycling in bed or just turning around and around."

Prozac-induced akathisia may also contribute to the drug's tendency to cause self-destructive or violent tendencies. Akathisia is very disturbing, especially if the individual does not realize what is happening. Akathisia can become the equivalent of biochemical torture and could possibly tip someone over the edge into self-destructive or violent behavior.

The *PDR* describes akathisia and numerous other abnormal neurological reactions as "infrequent" (occurring at a rate between 1/100 and 1/1000); but as we learned in studying tardive dyskinesia, psychiatrists

---

*This tendency to produce the very symptoms that it seeks to cure is similar to what we have seen with the neuroleptics. The neuroleptics initially suppress psychotic symptoms, but the long-term effect is to produce permanent psychoses that make it difficult or impossible to remove the patient from the drugs (chapter 4).

typically fail to notice neurological reactions in their patients. The June 1990 *Health Newsletter,* produced by the Public Citizen Health Research Group, reports, "Akathisia, or symptoms of restlessness, constant pacing, and purposeless movements of the feet and legs, may occur in 10–25 percent of patients on Prozac." The *Health Letter* also notes that Prozac can exacerbate parkinsonism, and attributes both the akathisia and the parkinsonism to interference with dopamine neurotransmission.

Lipinski also believes that Prozac causes akathisia by indirectly suppressing dopamine, eventually causing dopamine supersensitivity or hyperreactivity. Animal studies indicate that Prozac can suppress dopamine activity, and clinical reports confirm that, like the neuroleptics, it can produce not only parkinsonism and akathisia, but dystonias (muscle spasms of neurological origin).

We know that direct dopamine suppression by neuroleptics, followed by hyperreactivity, produces permanent neurological disorders, such as tardive dyskinesia, tardive akathisia, and even tardive dementia (chapter 4). What will the future show about Prozac's capacity to produce permanent neurological disease through its indirect suppression of dopamine?

The FDA and Prozac

When I ask patients or audiences, "How lengthy do you think the studies or trials were before Prozac was approved by the FDA?" most people guess several years or more. Aware of how long it sometimes takes to get FDA approval, some people assume that the drugs are tested for ten years. No one guesses the truth—that the Prozac scientifically controlled testing trials lasted a mere *five or six weeks.* Following that, the FDA is largely dependent on unscientific follow-up studies and anecdotal reports spanning a year or two. Once approval of the drug is then given, there is no reliable mechanism at the FDA for keeping track of dangerous effects that turn up with long-term use. Instead the FDA relies on information from the drug company itself. The FDA must keep track of so many reports that it scans them with a computer looking for unusual clusters of adverse effects. In my interviews with several past and present FDA administrators, it became apparent that long-term follow-up at the FDA is a low priority, largely because it is not demanded by the public and the Congress, which is more concerned with the initial approval process.

People assume that FDA approval and the widespread distribution of a drug—with many patients taking it for months or years—means that long-term studies have found it safe in regard to side effects, drug interactions, dependency, addiction, and withdrawal. Thus FDA approval grossly misleads the public, lulling it into an unfounded security.

The *PDR* also admits that Prozac's *effectiveness* has not been tested in controlled trials of "more than 5 or 6 weeks" and that "long-term" usefulness has therefore not been demonstrated. Yet by now many patients have been on the drug for more than a year, never imagining that it has not been tested or approved for long-term or continuous use.

Do the Antidepressants Accomplish Anything?

Despite the difficulty of showing any useful effect in the hundreds of studies thus far conducted, the antidepressants do have an impact on the mind.

Most obviously they reduce emotional responsiveness. This is why they are being used, however inappropriately, in a variety of severe anxiety disorders, such as insomnia, panic attacks, bulimia, obsessions and compulsions, various phobias in adults, and school phobia and attention deficit disorder in children. They are even used for chronic pain and for the control of aggression in brain-damaged and mentally retarded individuals. The blunting effect probably is due to a general toxicity as well as to the impact on specific neurotransmitter systems. Both the tricyclics and Prozac disrupt neurotransmission to the frontal lobes of the brain.

In many of their uses, the tricyclics are substitutes for the chemically related phenothiazine neuroleptics and their lobotomizing impact. Since the neuroleptics produce a more severe motor retardation—including a flat facial expression and restrained bodily movements—they would look as if they were worsening the symptoms of depression. Therefore the antidepressants, which cause less motor slowing, are preferred by psychiatrists as flattening agents for depressed people.*

Most antidepressants also have a tendency to rev up the brain, sometimes producing euphoria and more rarely delusions and hallucinations. These effects are most unwanted when trying to control an already excited "schizophrenic" individual. For that purpose, the stupefying, muscle-paralyzing effects of the neuroleptics are preferred.

The antidepressants also tend to produce an organic brain syndrome or delirium—the brain's response to generalized damage from any source, such as toxic drugs, viral encephalitis, or electroshock. It is characterized by memory difficulties, confusion, disorientation, impaired judgment, mood instability, and generalized intellectual malfunction. As we'll doc-

---

*Nonetheless, many patients on antidepressants do develop a zombielike reaction.

ument in the next chapter, this is exactly what happens in electroshock and provides the so-called antidepressant effect of that treatment as well. A patient typically is rendered unable to stay depressed during an episode of organic brain dysfunction, because depression requires a relatively intact brain and mind. Rendered either apathetic or artificially euphoric by brain dysfunction, the patient is evaluated as "improved."

In their mild delirium, patients themselves will say they are improved, due to the temporary high or euphoria associated with the initial stages of brain dysfunction and delirium. This is a familiar phenomenon that occurs frequently during the early stage of alcoholic intoxication. As in intoxication with alcohol, mild degrees of drug-induced delirium may be undetected by the patient or other observers and yet impair the individual's capacity to feel anything, including depression.*

In a study entitled "Confusional Episodes and Antidepressant Medication" in the July 1971 *American Journal of Psychiatry*, Robert Davies and a team from Yale examined the charts of 150 consecutive patients receiving relatively small doses of antidepressants on a thirty-bed intensive treatment psychiatric ward. They looked for symptoms of delirium, including "evening restlessness and pacing, followed by sleep disturbances" and progressing to "forgetfulness, agitation, illogical thoughts, disorientation, increasing insomnia, and, at times, delusional states."

The average drug-induced episode lasted a week, with a range of three to twenty days, which again is typical of shock treatment as well. It afflicted more than one-third of the patients over age forty, the average percentage of patients usually judged improved by antidepressant treatment. The authors themselves note that the onset of the acute organic brain syndrome—two to four weeks after the start of drug treatment—coincides exactly with the period when drug-induced relief from depression usually begins.

Unhappily, the authors completely fail to connect the brain dysfunction with the supposed recovery from depression. We shall find the same failure when we examine the relationship between brain dysfunction and supposed recovery after electroshock.[15]

In summary, the antidepressants probably have no specific antidepressant effect. Their clinical impact derives from any one of, or a combination of, at least four factors: (1) enhanced placebo effect, (2) emotional blunting, (3) an energizing or stimulant effect, and (4) the artificial euphoria or apathy associated with an organic brain syndrome. With it all, there is little evidence that they are of net benefit to depressed people.

---

*The patient's failure to recognize toxicity also will be discussed in regard to lithium and minor tranquilizers.

Dispensing with Antidepressants?

Depression is routinely treated by many psychotherapists working with individuals, families, and groups. Many psychotherapists wouldn't dream of prescribing a drug for anything so obviously psychological and spiritual in origin. They would resist blunting the passions of the already "out of touch" or suppressed person.

Even in a full-time lifetime general practice of psychiatry it's possible to offer help without ever starting a patient on antidepressants. Depressed people don't tend to hurt themselves when they have a good relationship with a therapist and some hope of improvement. I try to help individuals experience their feelings, to understand the sources of their despair, and to overcome hopelessness, while providing a caring, morale-building relationship and guidance toward more effective ways of living. Often this involves the client learning new, more positive values and a more daring, creative approach to life.

Nor do I think that I am more effective as a therapist than many others in the field. There are no "great therapists," only great clients. From my conversations with nonmedical therapists—such as psychologists, social workers, counselors, and family therapists—I find that many of them work successfully with severely depressed clients without ever referring them to a physician for drugs or electroshock.

Furthermore, the vast majority of people overcome depression without resort to any mental health services. They do so by virtue of their own inner strength, through reading and contemplation, friendship and love, work and play, religion, art, travel, beloved pets, and the passage of time—all of the infinite ways that people have to refresh their spirits and to transcend their losses.

Since the antidepressants frequently make people feel worse, since they interfere with both psychotherapy and spontaneous improvement by blunting the emotions and confusing the mind, since most are easy tools for suicide, since they have many adverse physical side effects, since they can be difficult to withdraw from, and since there's little evidence for their effectiveness—it makes sense never to use them.

Lithium

Probably because of toxicity problems, lithium is rarely prescribed by nonpsychiatric physicians and is therefore not among the most widely used psychotherapeutic agents. It accounts for considerably less than 3 percent of total prescriptions for psychotherapeutic drugs by all physicians.

Among psychiatrists, less than 10 percent of drug consultations concern lithium.

The commonly prescribed brand names contain "lith," as in Eskalith, Lithane, Lithobid, Lithonate, and Cibalith-S. Although some preparations are longer-acting, they are interchangeable in regard to their basic effects. Lithium carbonate is the usual form in which it is administered.

A Magic Bullet? Or Russian Roulette?

The promotional campaign for lithium began in 1970, the year the FDA approved it for psychiatric uses. The opening salvo was fired by NIMH in a booklet aimed at the media and the general public. Entitled *Lithium in the Treatment of Mood Disorders*, it called lithium "the first specific chemical treatment for a mental illness" and claimed that "it rarely produces any undesirable effects on emotional and intellectual functioning."

The NIMH booklet took a potshot at the neuroleptics, claiming that lithium, unlike the neuroleptics, does not produce a "pharmacological straightjacket" or "suppress the frantic emotional lability and hyperactivity of mania by wrapping the patient's entire mind in a cocoon of stupefaction." Never mind that other authorities at NIMH were denying those neuroleptic effects. This group wanted to promote the contrasting image of lithium as a magic bullet: "Only the symptoms are leached out while the rest of the personality remains unaffected."

In 1973, three years after the NIMH booklet, psychiatrist Ronald Fieve started a promotional blitz for lithium by making the media and medical conference rounds with his famous patient, Joshua Logan, by his side. Fieve, a well-known biological psychiatrist, was the director of research for the New York State Psychiatric Institute. Logan, sixty-four years old at the time, had been a producer and director of such Broadway hits as *South Pacific, Annie Get Your Gun,* and *Mr. Roberts.* Now he was offering himself as a demonstration of the efficacy of lithium in controlling his manic-depressive disorder. In earlier years he had done the talk show circuit in support of electroshock therapy.

Repeating the NIMH theme, Fieve told Diane Shah of the *National Observer* (July 7, 1973) that "most tranquilizers zonk a person out—puts them in a mental straightjacket. And they don't kill the mania, they just put it in chains. But lithium preserves normal mental and physical function and seems to get at the core of the illness by correcting basic biochemical imbalances."

In an article by Harry Nelson in the June 25, 1973, *Los Angeles Times,* and elsewhere, Fieve estimated that fifty thousand Americans already were receiving the drug. Fieve's goal was to put six million on the drug. Other lithium advocates had a still more grandiose and shocking vision —putting everyone in the United States on the drug.

How? With lithium in our drinking water.

Just Like Fluoride

Although the original research had been published in 1970 by Earl Dawson and others in *Diseases of the Nervous System*, the proposal for lithium in drinking water hit the press a few years later during the Fieve-Logan media tour. The researchers led by psychiatrist Dawson claimed to have found higher lithium levels in the drinking water of El Paso compared to Dallas. In El Paso, based on state mental hospital records, Dawson informed the press, "there are almost no mental illness admissions." Admissions to state hospitals were seven times higher where the lithium level was lowest in the water supply. Dawson's amazing conclusion is quoted in the July 7, 1973, *National Observer* by Diane Shah: "The lithium calms people in El Paso, makes them more cheerful, and gives them a more tranquil attitude toward life."

An October 15, 1971, *Medical World News* report picked up on the story and quoted Dawson as admitting, "Most of my reprint requests come from Poland, Czechoslovakia, Hungary and other Iron Curtain countries."

In his book Fieve concedes that lithium "probably" should never be added to the national water supply, and then he adds, "Nonetheless, the fascinating possibilities exist" (p. 220). Actually, the research was preposterous. The areas in Texas with high lithium concentrations in the water were also very rural, where state hospital admission rates are always lowest. * Furthermore, in psychiatry lithium is used at toxic or near-toxic levels, while the concentrations in the water were minute, much too small to influence the brain or mind. †

---

* State hospital admissions are largely proportional to *urban* poverty and homelessness, and to the willingness of hospitals to admit these people involuntarily (see chapter 3).
† Hardly anyone believes that lithium is such a panacea that its wide-scale use, even in clinically effective doses, could substantially reduce psychiatric admissions to hospitals. Nonetheless, the lithium-in-your-drinking-water proposal illustrates an extreme of biopsychiatric thinking that can only be restrained, like threats to liberty itself, by eternal vigilance. It was widely covered in the press, and other psychiatrists supported it.

A Harmless Natural Substance?

Today patients and the public frequently are told that lithium carbonate is a harmless metallic salt found "naturally" in the body and that its function in manic-depressive disorder is similar to the function of insulin in diabetes.

None of this is true, except that it is a metallic salt found in nature. So is lead. Like lead, it is a toxic metal with no known function in the body. Like lead, it appears in traces in the body simply because it's in the environment. Before the lithium PR campaign, the 1960 standard textbook *Goodman and Gilman's The Pharmacological Basis of Therapeutics* observed that lithium has "no biological function" and "the only pharmacological interest in lithium arises in the fact that [it] is toxic." While insulin actually functions to help the metabolism of sugar in the body, lithium does nothing so positive. Instead it interferes with nerve transmission in general, slowing down the responses of the brain.

While admitting that the mechanism of action of lithium is unknown, the *Comprehensive Textbook of Psychiatry* seems to approve of the misleading practice of telling patients that it corrects a biochemical imbalance: "Theories abound, but the explanation for lithium's effectiveness remains unknown. Patients are often told it corrects a biochemical imbalance, and, for many, this explanation suffices. There is no evidence that bipolar mood disorder is a lithium deficiency state or that lithium works by correcting such a deficiency" (p. 1656).

Lithium in Psychiatry

Within standard psychiatric practice, lithium has two generally approved applications: to help abort manic episodes and to help prevent their recurrence. Its other uses, such as the prevention of recurrent depression, are controversial even among avid biopsychiatrists and thus will not be addressed here.

In actual clinical practice lithium is not even the drug of choice for aborting manic attacks. While both the NIMH booklet and psychiatrist Fieve remark on how the neuroleptics create a chemical straitjacket and "zonk" the patient, the neuroleptics nonetheless remain the more commonly used agent for actually stopping a manic attack. Lithium doesn't work fast enough, sometimes taking several days or weeks to slow down the patient. Also, the toxic doses required to stop a manic attack are too dangerous.

Lithium's most established role in psychiatry is in long-term administration for prophylaxis when the patient is between manic episodes.

Even so, other drugs—such as the neuroleptics or the anticonvulsant Tegretol—are used for prophylaxis when lithium proves inadequate or too toxic. Any lobotomizing or sedating agent is likely to be found useful. None of this fits the "magic bullet" scenario, and the story of how lithium was discovered demolishes that image.

From Guinea Pigs to Hospital Patients

John Cade accidentally discovered the effect of lithium while injecting it into guinea pigs in his laboratory in Australia. Serendipitously he noticed that the guinea pigs became sedated and even flaccid. As he explained in the 1949 *Medical Journal of Australia*, "A noteworthy result was that after a latent period of about two hours the animals, although fully conscious, became extremely lethargic and nonresponsive to stimuli for one to two hours before once again becoming normally active and timid."

Notice that the animals became "extremely lethargic and unresponsive to stimuli." Does this sound like the discovery of a treatment specific for a "biochemical imbalance" in manic patients? It is, in fact, the now-familiar brain-disabling effect we first saw described in regard to the lobotomizing impact of the neuroleptics. Because this is so disillusioning, the typical textbook of psychiatry makes no mention of the many studies of lithium effects on animals, and the average psychiatrist knows little or nothing about it.

After this unexpected finding in guinea pigs, did Cade then set up a series of scientifically controlled studies in animals? No need for that, when he had ready access to human guinea pigs in the local state mental hospital. He quickly discovered that he could subdue hospital inmates as easily as he did the guinea pigs, making them into more docile inmates. He himself admitted in his pioneering report that the drug produced a nonspecific leveling effect:

An important feature was that, *although there was no fundamental improvement in any of them,* three who were usually restless, noisy and shouting nonsensical abuse . . . lost their excitement and restlessness and *became quiet and amenable for the first time in years.* (italics added)

Yet Cade would later call lithium a "magic wand" for mania.

For a miracle treatment lithium was slow in being accepted and promoted. There were two reasons. First, the drug companies couldn't patent an elementary metallic salt, so they did not see megabucks in promoting their own brands in a competitive market. Equally discouraging, perhaps, in 1949, the very year that Cade was first plugging lithium for mental patients, a small epidemic of lithium toxicity in humans was breaking out. A 1949 *Journal of the American Medical Association* report by A. C. Corcoran and others, entitled "Lithium Poisoning from the Use of Salt Substitutes," described how a few too many shakes of lithium chloride was causing dangerous and even fatal central nervous system toxicity.

Lithium's Effect on Normal Volunteers

From the start, drug experts promoted lithium as having no effect on normal volunteers. This position has been key to the claim that lithium cures a disease instead of intoxicating the normal brain. This theme is usually bolstered by references to a 1968 foreign journal report by Mogens Schou, perhaps the world's best-known lithium researcher.[16]

I was surprised to discover that the oft-cited Schou report was published in such an esoteric foreign journal that it was not even available in the stacks of the National Library of Medicine. Fortunately, Schou was kind enough to send me a copy of his article, which I have quoted from extensively in *Psychiatric Drugs: Hazards to the Brain*.

Schou and his two coauthors administered lithium to volunteers, but for too short a period of time to determine its effects. They then gave themselves lithium in doses within the therapeutic range for relatively short periods of one to three weeks.* Even though committed to the notion that lithium has no significant effect on "normal volunteers," their self-reports tell a dramatically different story. All three men were markedly emotionally flattened, especially when seen through the eyes of their families. In one case the family considered the blunting effect an improvement in Dad:

On other occasions responsiveness to the environmental stimuli was diminished; this was in one of the cases welcomed by the family ("Dad is much easier and nicer than usual"), while the families of the two other subjects complained about their being so dull.

The subjective experience was primarily one of indifference and slight general malaise. This led to a certain passivity. The subjects often had a feeling of being at a distance from their environment, as if separated from it by a glass wall. . . . Intellectual initiative was diminished, and there was a feeling of lowered ability to concentrate and memorize. . . . The assess-

---

*It is extremely unusual for psychiatrists to administer drugs to themselves as part of their research.

ment of time was often impaired; it was difficult to decide whether an event had taken place recently or some time ago. (Pp. 715–16)*

Despite these published observations, Schou himself would declare in a review article in the March 25, 1988, *Journal of the American Medical Association* that lithium counteracts abnormal moods but "interferes to a remarkably low extent with *normal* mood level and emotional reactivity."

The most in-depth research on the effect of lithium on normal volunteers was led by Lewis Judd, the recent director of NIMH, and reported in the *Archives of General Psychiatry* in 1977–79. A July 20, 1979, study showed a "general dulling and blunting of various personality functions" and overall slowing of cognitive processes. The normal volunteers were observed by trained mental health professionals as well as by a "significant other" in the volunteers' lives, such as a girlfriend or roommate. The significant others recognized lithium's dulling and alienating impact on their companions, including "increased levels of drowsiness and lowered ability to work hard and to think clearly." The trained mental health professionals—what did they observe? They were "unable to detect any behavioral changes in the subjects induced by lithium."

Mental health professionals are trained—but trained to what end? They conveniently are taught *not* to notice the damaging impact of their treatments. This is true whether we are talking about lobotomy, electroshock, or drugs.

Normal volunteers or patients taking lithium won't necessarily realize how impaired they have become. One reason why lithium serum levels must be taken periodically is that the drugged patients lose their judgment about their impaired state. † Frequently they don't notice or report symptoms, such as an obvious tremor or a skin rash. This inattention to harmful drug effects reflects the psychological indifference or apathy produced by the medication, a reaction that worsens with larger and more dangerous doses. Hardly the anticipated magic bullet!

Turning Down the Dial of Life

Studies of the impact of lithium on mental patients show the same mentally suppressive result found in volunteers. An October 1968 article

*The description is very similar to that of lobotomy, with its classic impact of reduced initiative and interest.

† Because of this drug-induced indifference, even to signs of toxicity, and because of the drug's negative impact on the brain, patients taking lithium must have their blood levels checked regularly in order to prevent potentially lethal reactions.

by William Dyson and Myer Mendelson in the *American Journal of Psychiatry* captures the lithium effect in graphic terms. Describing lithium's action upon patients who are high or hypomanic, they wrote:

It is as if their "intensity of living" dial had been turned down a few notches. Things do not seem so very important or imperative; there is a greater acceptance of everyday life as it is rather than as one might want it to be; and their spouses report a much more peaceful existence.

Turning down the dial of life! Getting people to accept life "as it is rather than as one might want it to be." Providing spouses a more peaceful existence. Many people would question these goals and the values inherent in them.

Lithium Toxicity

A recent report on noncompliance asks why a large proportion of patients, 43 percent in this study, stop taking their lithium. Michael Gitlin and his colleagues report in the April 1989 *Journal of Clinical Psychiatry* that patients most frequently stopped because of weight gain and mental impairment, with symptoms of "poor concentration," "mental confusion," "mental slowness," and "memory problems."

Consistent with its toxic effects on the nervous system, lithium causes a tremor in 30 to 50 percent of patients. Tremors can be a warning sign of impending serious toxicity of the brain, especially if it occurs along with other danger signals, such as memory dysfunction, reduced concentration, slowed thinking, confusion, disorientation, difficulty walking, slurred speech, blurred vision, ringing in the ears, nausea, vomiting, and headache. Muscle aches and twitches, weakness, lethargy, and thirst are other common signs of lithium toxicity. In the late stages of toxicity, the patient may become delirious and succumb to seizures and coma. EEG studies indicate an abnormal slowing of brain waves in a significant portion of patients routinely treated with lithium; the condition worsens with toxicity.*

---

*People who already have brain damage, as from electroshock or neuroleptic treatment; tend to become toxic more easily when taking lithium, probably because their brains have less functional reserve. Many sources recommend against combining lithium and electroshock. There are reports of life-threatening neurotoxic reactions when lithium is combined with neuroleptics, especially Haldol.

Newborn and Nursing Infants

If there was any doubt about the basic subduing effect of lithium, its impact on newborn and nursing infants should have put them to rest. In mothers receiving routine doses of lithium, it reaches the baby through the milk and makes them flaccid and apathetic. In pregnant mothers it crosses the placenta, impacting on the fetus and producing a newborn who is neurologically sluggish.[17]

Are There Permanent Mental and Neurological Effects?

The first indicator of generalized brain damage from any cause is often the subjective feeling of memory dysfunction. This awareness often develops far ahead of objective findings on neuropsychological or neurological tests. I initially expressed concern about memory impairment from lithium in my 1983 book on drugs. Three years later, concern about memory difficulties among lithium patients had become sufficiently widespread for the December 5, 1986, *Psychiatric News* to highlight research on the subject, in an article headlined LITHIUM AND MEMORY LOSS. Researchers were reporting "a major concern with respect to memory functioning." Patients on long-term lithium did more poorly on recalling numbers and on an information subtest of the Wechsler Memory Scale. Duration of exposure to lithium correlated with negative performance on a number of other memory measures. In addition, an unspecified but apparently significant number of patients reported memory difficulties.

The danger to memory sometimes goes unmentioned in textbooks, or it is dismissed. The *Comprehensive Textbook of Psychiatry* (1989) observes, "Patients may express concern about the effects of lithium carbonate on their learning, memory, spontaneity, or creativity. Although some impairment can be objectively delineated in detailed neuropsychological testing, most patients either do not experience this effect or do not find it unduly impairing" (p. 927). Yet as we've seen, many patients are so disturbed by these side effects that they stop taking lithium. Indeed, in a different section of the textbook it is stated, "Complaints of dysphoria, intellectual inefficiency, slowed reaction time, and lack of spontaneity are common, especially early in the course of treatment" (p. 1660). Meanwhile, others will be too blunted to complain.

One report raises the possibility of more severe mental deterioration on lithium. In 1985 in the French publication *L'Encéphale*, M-P Marchand presents two cases of "progressive intellectual deterioration" from lithium treatment and relates it to the drug's known toxic impact on cerebral functioning. While no body of evidence has accumulated to confirm this finding, I am gravely concerned that someday we will find ourselves confronting mountainous documentation for dementia due to long-term lithium exposure, much as we must do now in regard to the neuroleptics (chapter 4).

Other Lithium Side Effects

Many studies show that the *vast majority* of patients suffer from one or more side effects, the most common being thirst, dry mouth, metallic taste, excessive urination, weight gain, nausea and other gastrointestinal problems, sleep difficulties, fatigue or lethargy, poor coordination, tremor, and the various other neurological and mental effects already described.

Kidney problems associated with long-term lithium treatment have been the subject of much research and controversy. Lithium causes an increased excretion of water through the kidneys, and long-term use has resulted in pathological changes in the kidneys of some patients. Despite many studies, the relationship between lithium and kidney disease remains controversial and clouded, but the clouds are rather dark and ominous.

In a March 1989 review in the *Journal of Clinical Psychiatry*, James W. Jefferson of the Lithium Information Center at the University of Wisconsin responded to the question, "Does lithium cause kidney rot?" He answered:

Not exactly. While lithium is not a kidney-friendly drug, neither does it wreak the havoc on function and morphology [structure] that was suggested by studies in the late 1970s. It is well established that therapeutic amounts of lithium can impair renal concentrating ability, increase urine volume, and cause morphological abnormalities. . . . Patients can be told that while their kidneys may not win a beauty contest, they can expect them to function adequately for years. On the other hand, when long-term studies become very long-term, the result may not be as encouraging.

Most patients would not find these "beauty contest" remarks encouraging, and they are rarely given such a glimpse of the potential menace to their kidneys.

Lithium suppresses thyroid function, causing hypothyroidism and goiter, in up to 10 percent of patients. Hypothyroid symptoms of sluggishness can mimic or elicit depression, and the physician can mistakenly interpret the problem as a recurrence of depression requiring more of the offending medication.*

Much more rarely, lithium can produce hyperthyroidism, an over-activity of the thyroid gland. It also can produce an excessive output of hormone from the parathyroid gland, causing demineralization and weakening of the bones.[18]

Lithium raises the white-blood-cell count, and there are reported cases of leukemia in association with lithium treatment. Whether lithium actually produces leukemia and the seriousness of other reported blood abnormalities remains uncertain. Unhappily, these dangers frequently go unmentioned in authoritative sources.[19]

Skin rashes similar to psoriasis and acne frequently are caused by lithium; occasionally a rash persists long after removal from lithium. More than 10 percent of women may experience hair loss on lithium.

Perhaps as an aspect of its suppression of passion, lithium frequently reduces sexuality.

Twenty to 30 percent of patients taking lithium develop cardiac abnormalities as measured by electrocardiogram (EKG). Patients with arrhythmias should be cautious about taking lithium.

People Who Want Lithium

Patients should not take lithium under the mistaken impression that it is a specific cure for mania rather than a nonspecific brain-disabling agent. They should not be misled into believing that it is a natural substance in the body and that taking it is comparable to taking insulin for diabetes. Nor should they be led to believe it is harmless.

Earlier we saw that Joshua Logan traveled around the country promoting lithium with psychiatrist Ronald Fieve. Was Logan informed about the potential negative effects of lithium? We don't know, but in a letter to me Logan ridiculed the idea that the drug might harm his creativity. Yet his own doctor, Fieve, with coauthor Polatin, had described cases of suppressed creativity as early as 1971 in the *Journal of the American Medical Association (JAMA)*.

In the same *JAMA* article, Fieve declares that lithium is comparable in its specificity to insulin. That surely is misinformation. The key to Logan's promotion of shock treatment and then lithium probably lies in

*Other signs of hypothyroidism include dry and rough skin, hair loss, hoarseness, swelling of feet or lower legs, sensitivity to cold, and swelling in the neck (goiter). Because it is so frequent, the danger of hypothyroidism in lithium-treated patients requires careful warnings to patients.

a statement of astonishing candor that he made to the media: "It is much easier to take a pill than to think of even one self-revealing sentence."

Many patients with a history of becoming extremely high do want to take lithium. They certainly have the right to do so, and they will have little trouble finding a psychiatrist to provide it to them. But physicians and psychotherapists also should have the right to refuse to give toxic remedies, much as we reject giving alcohol or street drugs to patients who feel they cannot live without them.

We must ask ourselves whether drugs actually help people understand and take better control over their inner mental lives and their conduct, and we must ask ourselves whether the potential moral downside isn't too great. Taking psychoactive drugs on a regular basis readily becomes a symbolic gesture that interferes with personal growth and even fosters personal failure. The associated brain dysfunction also increases the individual's helplessness. Beyond that, we must be concerned about the long-lasting and permanent damage, known and unknown, that can result from these agents.

I don't doubt that some manic-depressive people have fewer mood swings as a result of taking lithium on a regular basis. But even greater numbers of people have fewer bouts of extreme emotion as a result of drinking alcohol, smoking cigarettes or marijuana, or overeating. Recently a patient consulted me after becoming manic when he stopped abusing alcohol, but I didn't encourage him to resume drinking beer. Instead I urged him to deal with himself and his problems, and he has transformed his life for the better without resorting to alcohol or lithium. Nonetheless, many persons feel so committed to "self-medicating" with alcohol that they will pursue it even when it becomes life-threatening. I don't believe that the desire to handle life through a psychiatric drug is essentially different from the desire to do it with alcohol, and I don't believe that physicians should look upon it more favorably.

To cast the problem of psychiatric drug use into the realm of drug use in general is more honest and realistic and should enable each person to make a more informed choice. In the meantime, drugs are being pushed by psychiatry and by the media.

Biomythology

In the world of modern psychiatry, claims can become truth, hopes can become achievements, and propaganda is taken as science. Nowhere is this more obvious than in psychiatric pretensions concerning the genetics, biology, and physical treatment of depression and mania. As we also found in regard to neuroleptics and so-called schizophrenia, biopsychiatric research is based too often on distortions, incomplete information, and sometimes outright fraud—at the expense of reason and science.

There are no known biological causes of depression in the lives of patients who routinely see psychiatrists.

There is no known genetic link in depression.

There is no sound drug treatment for depression.

The same is true for mania: no biology, no genetics, and little or no rational basis for endangering the brain with drugs.

The biomythology of depression denies the obvious causes of depression in the lives of most people who become depressed. Biopsychiatrists dare not look their patients in the eye for fear of seeing the psychological truth; they cannot look into their patients' hearts for fear of empathizing with them. Ultimately they must deny their own feelings in order to deny the feelings of others.

To treat a depressed person as a biochemically defective mechanism, and to blunt or damage the brain of the suffering individual, many biopsychiatrists approach the patient with an especially dehumanizing view. Out of this perspective grow extreme treatments like electroshock, the harrowing subject of the next chapter.

Chapter 9

"Shock Treatment Is Not Good for Your Brain"*

Well, what is the sense of ruining my head and erasing my memory, which is my capital, and putting me out of business. It was a brilliant cure but we lost the patient. It's a bum turn, Hotch, terrible.
> —*Ernest Hemingway, after ECT and shortly before he shot himself, quoted by A. E. Hotchner in* Papa Hemingway *(1967)*

As a neurologist and electroencephalographer, I have seen many patients after ECT, and I have no doubt that ECT produces effects identical to those of a head injury. After multiple sessions of ECT, a patient has symptoms identical to those of a retired, punch-drunk boxer. . . . After a few sessions of ECT the symptoms are those of moderate cerebral contusion, and further enthusiastic use of ECT may result in the patient functioning at a subhuman level. Electroconvulsive therapy in effect may be defined as a controlled type of brain damage produced by electrical means.
> —*Sidney Samant, M.D.*, Clinical Psychiatry News, *March 1983*

Electroshock in psychiatry involves the passage of an electrical current through the head and brain to produce unconsciousness and a convulsion.† When I mention to people that shock treatment is making a strong comeback, they often reply, "I thought that went out with *Cuckoo's Nest*,"‡ or "They did it to my grandmother and she was never the same.

---

*This title is borrowed from neurologist John Friedberg's book *Shock Treatment Is Not Good for Your Brain* (San Francisco: Glide Publications, 1976).

†Electroshock treatment (EST), electroconvulsive therapy (ECT), electrotherapy, and convulsive therapy nowadays all refer to the application of electricity to the head to produce grand mal convulsions. In the past convulsions were produced by other methods as well, such as insulin overdose, stimulant drugs, and gases.

‡The reference is usually to the movie based on Ken Kesey's novel *One Flew Over the Cuckoo's Nest* (New York: Viking Press, 1962) in which the hero, McMurphy, is forced to undergo electroshock.

I can't believe they are still doing it." Many people mistakenly believe that shock has been outlawed.

In reality, 100,000 or more Americans are being shocked each year, and the number is rising rapidly. In California, where elderly women are the most frequent targets of shock, three San Francisco hospitals* recently announced that they were starting to give the treatment—leading to a public outcry against it. A front-page headline in the November 28, 1990, *San Francisco Examiner* announced the controversy: CITY LOBBIED TO BAN SHOCK TREATMENT: EX-PATIENTS CALL PSYCHIATRIC TECHNIQUE "FRIGHTENING."

Two Survivors

Cynthia—an extremely intelligent young graphic designer who had taught courses in her field before completing her schooling—had been rendered permanently unable to teach or to work following a routine course of shock treatment (ECT). The ECT method used was state of the art, but her once-high IQ was now severely reduced and impaired.

Cynthia talked to me about what it was like to unexpectedly find herself with great gaps in her intelligence. Her entire identity was changed. Her previous intellectual sources of pride, pleasure, and entertainment were gone. Her precocious professional achievements were now forever beyond her grasp. Even her former friendships, based largely on shared intellectual interests, were gone. Nor could she recall and savor many of her previous accomplishments or her educational experiences. Worse still, Cynthia had lost more than portions of her memory and IQ. The brain damage put gaping holes in her intellectual functions that no one with a normal brain would ever have to endure, even if he or she were of below average intelligence.

Although there can be significant brain damage from shock treatment without it being detectable with modern brain-imaging techniques, Cynthia's CT scan did show shrinkage of the cortex of her frontal and temporal lobes. Neuropsychological testing also showed generalized brain dysfunction. The psychologist was courageous enough to attribute the damage to the ECT.

Cynthia was painfully aware of the harm done to her, but more often than not, brain-damaged patients tend to deny the degree of their memory loss and mental dysfunction. This is true whether the damage has resulted from medical treatment, disease, or accidental trauma. Denial of im-

*The three are St. Mary's Hospital, Pacific Presbyterian Medical Center, and the Langley Porter Psychiatric Hospital at the University of California, San Francisco.

pairment after brain injury is called anosognosia and is a very common finding.[1]

Manfred's attitude toward his ECT-induced mental dysfunction illustrates this principle. Manfred had become despairing a few years earlier following his wife's death and a psychiatrist had given him shock treatment. Now Manfred had brain damage to add to his psychospiritual loss.

Manfred tried to ignore or to make light of his mental dysfunction. His family and friends, however, reported that ever since shock treatment, he had severe memory blanks for events during the year or two prior to the shock, almost complete memory loss for several months around the shock, and difficulty grasping or recalling new information and ideas.

I evaluated Manfred, and my clinical impression was generalized brain dysfunction with memory impairment, relatively shallow emotional responses, poor judgment, difficulty with intellectual functions, and problems focusing his attention. He had dementia—global mental deterioration—caused by shock treatment.

Manfred wasn't exaggerating his brain damage. During our lengthy interview and preliminary psychological testing, Manfred's mental dysfunction gradually became apparent. His daughter, who was with us most of the time, became increasingly upset over the confirmation of her worst fears; but Manfred made silly jokes about his difficulties and went off on tangents, talking about relatively trivial matters.

I recommended more thorough neuropsychological testing, which confirmed the diagnosis of brain damage. I also talked privately with several of Manfred's friends, and they described how he had become a "changed person," with shallow feelings, inappropriate conduct, and obvious intellectual and memory problems. In particular, they said he no longer had the same mental acuity, ability to plan ahead, judgment, and insight in social situations. Thus he had symptoms of a frontal lobe syndrome (see chapter 3). Since he had previously earned an advanced degree and had been known for his remarkable memory, intelligence, and wit, the change was striking.

One close friend, a health professional, said he hadn't told Manfred about the obvious damage after ECT for fear of upsetting him. After all, there was no hope of significant improvement now that it was three years after the shock.

Only one person who regularly saw Manfred reported no damage to his brain or mind: his psychiatrist, the one who had ordered the shock treatment. He didn't even notice or record any memory loss.*

---

*I have found this time and again—everyone recognizes that the patient has been damaged, except the psychiatrist. Similarly, in a random selection of people, many are familiar with someone who has been "forever changed" by shock, except for psychiatrists, many of whom say they have never seen a bad outcome.

Survivors Take the Offensive

In 1989—while I was working with many ECT-damaged people like Cynthia and Manfred in my practice and reform activities—the American Psychiatric Association was busy issuing a new report, *The Practice of Electroconvulsive Therapy* (1990), and holding a press conference in support of electroshock treatment.[2] There was no hint that jolting the head with electricity might damage the brain, mind, or memory. The lengthy literature documenting brain damage from ECT, including animal and human studies, goes unmentioned (see ahead in this chapter).

Behind the shield of the APA report, the three San Francisco hospitals set up electroshock facilities on their wards. A group of outraged psychiatric survivors then convinced Angela Alioto, chair of the City Services Committee of the San Francisco Board of Supervisors, to hold a public hearing on ECT on November 27, 1990. The survivors and the committee invited me to San Francisco to generate media and public interest and to testify.

My presentation before the committee was countered by that of four doctors in favor of ECT. In a sense, the odds were four to one in favor of shock. But in another sense, the odds were twenty to none against the other doctors. The shock advocates were unable to produce a single patient to vouch for the allegedly lifesaving treatment; but the room was packed with outraged people who had signed up to bear witness to the damage done to them, their family members, or their friends. *

I was impressed by the thoroughness of Alioto's questioning of the shock doctors. During my testimony† she explained to me that she had been invited to witness a shock treatment. She would get to see the patient anesthetized, paralyzed by a muscle-blocking agent, artificially respirated, and then shocked with two electrodes across the forehead or on one side of the head. She'd get to see the technology applied to the *unconscious* patient. But while the patient's brain waves were being eradicated by an electrical storm, the outward signs of the convulsion—the twitches and

---

* Alioto challenged psychiatrist Glen Peterson, the leader of the shock lobby, to explain why not one patient had appeared at the hearing to support shock treatment, and he replied that patients found it too humiliating. Alioto suggested that patients would welcome the opportunity to publicize a supposedly lifesaving treatment if it were genuinely so helpful. In reality it is most difficult for patients to come forward when they have been injured by the treatment, because they must face not only the stigma of mental illness and shock treatment but also the stigma of brain damage. Nonetheless, many do take a public stand. The previous day I had shared one woman's personal struggle as she agonized over "coming out." She began by talking with columnist Rob Morse, who mentions her anonymously in "One Flies over the Board of Supes" in the November 27, 1990, *San Francisco Examiner*.

† My testimony was transcribed and published by Alice M. Earl in her newsletter, *Peer Advocate*, in an undated "Special Edition" in early 1991. It can be obtained by writing to the newsletter at P.O. Box 60845, Longmeadow, Mass. 01116–0845.

the spasms of the body—would be suppressed by the muscle-paralyzing agent.

I suggested to Supervisor Alioto that she'd learn much more if she insisted on seeing the *conscious* patient after a full series of shocks, and I volunteered to return to San Francisco to help guide her evaluation of the patients' mental condition after ECT. I explained that I was sure she would find that shock produces severe brain dysfunction.

Supervisor Alioto accepted my offer, but I doubted if we would get the opportunity to interview any shock patients. (We didn't). Shock advocates typically find excuses for not allowing potential critics to witness the actual effects of their assault on the brain.*

At the hearing I announced what was for me a new position—one that shock survivors had been urging me to take for twenty years. Instead of merely encouraging informed consent—including the patient's right to know shock's damaging effects before agreeing to the treatment—I came out in favor of banning ECT. For reasons that will become apparent throughout this chapter, I urged Supervisor Alioto to cut off city funds to any hospital trying to shock its patients. I called shock treatment an "electrically-induced closed-head injury" and an "electrical lobotomy."

At the hearings and to the media I explained that if a woman received an accidental shock in her kitchen, perhaps from touching her forehead against a short-circuited refrigerator, and fell to the floor convulsing, she'd be rushed to the local ER and treated as an acute medical emergency. If she awoke the way a shock patient does—dazed, confused, disoriented, and suffering from a headache, stiff neck, and nausea—she'd be hospitalized for careful observation and probably put on anticonvulsants for months to prevent another convulsion.[3] But on a psychiatric ward she'd be told she was doing fine and "not to worry," while the electrical closed-head injury was inflicted again and again.

Capitalism Versus Communism?

While shock is enjoying a vigorous promotional campaign by American psychiatrists, Soviet psychiatry has been taking a much dimmer view. In

---

*Reporters frequently are invited by Max Fink, the best-known shock advocate, to witness patients being given the treatment. I have urged media representatives to ask Fink to allow them to see his patients *after* they have received a full course of shocks. Under pressure, Fink has agreed, but with a catch. While he charges nothing for the media to watch a patient undergo the procedure, he decided to charge $25,000 for himself and $15,000 for the patient—a total of $40,000—for a single interview with the patient awake after a course of treatment. So far no one has taken up the offer, even when it was reduced on one occasion to $30,000.

The Structure of Psychiatry in the Soviet Union (1985), by Soviet psychiatrist Edward Babayan, shock is twice compared to another "brutal method," lobotomy. Animal tests at the USSR Academy of Medical Sciences have shown brain damage with nerve cell death from electroshock treatment. The Russian psychiatrist boasts that his country has placed grave limitations on the use of shock, while "in the USA, for example, it is very widely used and has become all but a repressive measure applied even to healthy people."[4]

As we shall see, teams of American researchers performed comparable animal experiments years ago, with similar findings, and then organized psychiatry immediately covered them up.

Celebrating Shock

Although it dates back to 1938 in Italy[5] and came to the United States soon after, electroshock treatment remains a revered symbol of authority in modern psychiatry. By promoting shock the new psychiatry reveals its ties to the old psychiatry and unabashedly defends this egregious assault on the patient. Thus when shock reached its fiftieth birthday in 1988, it literally was "celebrated" in an orchestrated fashion at meetings throughout the world, including the annual conventions of the American Psychiatric Association, the Society of Biological Psychiatry, the Royal College of Psychiatrists, and the International Psychiatric Congress. As if honoring a dead hero, shock's fiftieth birthday also was "celebrated" in an issue of the journal *Convulsive Therapy*, and "observances" were held at various hospitals that especially favor shock, such as the Friends Hospital in Philadelphia, the Oregon Health Sciences University, and Taylor Manor in Maryland. The festivities are lovingly described by Max Fink in "Fifty Years of ECT" in the May 1988 *Psychiatric Times*.

Promoting Shock

In 1975 at the annual meeting of the American Psychiatric Association, half a dozen leading advocates of shock met to found a group for the promotion of the procedure, including Gary Aden, who described the moment in the *American Journal of Social Psychiatry*.[6] Aden called the circumstances both exhilarating and depressing: exhilarating because legislative restrictions on ECT had been overturned recently in a California court case brought by Aden; depressing because further attempts at restrictive legislation were anticipated. The apparent purpose of the organization was to mount a campaign against the widespread public outrage over the increasing use of shock treatment. At one time named the International Psychiatric Association for the Advancement of Electrotherapy, it later was renamed the Association for Convulsive Therapy. The idea of a PR organization for a treatment immediately should raise issues about the scientific case for the treatment.

Three of the six founders would be involved in serious scandals in the next several years. Gary C. Aden, the cofounder and first president of the new organization, would agree to the revocation of his California medical license after being accused by former patients of sexually abusing them in an extremely sadistic manner (see ahead). H. C. Tien, a Michigan psychiatrist who founded an earlier organization, the American Society for Electrotherapy, would draw media attention in the late 1970s and early 1980s after I publicized his use of shock to obliterate and reprogram the mind of a woman to make her a more suitable housewife (see ahead). Former NIMH director Shervert Frazier would lose his professorship at Harvard Medical School after it was discovered that he had plagiarized four papers he had published between 1966 and 1975.[7]

The journal *Convulsive Therapy* was founded in 1985 with similar political motivations. Editor-in-chief Max Fink, in the send-off editorial, noted that "convulsive therapy is often attacked as 'intrusive and brain damaging,' and governmental agencies in some jurisdictions have attempted to interdict its use." He laments that teachers are "called on, with increasing frequency, to defend its use."

In the editorial Fink does not mention that his own research spanning several decades frequently had compared electroshock to traumatic injury of the head and brain, and that he often had asserted that brain damage and dysfunction are the cause of the so-called improvement (see ahead).

The Economics of Shock

If science is not the motivation behind the celebration of shock, then what is? An exposé by Vince Bielski in the April 18, 1990, *San Francisco Bay Guardian* quotes a nurse at a general hospital who reported, "The ECT ward made its profit for the year in the first quarter." The total bill for a month's stay with shock treatment was approximately $20,000. Most of the cost usually is covered by health insurance. As psychiatrist David Viscott observes in *The Making of a Psychiatrist* (1972), "Finding that the patient has insurance seemed like the most common indication for giving shock" (p. 356).

In California individual treatments cost $1,000, with the psychiatrist who pushes the button often making between $200 and $300,[8] although some state and federal insurance coverage may limit the payments to nearer $100. We can easily calculate the annual income a psychiatrist can generate by shocking an average of only five patients a week at a typical charge of $200 per treatment. Since he will shock each patient three times a week, he will do fifteen shock treatments each week. At that rate he will earn $150,000 a year.

The time invested by the shock doctor will hardly impinge on the rest of his week. Since each treatment takes only a few minutes, the doctor easily can do five in a hour, so it will take him a mere three hours per week to earn his annual income of $150,000.

If the shock doctor also visits his patients on the ward, he can make much more money. Hospital consultations, sometimes lasting only a few minutes, will be covered by insurance at a higher rate than is psychotherapy in a private office. If the psychiatrist sees each of his five shock patients three times a week at $150 per consultation, he can generate an additional $112,500, for a grand total of $262,500 a year, without using up more than a few hours' time. Such enormous financial incentives can wholly cloud the doctor's perception of whether or not shock is good for the patient. It's *too good* for the doctor.[9]

Glen Peterson is the psychiatrist most actively involved in lobbying for increased shock treatment in California. He says he shocks 10 to 15 percent of his patients. That relatively small portion of his practice easily could add up to a substantial annual income.

Shock survivor Leonard Frank provided me with a deposition given by Peterson in a lawsuit involving another doctor.[10] Under oath Peterson admitted that he had given one woman a total of 130 to 140 shock treatments, spaced once every few weeks, and that he still was continuing her regimen, with no apparent intention of stopping. If charging $200 per shock, he has already earned up to $28,000 for treating this one woman, not counting his various consultations with her.

Peterson claimed that shock doctors were already overregulated in California and needed no further controls; but giving this many shocks is something I have rarely seen over twenty years. Nor have I seen it recommended or sanctioned in the literature of the past couple of decades. It had been done in the early days of shock in state mental hospitals, when it was used for subduing lifelong, rebellious inmates. Furthermore, the woman already had received numerous ECTs before her exposure to Peterson, and Peterson admitted to using the highest possible electrical dose in her treatment.[11] When I cited the number of shocks given to the woman, Peterson—who testified immediately after me at the hearing—made no response to what I said. Such a large number of shocks is documented to cause severe brain damage and dysfunction in animal and human studies.[12]

There are ways for ECT advocates to make money other than by shocking individual patients. One of the leading shock promoters in the United States is Richard Abrams. He is a professor of psychiatry at the Chicago Medical School, the author of multiple books and articles on shock, a member of journal editorial boards, and an organizer of the 1985 NIMH/NIH Consensus Conference on ECT. He also had input into the 1990 APA task force report on ECT. Abrams defends shock doctors when they are sued, and he has been instrumental in bringing about the new trend of shocking elderly women (see below). In his 1988 book *Electroconvulsive Therapy,* he states that "increased age does not of itself increase the risk of ECT" and declares that "some of the most rewarding results with convulsive therapy are obtained in elderly debilitated patients."

Abrams also has been active in promoting Somatics, Inc., a Chicago firm that makes a shock machine called Thymatron. For example, he is coauthor of their "Thymatron Instruction Manual" and the 1988 Thymatron brochure, "What You Need to Know About Electroconvulsive Therapy," which describes ECT as very harmless.

But Abrams has another credential that he *never* lists when promoting shock, Somatics, or Thymatron. He does not mention this particular credential when he writes brochures in support of Somatics and Thymatron. *Abrams is president of Somatics, and he is a member of its two-person board of directors.* In a recent deposition as an expert witness, Abrams admitted under questioning that he makes approximately 50 percent of his income from Somatics, Inc. * Every time Abrams promotes shock or Thymatron, he promotes his own shock-machine business. †

Abrams is a close associate of Max Fink, and the two are among the most influential men in bringing ECT back to life. Fink works with Somatics, which sells videotapes narrated by him. Entitled "Informed ECT for Patients and Families" and "Informed ECT for Health Professionals," they sell for $350 apiece.[13]

Who Gets Shocked

While preparing for the hearing in San Francisco I reviewed the data on the twenty-five hundred shock patients reported to the state each year in

---

* Deposition of Richard Abrams in John R. Detoma vs. Richard E. Brohamer, in the Circuit Court of the Seventeenth Judicial Circuit in and for Broward County, Florida, no. 86–20906 CT, January 16, 1991, p. 155.

† I am reminded of the public disillusionment when it was disclosed that Bing Crosby owned a financial interest in a company whose orange juice he was promoting on television. Abrams's duplicity, of course, has far more serious ethical ramifications. Crosby wasn't presenting himself as an unbiased scientist, he wasn't promoting orange juice as a scientifically proven health cure, and orange juice doesn't cause brain damage.

California. Since the data collection began over a decade ago, more than two-thirds have been women. Still more ominous, in recent times there has been an escalating percentage of elderly ECT patients. In 1977 only 28.7 percent of all patients were age sixty-five or older, but by 1983 it had leaped to 43.1 percent, and finally to 53.1 percent in 1988.[14] This means that *elderly women are among the most frequent victims of shock treatment in California.* The sexist and ageist implications of this national trend cannot be overlooked.

At the hearing I emphasized the vulnerability of older women, many of whom are alone, many living in relative isolation, and many barely making ends meet. I talked about the need to provide these individuals with psychosocial and economic support, with nutrition and medical care, and with friendship and love; but not with electrically induced closed-head injury. I also emphasized the vulnerability of these elderly women to being pushed or cajoled by their doctors into getting shock treatment. Frail, despairing, desperately needing emotional support, elderly women often have no one to defend them or to stand up for them, and they are unlikely to find the strength in themselves to defy their doctors. Sadly, those whose lives are least treasured in the society are those most likely to be afflicted with psychiatry's most destructive treatments. Concluding my testimony I compared the shocking of these patients to elder abuse in general, a theme that the press chose to pick up.

In defense of shocking the elderly, the psychiatrists at the hearing stated that antidepressants are often lethal in the elderly, requiring the alternative of ECT. The truth is that while antidepressants are especially dangerous to older people, so is electroshock. Reports are coming in that the elderly are far more sensitive to shock's damaging effects, including brain damage and dysfunction (see ahead). This is not surprising; the older brain is more fragile.

The national trend toward shocking the elderly, as well as the tunnel vision of biopsychiatrists, is exemplified in a November 1990 *Psychiatry Times* article entitled "ECT Safe and Effective Treatment for Elderly Psychiatric Patients." The report is especially important because psychiatrists can read it for continuing medical education (CME) credits.* The author, Donald Hay, discusses antidepressants and ECT, often recommending ECT as the *first* approach for depressed elderly patients. There is no mention whatsoever of any method of help other than drugs or shock for the depressed elderly. This illustrates the principle that your doctor's condition, rather than your own, determines whether or not you get drugged and shocked.

---

*CME credits are required for membership in national organizations, such as the APA, and for licensure in some states.

In pushing ECT for the elderly Hay makes no mention of the typical psychosocial and economic stresses that cause despair and hopelessness among the elderly. It's as if the elderly have no *reasons* for being dreadfully unhappy. He gives no hint that psychotherapeutic, social work, volunteer, family, or community interventions might help isolated, frightened, despairing, frequently unloved old people.

For the biopsychiatrist like Hay, the elderly live in a psychosocial and spiritual vacuum, needing drugs and shock to correct their presumably abnormal brain chemistry. Indeed, Hay recommends ECT for patients already suffering from *severe brain disease*—a certain formula for causing them even more extreme memory loss and mental dysfunction. He even wants to shock patients who are suffering from drug-induced akathisia, dystonia, parkinsonism, and tardive dyskinesia (see chapter 4), thereby compounding their doctor-induced neurologic disease with still more of the same. Although Hay doesn't discuss it, the ECT-induced brain dysfunction would certainly stop the patients from complaining about their iatrogenic neurological disorders.

Hay finds virtually no contraindications to imposing ECT on the elderly. He notes that the elderly may refuse to accept the treatment and thus recommends, where legally possible, doing it against their will. The effect is to give a carte blanche for shocking older people and immunity from legal recourse once the damage is done. Any psychiatrist can at least try to wave this article in court in self-defense, claiming "I acted according to accepted medical standards," without regard for the harm he or she has done.

The official report produced by the American Psychiatric Association, *The Practice of Electroconvulsive Therapy* (1990), strongly supports ECT for the elderly, citing a successful case involving a 102-year-old patient. Nonetheless, it acknowledges that the aged suffer "an increased likelihood of appreciable memory deficits and confusion during the course of treatment." The report also notes that it is harder to cause a convulsion in the elderly, *and therefore more electrical current must be used.*

Reports like Hay's and the 1990 whitewash published by APA (see ahead for further discussion) have reinforced my recent decision to support a ban against ECT. Clearly, psychiatry cannot be trusted to warn patients about the dangers of shock treatment, and once the treatment has taken effect, the patient is rendered unable to protest.

How Many Patients?

In my 1979 medical book *Electroshock: Its Brain-Disabling Effects*, I described the upswing of ECT and estimated that shock was being given to about 100,000 persons a year in the United States. This corresponded roughly with the APA estimate of over 88,000 per year in its 1978 *Task Force Report on Electroconvulsive Therapy* (see table 3 on p. 47), and now my estimate has been generally accepted. Even without an increase in the rate of shock treatment, a million or more people will be subjected to it in the coming decade.

The numbers of people shocked will escalate if the current promotional campaign continues to meet with so little scrutiny or opposition. Most unfortunately, these promotional efforts are being abetted by NAMI, the parent group that so avidly supports biopsychiatry. The summer 1990 issue of *The Journal* of the California Alliance for the Mentally Ill (CAMI), the largest state branch of NAMI, devotes several articles to supporting shock. The featured testimonial is not from a patient but from an "Anonymous Father." Indeed, ECT testimonials are almost always from someone other than the patient.

The Impact of Shock Treatment

Electroshock or electroconvulsive therapy involves the passage of an electrical current through the brain of the patient to produce a grand mal or major epileptic seizure. Sometimes the two electrodes are placed over both temples (bilateral shock) and sometimes over one side of the head (unilateral).

The shock induces an electrical storm that obliterates the normal electrical patterns of the brain, driving the recording needle on the EEG up and down in violent, jagged swings. This period of extreme bursts of electrical energy often is followed by a briefer period of absolutely no electrical activity, called the isoelectric phase. The brain waves become temporarily flat, exactly as in brain death, and it may be that cell death takes place during this time.

A shock-induced seizure is typically far more severe than those suffered during spontaneous epilepsy. In earlier times, when the shock patient's body was not paralyzed by pharmacological agents, it would undergo muscle spasms sufficiently violent at times to crack vertebrae and break limb bones.

The Acute Organic Brain Syndrome or Delirium

Typically the treatment is given three times a week for a total of at least six to ten sessions. After several sessions of shock, the patient awakens in a few (or sometimes many) minutes in a state of apathy and docility.

There will be some memory loss and some confusion and often a headache, stiff neck, and nausea. As the course of shocks progresses, the patient's apathy, memory loss, and confusion increase. Judgment and general mental function become impaired. Sometimes the patient becomes temporarily giddy or artificially high. This generalized mental and emotional dysfunction is called an acute organic brain syndrome or delirium—the brain's typical response to severe stress or damage. Less frequently, extreme states of delirium develop in which the patient appears grossly psychotic, with hallucinations and delusions.

Even exponents of shock treatment usually admit in their professional publications that many or all shock patients develop an acute organic brain syndrome. In his 1988 book *Electroconvulsive Therapy*, shock advocate Abrams says of all forms of shock treatment: "A patient recovering consciousness from ECT understandably exhibits multiform abnormalities of *all* aspects of thinking, feeling, and behaving, including disturbed memory, impaired comprehension, automatic movements, a dazed facial expression, and motor restlessness" (pp. 130–31).

In *Multiple-Monitored Electroconvulsive Therapy* (1981), Barry Maletzky points out that it "usually" takes two to four weeks for the EEG to return to normal after ECT; "However, some abnormalities may persist several months or longer and are considered to be poor prognostic signs" (p. 136). Some studies show that many patients never recover normal EEGs following shock treatment.[15]

There's No Question About Brain Dysfunction

Because shock treatment routinely causes an acute organic brain syndrome or delirium, the question is not whether shock can cause brain dysfunction. *Shock treatment always causes severe brain dysfunction.* The only legitimate question is, "How often is recovery complete?"

From what we know of head injury, we expect a high percentage of chronic impairments following other types of trauma much less severe than that incurred during ECT. In *Neurology: Problems in Primary Care* (1987), James Bernat and Frederick Vincent point out that "many patients following minor head trauma complain of difficulty with concentration, memory loss, dizziness, and headache" (p. 573). While some may be reacting psychologically, "as many as 50% of such patients studied with neuropsychiatric testing have demonstrated organic cognitive deficits."*

---

*These patients have "minor head injury," typically without loss of consciousness, seizures, disorientation, or confusion. This is a much less traumatic state than that of post-ECT patients.

It is recognized in neurology that even mild head injury frequently results in lasting, debilitating problems, such as memory difficulties, deficiencies in focusing and maintaining concentration, and loss of problem-solving skills. Frequently the person feels "changed" in a fundamental and catastrophic fashion. Often there is a frontal-lobe syndrome with loss of interest or emotional intensity, difficulties with abstract reasoning and planning, and so on. These responses to head injury are described vividly by Paul Chance in "Life After Head Injury," in the October 1986 *Psychology Today*.[16]

In their books, articles, and public statements, shock supporters, including the American Psychiatric Association, often ignore the vast literature on the damaging effects of even minor head injury. An exception (see ahead) is advocate Max Fink, who believes that shock treatment works by causing the typical aftermath of closed-head injury.

Evidence for Permanent Brain Damage

Brain damage from shock is amply demonstrated by animal research. Research conducted on dogs, cats, and monkeys in the 1940s and 1950s was so convincing that the search for further evidence came to a halt. Nonetheless, leading shock advocates, like Lothar Kalinowsky, claimed in their reviews that the animal research showed no damage. To the dismay of those of us who independently read the original investigations, most animal studies turned out to provide unequivocal proof of brain damage.[17] For example, in 1952 Hans Hartelius published a book-length report, "Cerebral Changes Following Electrically Induced Convulsions," as a supplement to *Acta Psychiatrica Neurologica Scandinavica* (vol. 77). He found scattered cell death and small hemorrhages in the brains of cats following relatively small doses of shock. Almost without exception, merely by examining their brains microscopically, he was able to predict which animals had been shocked.

Having first claimed that the early animal studies were negative, shock doctors instead now claim that these studies are too old or too flawed to count. If the studies showing brain damage were indeed outdated, it would be up to the shock doctors to stop using such a patently dangerous treatment while awaiting new studies with large animals, like dogs or monkeys. However, the older studies are not outdated, since they used less current than that applied to humans in modern ECT.

There is no reason to believe that modern shock is safer. The electrical stimulation must, in fact, be stronger nowadays, since the patients are sedated, and sedation makes it more difficult to convulse the patients. Cell death and widespread small, and sometimes large, hemorrhages are confirmed by human autopsy studies. Other evidence for persistent brain-damage is found on EEG studies, neuropsychological testing, some brain-scan studies, and many clinical reports.[18]

The damage is caused by several factors that have been studied by direct examination of animal brains subjected to very small electrical stimulation: first, mechanical and heat trauma from the electric current; second, spasm and breakdown of blood vessel walls as the electricity travels down the vascular tree; and third, to a much lesser extent, the convulsions.[19]

Nowadays shock doctors are very sensitive to public and professional opinion, and therefore they maintain that the treatment is relatively harmless and that its method of action is unknown. But in the first couple of decades of use, many shock authorities boldly declared that the treatment works precisely by damaging the brain and that brain-cell death is the key to successful treatment.[20]

In April 1946 psychiatrist P. H. Wilcox complained in *Diseases of the Nervous System* that "there is a prevailing assumption that therapy of certain types of mental diseases must or can be accomplished only by destroying brain cells . . ." and that "this belief has become sufficiently current so that it is not unusual to hear prominent psychiatrists and neurologists express the opinion that improvement from any of the shock therapies in certain mental conditions must necessarily depend upon brain tissue destruction."

The Damage Is the "Cure"

To the extent that it works at all, shock has its impact by disabling the brain.[21] It does so by causing an organic brain syndrome, with memory loss, confusion, and disorientation, and by producing lobotomy effects. For a few days or weeks the patient may be euphoric or high as a result of the brain damage, and this may be experienced as "feeling better." In the long run the patient becomes more apathetic and "makes fewer complaints."

Max Fink acknowledges that denial and euphoria are directly correlated to the degree of brain damage* as it is demonstrated by *abnormal* brain wave patterns and other signs of dysfunction; brain dysfunction is not, in Fink's own words, a "complication" or "side effect" but the "*sine qua non* of the mode of action." Clearly describing a patient with an organic

---

*In some later papers and books the phrase *brain damage* is discarded and the euphemism *altered state of brain function* is used instead; but the import of what is said remains the same.

brain syndrome following shock treatment, Fink declares that when a patient becomes "jovial and euphoric, denies his problems and sees his previous thoughts of suicide as 'silly,' a rating of 'much improved' is made." Fink declares that the basis of improvement is "similar to that of craniocerebral trauma" or head injury.[22] Finally, in the January/February 1978 issue of *Comprehensive Psychiatry*, Fink makes a statement that could have been attributed to those of us who oppose shock: "The principal complications of EST are death, brain damage, memory impairment, and spontaneous seizures. These complications are similar to those seen after head trauma, with which EST has been compared."[23]

Fink's viewpoint is consistent with my own—that shock produces brain damage and dysfunction with denial and anosognosia.[24] This enables both the doctor and the patient to make believe that the patient has neither brain dysfunction nor personal problems.

That shock works by damaging the brain and by making patients more simpleminded, less self-aware, and docile is such an obnoxious idea to most people that the theory is never presented to the public or repeated in court, even by its main proponent, Max Fink. In public Fink states that shock's mode of action is unknown and that it may correct biochemical imbalances. When interviewed for a magazine article on shock treatment in 1989 Fink declared, "I can't prove there's no brain damage. I can't prove there are no other sentient beings in the universe, either. But scientists have been trying for thirty years to find both, and so far they haven't come up with a thing."[25]

ECT and Women

Survivors of ECT, their friends, and their families consistently report serious memory difficulties following ECT. And, as we shall see, some doctors actually use ECT purposely to erase memories.

In a startling report in a 1988 issue of *Research in the Sociology of Health Care* (7:283–300), Carol Warren studied ten women, including their family relationships, following shock treatment. Many of the patients thought that the erasure of memory was the actual intent or purpose of shock treatment. As one woman put it, "I can't remember a lot of things—but I'd rather not." Another woman, who felt rejected by her father, said, "I want to forget." Other patients resented losing their memory for what had happened in their lives to cause their problems. One woman felt the shock was given to her specifically to make her forget her resentment toward her husband for having committed her.

While the women were divided on the benefit of forgetting their problems, they "uniformly disliked the loss of everyday memory, as well as associated effects such as losing one's train of thought, incoherent speech or slowness of affect. What specifically was forgotten varied from matters of everyday routine to the existence of one or more of one's children. . . ."

The loss of everyday memory indicates ongoing memory dysfunction. Combined with "losing one's train of thought," "incoherence of thought," and "slowness of affect," we have convincing signs of dementia—chronic deterioration of the brain and mind. Such patients, when referred for neuropsychological testing, almost invariably will be diagnosed as suffering from dementia or a chronic organic brain syndrome. That the patients do not recognize the significance of their losses is again typical of serious brain damage and dysfunction. That Warren reports these symptoms without discussing their importance adds to their significance. Had she been on the lookout for signs of dementia, even more may have surfaced. The disclosure of several such cases in a small sample strengthens my concerns about ECT's severely damaging effects.

Forgetting the names or even the existence of other people was especially perplexing. One of the women never again felt that her child was her own. Warren comments on the irony that the same patient might be given shock to forget her memories and psychotherapy to recall them. Psychotherapy, of course, can do little to help recover memories lost through physical trauma and damage to the brain.

Some of Warren's most chilling observations concerned the viewpoint of husbands and other family members about the patient's memory loss. A husband said of the shock treatment, "They did a good job there," because his wife's long-term memory loss spanned the period of conflict with him when she was depressed. A patient who had been molested as a child by her mother's brother explained that her mother denied it and wanted her to have "the full treatment" to "make me forget all those things that happened."*

Three of the ten women lived in dread of ECT for years afterward; and therefore they refrained from expressing any angry feelings toward their husbands, for fear of being sent back to the hospital for involuntary shock treatment. One said, "Shock treatment is a helluva way to treat marital problems—the problems involved both of us." This confirms my impression that many shock survivors are too afraid to report their resentment of the treatment to anyone, and especially to the people they have reason to fear, such as their husbands—and their psychiatrists.

---

*ECT probably functions to suppress memories of and protests against physical and sexual abuse in many women. In *Women and Depression: Risk Factors and Treatment Issues* (1990), by the American Psychological Association National Task Force on Women and Depression, it is confirmed that a high percentage of depressed women suffer from past molestations (see chapter 14).

Making Peggy Into Belinda

Not all shock doctors deny ECT's damaging effects on memory. H. C. Tien from Michigan has utilized it to erase memory and personality. In one case he reprogrammed a woman into a more docile mate, reminiscent of the Stepford wives, from the movie of the same name in which the men in a community murdered women and used their bodies to make "ideal wives." Nor was Tien's work done in obscurity. It was reported in detail in the November 1 and November 15, 1972, issues of *Frontiers in Psychiatry*, a Roche Laboratories (a pharmaceutical company) free handout sent to all psychiatrists in the country.

Tien, a self-styled "family psychiatrist," purposely used the older methods of shock to "maximize memory loss—and for a very good reason," which was to eradicate the woman's identity or personality in order to reprogram it. Tien believes that the "memory loosening" and the "infantile" state produced by the electroshock make the patient amenable to drastic change. A relative helps reprogram the patient's personality according to a "blueprint" worked out prior to the shock.

Verbatim dialogues with Tien and a married couple dramatize how the wife believes, before her shock treatment, that she wants to leave her husband. She doesn't love him, he is never home, and he beats her in front of the children. Under threat that her husband would try to get custody of the children in a divorce, the wife, Peggy, agrees to undergo the treatment. After each ECT Peggy regresses to a childlike state and is "reprogrammed" by her bottle-feeding husband to believe that her past personality was bad and that her new one is "good." She assumes a new first name, Belinda, to signify the change.

Incidentally, Tien tells us, she became "paranoid" during the first treatment, accusing those around her of harming her; but then she submitted to a second series of shock. Afterward: "Belinda is more balanced, more mature and adaptable in social situations than Peggy was. Now, as Belinda, her marriage is reasonably stable."

Tien calls his method ELT, explaining that E is for electricity, L is for love, and T is for therapy.

Except for my own 1979 book, I am unaware of criticism of Tien and his technique from the psychiatric profession.

With a Little Help from the CIA

Tien isn't the only psychiatrist to use shock to eradicate memories and even identities, usually those of women. In his book *The History of Shock Treatment* (1978) shock survivor Leonard Frank made probably the first public disclosure of the work of D. Ewen Cameron of Canada, who assaulted patients with massive drug doses, bizarre forms of conditioning, and what he called depatterning treatment. Cameron was professor of psychiatry at McGill University and the Allen Memorial Institute in Montreal. As president of the American Psychiatric Association (1953) and as the first president of the World Psychiatric Association, Cameron was one of the most revered and rewarded psychiatrists on the international scene.

Cameron subjected patients to twice-daily doses of six electroshocks, one after another, to maintain the individual in one prolonged stupor. Typically thirty to forty or more shocks were given in this blockbuster manner during his experiments on more than fifty patients in the late 1950s and early 1960s.

The result of this devastating treatment was a severe delirium; patients would lose their sense of identity and sometimes become delusional. Robbed of virtually all memory, the patients became completely focused on present sensations and feelings. With much or even all of their lifetime memory bank obliterated, six months would be taken to reprogram them with new memories of themselves and a more docile personality.

Around the time of Frank's disclosures about Cameron's treatments, Cameron's work suddenly became a major scandal. The outcry wasn't directed at the extreme treatments themselves, which were similar to numerous other regressive shock techniques, variations of which still are practiced in the United States (see below). What made Cameron suddenly newsworthy was the disclosure in newspaper reports and books that he had been secretly financed in part by CIA funds.

Eager to learn how to "brainwash" people and to wipe out their memories, the CIA found a willing ally in Cameron. Although Cameron was doing regressive shock on his own initiative as routine clinical practice, he accepted the CIA funds. His grisly, shameful methods, and their CIA funding, were documented in detail in John Marks's 1979 book *The Search for the 'Manchurian Candidate.'* In 1988, with Cameron deceased, some of his victims divided $750,000, individually receiving relatively small payments in a settlement from the CIA.[26]

I located one independent follow-up study of Cameron's shock treatments, by A. E. Schwartzman and P. Termansen in the April 1967 *Canadian Psychiatric Association Journal*, and directed Marks's researcher to it. It discloses severe chronic memory problems persisting many years after treatment. In their sample, 63 percent of patients still felt dependent on others for recalling aspects of their past. Sixty percent reported losses of memories spanning six months to ten years prior to the treatment. Except for the typical denial of symptoms that occurs with severe brain damage, undoubtedly many more would have reported serious lasting effects. In addition, 75 percent were found to suffer from "unsatisfactory or impoverished social adjustment."

Ironically, it is Cameron himself who waxed as eloquent as anyone in describing how important memory is. In the May 1963 *British Journal of Psychiatry* in wrote:

Intelligence may be the pride—the towering distinction of man; emotion gives color and force to his actions; but memory is the bastion of his being. Without memory, there is no personal identity, there is no continuity to the days of his life. Memory provides the raw material for designs both small and great. Thus, governed and enriched by memory, all the enterprises of man go forward.

One of Cameron's patients, the wife of a Canadian politician, permanently lost all of her sense of self—memories and personality—for her entire life prior to the treatment.

Long before the scandal and lawsuits surrounding CIA sponsorship, Cameron wrote in graphic detail about his own work in major peer review journals, including the *Canadian Medical Association Journal* (January, 15, 1958) and *Comprehensive Psychiatry* (February 1960 and April 1962). And, as we have seen, a follow-up was published in 1967 describing the fate of his victims. Cameron's extravagances were not the product of CIA financing or influence. Cameron already was carrying out his shock tortures before the CIA became interested. He would have carried on his work with or without the CIA, which never gave him more than $20,000 per year. Posthumously he would have remained one of the most renowned leaders in the history of psychiatry, except for the disclosure of his CIA connections. The irony is that the adverse publicity focused mostly on the CIA funding rather than on the most scandalous fact of all—that Cameron and his brutalities, although well known throughout the profession, were never criticized by mainstream psychiatry.

Nor was Cameron alone in inflicting sufficient amounts of shock to reduce patients to helpless, dilapidated, and demented human beings. In 1957 in the *Psychiatric Quarterly*, an official journal of the New York State Department of Mental Health, Glueck and his colleagues at Stoney Lodge, a private hospital in Ossining, New York, described giving shock until the patient became demented, unable to talk, lapsed into "utter apathy," and "behaves like a helpless infant, is incontinent of both bowel and bladder functions, requires spoon feeding and at times, tube feeding." It required a total of seventeen to sixty-four closely spaced treatments. Stoney Lodge continued these treatments at least until the 1970s, when I began to publicize them.

In *Multiple-Monitored Electroconvulsive Therapy* (1981) psychiatrist

203

Barry Maletzky advocates and utilizes a contemporary version of intensive ECT called MMECT (multiple-monitored ECT). Patients are kept unconscious and almost continuously in a state of convulsion by several shocks in a row in each treatment session. As many as five seizures are induced in a period of up to fifty minutes of sustained convulsion. Several sessions are administered. According to the 1990 APA task force on ECT, a "substantial minority" of practitioners use the method.

The field of medicine is well acquainted with the effects of multiple, continuous seizures on the brain, whether these seizures are spontaneous, as in some forms of epilepsy, or caused by injury to the brain. A patient who suffers several convulsions in a row without regaining consciousness is defined as being in status epilepticus, which is recognized in neurology and medicine as a severe medical emergency requiring immediate intervention before it produces permanent brain damage.[27]

Further Evidence of Memory Loss and Memory Dysfunction

There is no way to get access to large numbers of shock patients for controlled studies except through the shock doctors themselves, and so meaningful scientific studies are few and far between. However, in the 1940s and 1950s I. L. Janis, a Yale psychologist, using controls, studied the effects of routine shock treatment on the recollection of personal memories. He found considerable losses at several weeks and then at a follow-up one year later.*

More recently, several shock doctors have found that a large percentage of ECT patients report significant memory blanks and continuing memory dysfunction years after shock treatment.[28] In a study by Larry Squire and Pamela Slater in the *British Journal of Psychiatry* in 1983 (pp. 1–8), patients questioned seven months after shock treatment reported memory loss spanning, on the average, a block of twenty-seven months surrounding the treatment. In another survey of routine shock patients in Scotland, by C. P. L. Freeman and R. E. Kendell in the *Annals of the New York Academy of Sciences* (vol. 462, 1986), patients returned to the hospital to be questioned face-to-face by the doctor who gave them the treatment. As Freeman and Kendell admit, patients might feel intimidated about criticizing shock under such conditions. Nonetheless, 74 percent men-

---

*See I. L. Janis, "Psychological Effects of Electric Convulsive Treatments," *Journal of Nervous and Mental Diseases* (May 1950), and a more complete review of his publications in P. Breggin, *Electroshock: Its Brain-Disabling Effects* (1979).

tioned "memory impairment" as a problem following shock treatment and "a striking 30 percent felt that their memory had been permanently affected."

In the same 1986 *Annals of the New York Academy of Sciences*, a team led by psychiatrist Richard Weiner of Duke University attempted to test for loss of personal subjective recollections of past experiences, because they are "most consistent with the nature of memory complaints by ECT patients themselves." Their memory inventory spanned several years prior to the shock and the testing. This was perhaps the first such study carried out in the several decades since those of Janis. Despite a strong bias toward shock treatment, the group found "objective personal memory losses." These lasted the duration of the study—six months—after bilateral ECT.

Older ECT Patients

Because of the growing tendency to shock older people, it is important to understand their greater vulnerability to ECT-induced brain damage and dysfunction. Ongoing memory function is the subject of a study entitled "Cognitive Functioning in Depressed Geriatric Patients with a History of ECT," by Helen Pettinati and Kathryn Bonner, in the January 1984 *American Journal of Psychiatry*.[29] Among the older patients, performance was decreased on a test specifically aimed at disclosing "organic brain dysfunction" or "confusion." Short-term memory was impaired in both the older and the younger groups. As expected, age plus shock treatment produced the most deficits—a grave warning to those who are promoting shock treatment as ideal for the elderly.

In "The Safety of ECT in Geriatric Psychiatry," by William Burke and his associates, in the June 1987 issue of the *Journal of the American Geriatrics Society*, it was found that ECT complications increase with age. Six of eight patients over seventy-five years of age had "some untoward event." The "common complications" included "confusion, falls, and cardiorespiratory problems."[30]

Gary Figiel and his colleagues, in "Brain Magnetic Resonance Imaging Findings in ECT-Induced Delirium," in the winter 1990 issue of the *Journal of Neuropsychiatry*, found that 11 percent of elderly patients developed an especially severe reaction characterized as delirium. They note concerns that elderly patients "may be at relatively high risk for developing encephalopathic side effects from the treatment."*

---

*"Encephalopathic" refers to degenerative disease of the brain.

The American Psychiatric Association's 1990 Task Force

The APA's 1990 task force report, *The Practice of Electroconvulsive Therapy*, discusses and dismisses brain damage and memory loss from ECT —but without mentioning the relevant literature cited in the text and endnotes of this book, and in much greater detail in my 1979 textbook. For example, it does not refer to Hans Hartelius's definitive investigation of brain damage in cats or, for that matter, any of several other such animal studies by well-known American groups. Nor does it mention Janis's classic research on memory loss or Larry Squire and Pamela Slater's more recent research, although both are very well known in the field. Helen Pettinati and Kathryn Bonner's report on shock treatment of the elderly goes unmentioned. My publications, and those of John Friedberg and others, are not mentioned. Indeed, almost every article pertinent to memory dysfunction and brain damage is omitted from this latest APA report, including several that previously appeared in the two most widely used textbooks written by the advocates themselves.[31] Even the APA's own previous task force report on *Electroconvulsive Therapy* (1978) contains more information on memory loss. In psychiatry, "science" often goes backward!

The one negative study cited in the APA report is irresponsibly misrepresented. The task force declares that C. P. L. Freeman and R. E. Kendell found that "a small minority of patients, however, report persistent deficits" in memory. Freeman and Kendell, as already described, found that 74 percent of patients reported memory impairment and that a "striking 30%" said that their memory function was permanently impaired.

One must conclude that the APA report carefully paints an unblemished portrait of ECT in order to promote the treatment and to protect psychiatrists against malpractice suits. Thus the report was introduced at a press conference for the general media in late 1989 while still in the form of an unpublished manuscript.*

Evidence for Efficacy

A thorough review of the shock literature shows that there are no controlled studies indicating any "beneficial" effect beyond four weeks. Most show little or no improvement at all. The point was proven at the 1985

---

*By holding a press conference based on the unpublished version of the report, they gained national news coverage without fear of rebuttal from critics of the treatment, who had been refused access to the manuscript.

Consensus Conference on Electroconvulsive Therapy held by NIMH and NIH, at which psychologist and attorney Edward Opton, Jr., presented his review.* When none of the assembled shock doctors could provide any contradictory evidence, his conclusions were accepted in the Consensus Conference panel report, "Electroconvulsive Therapy," published in the October 18, 1985, *Journal of the American Medical Association*.

The four-week limit to treatment effectiveness is critical in two ways. First, it tends to confirm the brain-disabling hypothesis. Four weeks is the approximate period of time during which the patient's brain dysfunction, with associated euphoria or apathy, is most severe. Second, only four weeks of "relief" is very short considering the grave risks involved.

At the November 27, 1990, hearings in San Francisco, psychiatric survivor Wade Hudson reviewed the literature on electroshock, again focusing on controlled studies in which shock is compared to placebo in the form of simulated or "sham shock"—a mock shock procedure without the delivery of the electric current. The most recent relevant publication was by Timothy Crow and Eve Johnstone, "Controlled Trials of Electroconvulsive Therapy," in the 1986 New York Academy of Sciences proceedings, entitled *Electroconvulsive Therapy: Clinical and Basic Research Issues*. Crow and Johnstone confirm the power of placebo: simulated ECT resulted in "substantial improvements." They found only a slight and inconsistent tendency for ECT patients to perform better on a few test protocols for depression, and that was limited to the first month. They conclude, "Whether electrically induced convulsions exert therapeutic effects in certain types of depression . . . has yet to be clearly established."† After more than fifty years there is still no meaningful evidence that this dangerous treatment has any beneficial effect.[32]

Shock as a "Lifesaving" Treatment

As drastic as it is, does shock have some merit as a lifesaving treatment for suicidal people? Shock doctors frequently make that claim. But when confronted at the Consensus Conference they could cite only one paper in support of their thesis: David Avery and George Winokur's "Mortality in Depressed Patients Treated with Electroconvulsive Therapy and An-

---

*Opton's report was excluded from publication in the proceedings of the NIMH Consensus Conference. NIMH promotes all biopsychiatric treatments, including ECT.
†This is a most remarkable conclusion from the heart of the establishment, and it, too, was omitted from the APA task force report.

tidepressants" in the September 1976 *Archives of General Psychiatry*. One of them even read the abstract of the paper to the audience in a manner too rushed to be comprehensible. This was not the first time I'd seen the specter of this paper raised, and so I pulled it from my files at lunchtime and distributed copies at the conference. What the paper actually says is the opposite of what the shock advocates claim: "In the present study, treatment was not shown to affect the suicide rate" (p. 1033).[33]

Despite the ease of studying suicide—one must merely follow up the patients and count the suicides—there is no published evidence whatsoever that electroshock helps. Instead, some clinicians, including neurologist John Friedberg and myself, are familiar with people who have killed themselves in despair over their brain damage from shock treatment, and we know many others who suffer lifelong despair. Happily, I also know a number of survivors who have recognized the damage but triumphed over it to lead full, rich lives—often as activists against psychiatric abuse.*

The Safety of the "New" Shock Treatment

The most highly publicized alleged improvement is called modified ECT. It involves sedation, muscle paralysis, and artificial respiration. Despite the PR, this method is not new at all: I administered it more than twenty-five years ago in the early 1960s during my training at Harvard.[34] Furthermore, modified shock, of necessity, is *more* dangerous. First, the hazards of general anesthesia and muscle-paralyzing agents are added to those of the shock. Second, the intensity of current must be greater to overcome the anticonvulsant effect of the short-acting sedative that is injected immediately prior to the shock. In addition, patients in modern psychiatric hospitals frequently receive other medications, such as sedatives and minor tranquilizers, which further raise the seizure threshold. Furthermore, patients too often receive neuroleptics, antidepressants, and especially lithium, all of which can worsen the impact of shock.

Modified ECT wasn't introduced to reduce brain damage, since the shock doctors used to believe that the damage was therapeutic. The purpose of the modifications was to prevent fractures from muscle spasms.

---

*Shock advocates frequently suggest that the eloquence of survivors like Leonard Frank is evidence that shock is not permanently damaging. I have known Leonard, and several other eloquent survivors, for almost twenty years, and I can vouch for the struggles they have undergone to recover as much as possible from the damage. These individuals are living proof of the capacity of the human being to triumph over brain damage and dysfunction. It seems cruel and self-serving for shock promoters to deny both their suffering and their heroic efforts to live life to the fullest despite their iatrogenic handicaps.

The claim that modified ECT reduces brain damage is a very recent public relations twist and has no validity whatsoever.

Another alleged improvement involves the use of differing types of electrical stimulation. But the relative safety of these innovations is controversial, and most of them have been around for decades. Besides, a great deal of shock is done at the same or higher energy levels used in the 1940s. The electrical current must in any case be sufficiently disruptive to produce a convulsion. Sometimes, if the patient is slow to "improve," an older machine will be brought in or the shock doctor will flip off the switch that protects the patient from especially high current intensities. While they won't admit it, many shock doctors act on the old axiom that the brain damage does the trick.

Sacrificing the Right Brain

Another supposedly less harmful innovation is the placement of the two electrodes over the same side of the head—unilateral electroshock treatment. It is applied to the so-called nondominant or nonverbal side of the brain to focus the energy away from the verbal centers. In right-handed people the nonverbal side is usually, but not always, on the right. For a variety of technical reasons, this form of shock is potentially more dangerous than traditional bilateral shock.[35]

Why do shock advocates promote unilateral, nondominant shock? It's relatively easier for doctors to overlook harm done to the nonverbal side, because the patient can't speak about it. However, to people who use visual skills—such as homemakers, scientists, engineers, photographers, or artists—damage to the nondominant side may be more functionally devastating than damage to the more verbal side, even if the patient cannot communicate about it.[36]

The nonverbal side of the brain is involved in myriad subtle functions that are critical to a full, effective, happy life. Thomas Blakeslee describes these nondominant brain functions in his very readable book *The Right Brain: A New Understanding of the Unconscious Mind and Its Creative Powers* (1983). They include the creative faculties, such as imagination and the use of metaphor; visual and spatial capacities, as well as musical and motor abilities, such as coordination, dance, and athletics; the quality or vibrancy of personality; initiative and autonomy; and insight.

It's ironic that modern psychology currently is placing so much emphasis on the importance of developing right brain function at the very moment that shock doctors are trying to tell us that we can more easily afford to sacrifice right brain function to repeated jolts of electricity. Notice also that the functions of the nondominant side mirror those of the frontal lobes—for example, initiative, autonomy, and insight—so that nondominant shock is potentially more lobotomylike than regular shock.

The FDA, the APA, and ECT

Organized psychiatry realizes that shock cannot withstand scrutiny. In 1979 the FDA put shock machines into Class III, which means demonstrating "an unreasonable risk of illness or injury." Class III is the most restrictive category for medical devices and would have required manufacturers to provide premarketing data on safety and effectiveness.[37] This probably would have necessitated renewed animal testing.

Led by the American Psychiatric Association, psychiatry lobbied to have that decision reversed, and it succeeded. The FDA gave notice of its intention to reclassify shock machines into Class II, approving them as safe and efficacious and requiring no testing. It was a clear-cut illustration of psychiatry's lobbying strength at FDA.

A group of several hundred outraged shock survivors, organized by Marilyn Rice, began pressuring the FDA to maintain its earlier classification of the machines as dangerous and in need of testing. Most of the mail received by the FDA came from shock survivors testifying to the damage done to them.[38] The APA responded with its 1990 report claiming that the treatment is virtually harmless.

In September 1990 the FDA proposed a compromise that has satisfied neither side.[39] It would classify the machines as safe (Class II) for depression, but not for other disorders. The ruling permits shock machines to be used with impunity as long as the patient is diagnosed as very depressed. This will provide little protection to patients, since manipulating diagnoses to fit the treatment is commonplace in psychiatry. But it might open the way to more frequent malpractice suits against shock doctors when and if it can be shown that the patient failed to meet the proper diagnostic standard.

The FDA-ECT story illustrates how psychiatry places self-interest above both scientific inquiry and the well-being of its patients, as it stifled an examination of its treatment and rejected the outcry from the survivors. The story also confirms that the FDA has a greater commitment to placating psychiatry than to monitoring it (see chapter 15).

What Many Psychiatrists Believe About Shock

Meanwhile, a large percentage of psychiatrists privately believe that the treatment is brain-damaging. How do we know? In a survey published in the earlier APA task force report on ECT (1978, p. 4), psychiatrists were asked, "Is it likely that ECT produces slight or subtle brain damage?" Forty-one percent voted yes and only 26 percent voted no.

Shock Doctors Strike Back

In her 1972 book *Beyond the Couch* psychiatrist Eileen Walkenstein asks, "Who will doctor their patient's brain cells, killed forever by these brain cell murderers?" As a resident in psychiatry she was required to give the treatment, but she "could not, *would not* push those buttons and damage and destroy an already tormented soul." What could she do? At the last minute she invented a research project as a substitute for her tour of duty on the shock ward, and thankfully, it was accepted. "My time on the shock wards was to be spent on my own project. . . . I would not have to electrocute a single person!"

Walkenstein was fortunate to escape giving shock without risking her career. In chapter 1, I mentioned the young psychiatrist who recently submitted to giving shock on threat of being fired from a university training program. In my own second year of residency, another young psychiatrist who refused to give shock was fired and his career ruined.

John Friedberg, who practices neurology in Berkeley, California, was the first physician to take an effective public stand against shock treatment, and he, too, paid the price. As a neurologist in training Friedberg wrote an article critical of shock treatment for *Psychology Today* (August 1975), and he was fired. It looked as if his medical career was destroyed, until he was invited to finish his training in Portland, Oregon, where Robert Grimm was director of neurological training at Good Samaritan Hospital. Grimm, who is both a clinician and a scientist, is one of the few neurologists to dare to make criticisms of both psychosurgery and shock.

Friedberg went on to write the book *Shock Treatment Is Not Good for Your Brain* (1976). At the time he thought he might never get another chance to do such a book, so he wanted the title to tell the whole story to people who might not have the time or inclination to read it.

In a recent personal interview, Friedberg shared with me his disillusionment with the profession when he reviewed the animal literature and discovered, contrary to the shock doctors' claims, that the key studies all showed brain damage. Yet his medical knowledge informed him it could be no other way; bypassing the brain's protective coverings with a jolt of electricity was bound to do damage. With eloquence he explains,

The brain was packaged by nature to be incredibly protected, much more so than any other organ in the whole system. It's got hair on the outside, skin, a little bit of fat, then the bone of the skull which is very thick. The only part of the human that's an exoskeleton is the skull to encase the brain. Then it's floating in spinal fluid as additional protection against injury, and it's encased in this very delicate Saran Wrap–like material. And then there's the tissue of the brain itself which is probably as vulnerable as any tissue in the whole body. It has to be very gently treated. No wonder the pathologists concluded that electroshock consistently caused some brain damage.

Why Would They Do It?

The economic and political motives behind shock have been discussed; but is there something more personal motivating these doctors?

More than three decades ago two well-known psychiatrists, David Abse and John Ewing, published a study of the motives of biopsychiatrists. Entitled "Transference and Countertransference in Somatic Therapies," it appeared in the January 1956 *Journal of Nervous and Mental Diseases.* Due to organized psychiatry's emphasis on maintaining its image, the article could never get published nowadays in a professional journal. Abse and Ewing's several-page analysis of "The Attitudes of Shock Therapists" draws a picture of men expressing thinly veiled hatred and violence toward their victims. Abse and Ewing find "unconscious guilt" in the doctors' facetious, inappropriate jests about shocking patients. Some of the typical quotes they cite from shock doctors are "Let's give him the works," "Hit him with all we've got," "Why don't we throw the book at him," "Why don't we put him on the assembly line," and "The patient was noisy and resistive so I put him on intensive EST three times a week."

Two shock-doctor comments struck me as especially revealing. In one case the psychiatrist told the husband of a patient that the treatment would help his wife by virtue of its effect as "a mental spanking." In another case a doctor decided, "She's too nice a patient for us to give her EST."

The authors conclude, "Clearly, the main attitudes expressed are those of hostility and punishment" in regard to giving electroshock. Frequent jests were seen as "the therapist's reaction against the sadistic implications of shock treatment."

Abse and Ewing also document the use of shock as a threat against difficult patients. Personnel on the hospital wards would warn, "You will go on the shock list." The authors found this generally limited to "junior attendants who are enjoying a new-found sense of power" and who desire an "unconscious participation in the 'omnipotence' of the shock therapist."

Most depressed patients feel very guilty and self-punishing, leading some to commit suicide. Abse and Ewing suggest that patients who feel improved by shock probably experience themselves as undergoing punishment for their sins. "It seems probable therefore that even the most organically [biologically] minded shock therapist unconsciously allies himself with the punitive super-ego of the depressed patient."

Shock was widely used by psychiatrists in Nazi Germany. Benno Muller-Hill, a German professor of genetics, provided me the opportunity to look into the souls of those doctors through a remarkable article—which he located and helped to translate—that explores the dreams of shock doctors. Here is one of their characteristic dreams of violence and fear of retaliation:

I was commander of German shock troops who were attacking the French Maginot Line. My soldiers and I were wearing shock machines on our backs instead of our army packs. The electrode was like a flame thrower which we merely had to point toward our enemies. We destroyed all life in front of us, including the plants. The most horrifying part of the dream was that the corpses of our enemies behind us were still moving in epileptic seizures and I had the horrible feeling that they would roll upon us and crush and choke us. The dead behind us were more disquieting than the still living enemies in front of us.[40]

We cannot, of course, read the minds of modern shock doctors, but we continue to get some frightening hints. Before Glen Peterson took over the task from him, the leading public advocate of shock in California was Gary Aden. As already described, Aden was a founder and the first president of the International Psychiatric Association for the Advancement of Electrotherapy (now the Association for Convulsive Therapy). Aden's promotion of shock is praised in Rael Jean Isaac and Virginia C. Armat's book *Madness in the Streets* (1990). What Isaac and Armat fail to mention about Aden can be found in a newspaper account dated September 27, 1989, in the *San Diego Union*: "Dr. Gary Carl Aden, 53, of La Jolla gave up his medical license effective September 8 after allegations that he had sex with patients, beat them and *branded two of the women with heated metal devices, including an iron that bore his initials*" (italics added).[41]

In another story a patient describes Aden as drugging her with a hypodermic before sexually abusing her and beating her with a riding crop.[42]

Aden was permitted to forfeit his license without admitting guilt. He was not subjected to being psychiatrically diagnosed or treated involuntarily, nor was he criminally charged.

When California limited the number of shock treatments that could be given to a patient in a single year, psychiatrists protested vociferously. Afraid that psychiatrists would try to get around the limitation on electrically induced convulsions by giving nonconvulsive shocks, the regulations of the Department of Mental Health further stipulated that even shocks that did not cause convulsions must be counted. The departmental director, psychiatrist Michael O'Connor, declared that this was necessary to prevent doctors from administering an unlimited number of treatments. Outraged that a psychiatrist would order such constraints on ECT, Isaac and Armat comment in *Madness in the Streets* that O'Connor's attitude "assumed that psychiatrists would pass electricity into people's bodies merely to satisfy their sadistic impulses."*

The Survivors Fight Back

With the profession managing to control and even purge itself of critics and criticism, the main resistance to shock has come from those who have been damaged by it. Some have chained themselves to the gates or entrance doors of hospitals reputed to be shock mills. Leonard Frank also has debated shock doctors at their meetings and has written *The History of Shock Treatment* (1978) as well as the recently published comprehensive critique of ECT, "Electroshock: Death, Brain Damage, Memory Loss, and Brainwashing."[43] He was a founder of the national patients' rights movement and remains a heartening example to hundreds of survivors. Other survivors endure the stress of going on radio and television and of picketing the annual meetings of the American Psychiatric Association. Some have written about undergoing shock, like Janet Gotkin, with her husband Paul, in *Too Much Anger, Too Many Tears: A Personal Triumph Over Psychiatry* (1975). Marilyn Rice has become a watchdog of the FDA when it fails to perform its watchdog duties.

Most dramatically, one man—who was electroshocked at the age of six—managed for a few brief days to halt the use of shock in one of America's cities. Ted Chabasinski was a shy child genius growing up in a poor and dysfunctional family when a social worker removed him from his home and placed him in the psychiatric system. Soon he was subjected to shock treatment at the hands of one of the most famous child psychiatrists of all time, Loretta Bender.

Young Chabasinski was so confused and terrorized by the treatment that he inadvertently helped to maintain his long odyssey within the state

---

* According to Isaac and Armat, the APA and many psychiatrists protested that limiting the number of shocks a doctor could apply to a patient in a year "would lead to psychiatrists using higher levels of electricity (thereby causing more memory loss)" (p. 392).

mental hospital system. When the doctors asked the little boy "Do you hear voices?" he would dutifully reply yes, hoping to please his captors and to avoid further shock.

After being discharged from Rockland State in his teens it took Chabasinski several years to build a life for himself. In 1971, like so many other survivors, he joined the newly burgeoning ex-inmate movement in California and received enormous moral support from it. Eventually he went to law school and is now a practicing attorney and patients' rights advocate.

In 1982, before gaining his law degree, Chabasinski organized what eventually became the Berkeley ban, a citizens' movement aimed at stopping electroshock in Berkeley and specifically at Herrick Hospital, a general hospital with a psychiatric ward. An overwhelming victory was won at the polls as the people of Berkeley voted yes on a proposition to say no to shock. But within a few weeks the American Psychiatric Association had obtained a court order overturning the vote. Eventually the case was won by organized psychiatry, but for forty-one days in the winter of 1982 there was a "power outage" at Herrick.

As far as anyone knows, that was the only time anywhere in the world that shock treatment actually was banned. The following year Herrick Hospital shocked more people than ever before, and it is still going strong.

A few weeks ago, I had little positive with which to conclude this chapter. Shock treatment is on the rise, and elderly women are being targeted. The number of people subjected to shock is surpassing 100,000 per year in America, and it will keep on climbing unless the public takes an effective stand against it. But as I described earlier in the chapter, there has been a series of encouraging events in California. As a result of reports that three more hospitals were starting to give shock in the San Francisco area, there were protests, public hearings, and surprisingly favorable media coverage of efforts to stymie the shock doctors. Led by Supervisor Angela Alioto, the Board of Supervisors of San Francisco (the city's governing body) has passed a resolution declaring its opposition to the "use and financing" of ECT. It also urged the state legislature to strengthen the requirements for informed consent, including my suggestion that potential patients be exposed to audio or video tapes by professionals who view ECT critically. On February 20, 1991, Mayor Art Agnos signed the resolution. While this resolution will not stop ECT in San Francisco, it is very encouraging to those of us who oppose the treatment, and hopefully will lead to further governmental actions around the country.

Part III

"Anxiety" Overwhelm and the Minor Tranquilizers

Chapter 10

Understanding the Passion of Anxiety Overwhelm: Panic Attacks, Depersonalization, Phobias, Obsessions and Compulsions, Addictions, and Eating Disorders

People wish to be settled; only as far as they are unsettled is there any hope for them. . . . He has not learned the lesson of life who does not every day surmount a fear.
—*Ralph Waldo Emerson (1841)*

Bless your uneasiness as a sign that there is still life in you.
—*Dag Hammarskjold (1956)*

. . . anxiety has no more survival value than a tension headache. Its elimination would be a blessing.
—*Biopsychiatrist Donald W. Goodwin (1986)*

Rana Lee remembers the time she went to her doctor because her husband was beating her. The doctor, she told a congressional committee, "prescribed 10 milligrams of Valium three times a day to calm me down. . . . He refilled it for five years, with no questions asked."
—Washington Post Health, *January 3, 1989*

In its effort to open new markets, organized psychiatry has made anxiety its promotional campaign theme of the 1990s.* Estimates from "official sources," such as NIMH, have declared anxiety America's number-one

---

*The politics of anxiety will be discussed in chapters 11 and 15.

health problem, one that afflicts 8 percent of the population. Three million Americans are said to suffer from panic disorder or recurrent attacks of anxiety, while eleven million suffer from such variations as phobias, obsessions and compulsions, and chronic levels of apprehension and dread. The NIMH "educational" campaign defines anxiety as a medical condition and promotes drugs as the preferred treatment.[1]

Evolution of a "Panic Disorder"

Alice sought psychotherapy following her decision to leave her husband. A woman in her thirties with two young children and a small business that was marginally supporting her, she was vulnerable to all of the anxieties that go along with separation and divorce.

One afternoon, several weeks after beginning therapy, she experienced a sudden attack of "sickness" on the subway on the way to see her divorce lawyer. She got "chills like hot flashes" and at first thought "I'm going through early menopause." When she got off the train at the next stop, she immediately felt fine; but to her dismay, it began again the instant she got on the next train.

During her initial panic attack Alice felt intense anxiety, trembling, clamminess, and a sense of dread that "something absolutely horrible was going to happen." It felt, for a moment, as if somehow she might be annihilated. But in subsequent episodes she increasingly focused on one theme—her fear of vomiting in public. With humor, in retrospect, Alice describes how the terror distorted her sense of reality. She would look around the subway car and see nothing but "expensive camel hair coats—a sea of camel hair coats," all the potential targets of her nausea.

Within a short time her anxiety attacks began to erupt in many other public places, from department stores to church. She would buy only a few items at a time at the supermarket in order to rush through the express lane.

At the time in her life when her anxiety attacks began, Alice was feeling a great fear of being alone. "I'd feel different from everyone else. Everyone else looked content and prosperous like they were normal. My life was different—isolated and alone."

In therapy we immediately began to try to understand what was going on. We agreed it was important that the first episode started on her way to her attorney to discuss the most threatening aspect of her life, the conflict with her estranged husband. We talked about how difficult it is for women in general to stand up for themselves, and I encouraged her to look at the problem in a context of women's issues. She learned to handle anxiety by turning it into manageable fears, such as "I'm frightened of dealing with my husband, but I have a good plan and a good attorney to help me." She became more able to identify the fears underlying the apparently irrational anxieties and then to develop and to implement solutions to the problems. "Instead of losing your head when the anxiety begins," I suggested, "become as rational as you can and focus on the real problems."*

Because Alice felt so "different" from other people, we talked about how natural it is to experience any number of "symptoms" during a period of separation and divorce. I told her I'd never known a person who didn't feel as if he or she was coming apart during such times. I shared my own personal reactions to undergoing separation and divorce, and we laughed together at the seemingly irrational ways we humans respond to stress.

In retrospect Alice felt that it was especially important that I never treated her as if she had a mental illness. In contrast, when she told a close friend about her episodes of anxiety, the woman blurted out, "You're not becoming one of 'them'"? The "them" referred to people shown as examples of "panic disorder" on a TV report about the latest psychiatric theories of anxiety. The notion of having a psychiatric diagnosis was frightening; it made Alice think she was abnormal. She explained to me, "But you made me feel like a normal person going through a hard time. That meant a lot to me."

We talked about panic attacks as sending a message that life seems overwhelming, and we worked specifically on how to handle each of the stresses in her life by developing her business, locating emergency financial resources, developing a network to help with her children, and expanding her social life. We also talked about her vulnerability to anxiety from her childhood experiences.

Within a few months the panic attacks had subsided completely. Alice dates the turning point to the evening she met Warren, a man who immediately struck her as kind, gentle, and caring. "After my first night with Warren," she recalled, "I felt a million times better and the attacks started to ease up right away." Overcoming many fears, she also was learning to promote her business, and soon she was putting money in her savings account. "It was my change in circumstances that helped the most," she recently said. "Where the therapy helped was in showing me how to change my circumstances—how to take better care of myself, how to reach out to people, how to market myself and my services in business."

Therapy also helped give her the courage "never to quit doing things," no matter how frightened she got. I had told her that panic attacks are like wild beasts—if you give in to them the moment they start threatening you, they get more and more ferocious. Our talks together encouraged her to feel like a "member of the human race."

"If it happened to me again," Alice says, "I'd think about what I'd have to change—what I'd have to do for myself in my life. I don't think it's at

---

*While I felt that these methods of handling anxiety were critical to her improvement, Alice, as we'll see, believes that my help in bettering her overall life was far more important. Clients often differ from therapists in their analysis of what helps, and it's important for therapists to listen to what they are being told.

all a chemical thing. I don't think my chemistry changed that day on the subway train." In retrospect her panic attacks seemed like "the accumulation of a year of panic" generated by the separation and divorce.

Anxiety, Guilt, and Shame

How a person deals with anxiety can determine the course of his or her life. People who will "do anything" to avoid anxiety often become helpless avoiders of life. People who are willing to think and to act despite anxiety, people who face anxiety as something to be understood and conquered, are likely to overcome many of life's challenges. Since anxiety is a signal of overwhelm, it is not something to be gotten rid of, but something to be understood and then overcome through personal growth and change.

I conceive of the various negative, self-defeating emotions—guilt, shame, and anxiety—as stemming from childhood fear and helplessness. [2] In discussing so-called schizophrenia we found that shame focuses on our feelings of impotence, weakness, and worthlessness. When ashamed or humiliated we feel victimized by powers greater than ourselves. In comparison to others, we are made to feel like "nothing," like an "utter zero." We become very sensitive and vulnerable to any slight directed toward us. In discussing depression we found that guilt focuses on our feelings of being bad—our power to do harm and even evil to others. Feelings of blame are directed toward ourselves rather than toward others, and anger is directed inward rather than outward. We look within for any sign that we are evil. In anxiety we tend not to blame anyone or anything, and we have no place to direct our attention or our anger. Instead we collapse into a "know-nothing" helplessness, a pure overwhelm with no assigned cause for the problem. In other words, anxiety is an overwhelming emotional turmoil, unawareness, or confusion for which we can locate no cause. We cannot act at all, because we have no idea what is going on.

First and foremost, the anxious person must marshal every bit of will-power to regain rational control and to focus his or her attention on overcoming helplessness.

It's important never to let anxiety motivate our choices or control our actions. When anxiety dictates terms to us, our lives grow narrow indeed. We should attempt, instead, to dispel and defuse anxiety with an understanding of its origins, while guiding our lives with more reliable values, such as reason and love. In the case of mind-numbing anxiety, it's especially useful to focus attention on remaining rational and on identifying any real threats. The goal is to dispel the helpless confusion and know-nothingness and to replace it with conscious, working principles.

Melissa's Triumph Over Anxiety

Melissa at age twenty-five had an undergraduate degree in accounting and was working as an assistant bookkeeper, a job she found boring and without a future. She also had a boyfriend, an alcoholic who gave her little love and no security. Her true love was laboratory science, but the closest she came to it was looking longingly at a *Scientific American* or *Science News* in her spare time.

Melissa had told her first psychiatrist, "I'll be sitting at my desk in the library and all of a sudden I'm frightened to death. I've got to get up. I've got to get away from the whole building. But of course, I can't; I work there. Sometimes I'll try to hide in the record room for awhile. But it doesn't really matter what I do. I start breathing fast and I can't catch my breath. If I try to stand up, I'll see spots and start to faint."

She explained that the panic attacks could strike her anywhere, and so she'd begun to restrict her life. They had been going on for months, and her body was showing signs of chronic stress: headache, backache, numbness in her face from clenching her jaw, a frightening tightness in her chest, fatigue. She was having trouble falling asleep and staying asleep. She was losing too much weight. "Battle fatigue," she called it. "But I don't know what the hell I'm fighting." Melissa's psychiatrist told her that she had a physical problem—a hyperactive nervous system—and he prescribed Valium to "smooth out the nerves." But when Melissa got home she decided that drugs couldn't solve her problems, and she looked for another doctor.

After hearing Melissa's story, I suggested, "You're preoccupied with the symptoms. All you want to talk about is getting relief from them. And I can understand that, but it's not the answer. You're in such a state because you don't know how to control your mind or your life; you've got to learn to be in charge of yourself in a way that really works for you. We've got to stop talking about the symptoms long enough to talk about new approaches to your life." Melissa had no preparation for dealing with life's challenges. Her mother was helplessly preoccupied with physical problems and personal feelings of inadequacy. She worried herself "to death" over any risk Melissa took. Her father didn't envision women as potentially strong and able. As a child, when Melissa had asked for a chemistry set, he had laughed at her.

Caught between the strength of her true spirit and her dread of facing life's challenges, Melissa had begun to "come apart at the seams." She would end up in a state of helpless panic. It was as if her psychospiritual state had a fracture down the middle—a gaping disparity between how she wanted to live and how she was living. She learned to deal with this fissure in her personality by being emotionally stupid or confused about herself.

I reminded Melissa again and again that the goal was to learn to control her life more rationally.

"I can't even control my body anymore! And I feel like I'm losing my mind."

It's now several years later—and she hasn't had a panic attack or severe anxiety in a long time. I asked her if she'd mind telling me, in retrospect, what had helped her to overcome her panic attacks and chronic anxiety.

"I remember how frightened I used to be about making any choices, and I remember one day how you told me that very few choices in life are irrevocable. I learned that I could make a choice, try it out, and move in another direction if it didn't work out. It wasn't all life and death like my mother said. I could find my way step by step.

"I also learned to take control of myself, my body, my life. You kept reminding me to look for what was truly frightening me when I began to feel anxious. I learned to identify what was actually upsetting me, so I could deal with it. A woman doesn't have to be helpless, despite what my father always said."

Gradually Melissa learned to welcome thoughts that guided her toward successful actions and to reject thoughts that insisted she was helpless and dependent. She learned to relate to other people in the same way, rejecting some of her more helpless companions in favor of new people who lived successfully and would encourage her in the same direction. Especially she learned to spot signals from her parents that communicated fear and help-lessness to her. Again and again I emphasized that anxiety is a reaction of emotional stupidity in the face of inner stress. She had to insist to herself, over and over again, that she could make sense out of her feelings and then find the courage to make the next step in life.

"Oh, yeah," she added. "I had to get out of the victim role. I had to stop feeling that everything unfair on earth was being done to me, and instead that I could actually direct my life. That was why I was able to tell my boyfriend to leave. And why I was able to go back to school."

Melissa obtained an advanced degree in science and now works for a respected research institute.

An Ethical Journey

Life is an ethical journey in which we find our way by assuming as much responsibility for the conduct of our lives as possible. This is self-determination. When we lapse into psychological or learned helplessness and stop taking charge of our lives, we become the victims of our emotional reactions.

Refusing to be guided by guilt, shame, and anxiety is a major step toward making room within oneself for reason and love. Once a person refuses to empower self-destructive feelings, they tend to wither with time. But if we pamper them, it's like throwing steak to wild dogs; they grow in their demands and their boldness. In short, one goal of life is to supplant guilt, shame, and anxiety with rationally chosen ethics, reason, and love.

Looking at the childhood origins of painful emotions and reexperiencing their initial impact on us can help us transcend these emotions. Knowing how we were made to feel ashamed, guilty, or anxious in childhood helps us reject being guided by these emotions as adults. We learn to say to ourselves, "I'm not really feeling guilty or anxious over this immediate event; I'm reacting from those old sources in childhood" or "I don't have to panic right now; this is a terror from the past."

Seeing the childhood origins of guilt, shame, and anxiety discredits them as guidelines for mature living. Once we discover that these emotional reactions slammed us around at the age of five, they no longer seem appropriate in adult deliberations.

Life is complex and so are we, and we don't always experience guilt, shame, or anxiety in a pure form. Often they are mixed together and sometimes they can rear up in succession in a matter of moments. The common element in each will be the feelings of fear and helplessness, frequently of childhood origin. The common goal is not to cave in to the emotion and instead to take charge of oneself.

In *Managing Your Anxiety* (1985) Christopher McCullough and Robert Woods Mann invoke the ethics of freedom and responsibility in overcoming helplessness. Self-defeating fears, such as phobias, "are a natural consequence of being afraid of our own freedom to exist as a unique being or separate person." People who are chronically anxious often *seem* to be highly responsible, even to a fault. They may, for example, worry a lot about whether or not they are "doing right." But they need to be more honest with themselves and more self-directing. According to McCullough and Mann, "If we are a truly responsible person, we see clearly that we are accountable only for *the foreseeable results of our own choices and actions*—and not for what other people feel, think, or do." In other words, autonomy and self-determination are key in overcoming anxiety.

Depersonalization and Derealization

Intense anxiety can cause a sense of unreality in how we feel about ourselves, others, or the world. We feel "different" or "changed" (depersonalization), or other people and our surroundings seem "far away" and "unreal" (derealization). While psychiatrists do not consider these to be psychotic reactions, individuals who suffer depersonalization and derealization often feel as if they are going mad. Their experience frequently is dominated by anxiety, but with heavy doses of guilt and shame as well.

These dread reactions can result from childhood abuse, often of a physical or sexual nature, or they can follow on the heels of adult trauma, such as combat or a severe accident. These origins suggest that depersonalization and derealization are defenses against severe painful emotion. They also can result from overwhelming internal stresses, such as a childhood identity that cannot confront the real adult world. Depersonalization is a common experience.

DSM-III-R suggests that a mammoth 70 percent of young people may experience some degree of depersonalization at least once. We are dealing with a human experience, one that exists along a continuum from commonplace to extraordinary. The *New Harvard Guide to Psychiatry* (1988) states that "depersonalization is not only common but should not be viewed as evidence of emotional illness," unless it is severe and persistent. Oh, that this textbook would say that about all forms and all degrees of human distress. The severity or persistence of a psychospiritual crisis does not turn it into an "illness." Psychological and spiritual crises are better seen as opportunities, even when the opportunity seems to have been lost. As long as people remain alive, so does the hope for personal growth.

Selma Loses Herself

Looking at Selma from the outside, she was the least likely person to be harboring the potential for a great inner drama of seeming madness. She had reached her first year of college without consciously experiencing a great deal of emotional turmoil. Outwardly lighthearted and good-natured with a very sweet nature, she had many casual friends in a wide social circle. The only flaw in her social résumé, if anyone had noticed, was the lack of a truly intimate or close friend.

Selma was black, and her family was first-generation middle class. They were determined to be very middle class, and all of their behavior was measured against acceptability in the eyes of Selma's grandmother, a Baptist minister's wife.

Selma's first year of college did not start out especially remarkably, except that she met a young man and became seriously involved with him. Then "it" happened. During a disagreement with her boyfriend one night, she abruptly became unaccountably anxious. There was a split-second sense of something cataclysmic befalling her, and then she became "dead inside." At first she thought her boyfriend had put a drug in her drink. Then she thought she was awakening from a bad dream. She grew afraid that she was going crazy.

By the time she arrived in my office about a month later, she was frightened to the core. Yet she could hardly describe what was the matter. "I'm changed," she blurted out. "Do you understand? Changed!" She said "changed" as if something diabolical had happened to her, as if the devil himself had taken her over. And she did briefly entertain the idea that she was possessed, a possibility with some precedent within her culture.

Like most people who undergo this dread experience, Selma felt certain that no one else had ever been through it. She felt as if no one else on earth could survive such feelings of emotional estrangement. She saw herself doomed in some unspeakable fashion to a life hardly human. Selma's loss of self at times became a disconnection from her own body: "It's like I'm not even in the room with you." And then in still more pain: "I'm not even in the room with myself! I'm having feelings, but they're not my feelings, or it's not me feeling them . . ."

When I first tried to get Selma to talk about herself and her family life, it came out like an advertisement for the "American way." "I have a perfect boyfriend. A perfect family. A perfect life. Why is this happening to me?"

She had never rebelled against her parents or challenged any of their values. Her family was supposed to be conflict-free. She never faced painful issues of love and rejection, because passions were always muted in her family. She had been taught to skate on the surface of life, and now the ice was breaking under her. Emotions and needs long suppressed were demanding attention, and she could only take flight from them into the strange and frightening new reality.

In the early sessions her emotional repertoire was limited to anxiety and the depersonalization that accompanied it. As I urged her to talk over a period of weeks, more complex feelings came out about her boyfriend, her family, and her life. She especially felt angry; and then she felt guilty and anxious whenever the anger surfaced.

The depersonalization had begun the night of the fight with her boyfriend. She had hinted to him that she wanted to break up. Just a hint. Nothing in her life had prepared her for handling the pain she saw in his face. His pain—her guilt about it—was unbearable to her. And nothing had prepared her for the fear of being on her own at college without a boyfriend. She declared, "I'll never find another man ever again in my whole life."

Selma couldn't talk with her parents about her involvement with her boyfriend. Newly risen from the inner city, Mom and Dad would panic at any hint that she might get pregnant before finishing college. Nor would they understand how she could have psychological problems. Selma was afraid that her family would worry about what they had done wrong—and so she told them as little as possible.

Each time she found a new emotion within herself, Selma grew ashamed and guilty over it. Her shame reactions heaped ridicule on her: "Who do you think you are? Better than your parents? Someone special? You don't deserve any more attention than anyone else." Then the guilt set in: "You're bad to hurt your boyfriend by leaving him. And you're a wretch for making your parents suffer." Then anxiety: "It's happening again, and I don't know why or what it is . . ." The anxiety would bring the depersonalization flooding over her again.

Then one session, after several weeks of hard work, she abruptly announced, "Of course, I'm changing. I need to change!"

No longer fighting the shattering of her old reality, she took an active hand in creating something new from the chaos. Thus Selma took the single most important step for a person undergoing severe emotional turmoil—she resolved to come out of it a stronger, more determined person, one with the courage to face her feelings and to fulfill her genuine aspirations.

Selma became able to hold her boyfriend at a distance while deciding how she genuinely felt toward him. She was able to tell her parents, "I am going through hell, but I'm going to get through, and I'd like to tell you about it." By the end of the school year, hell had been left a long way behind her.

How would the modern psychiatrist treat Selma? Most probably with medication. Very few would approach her depersonalization reaction as an opportunity for new growth in a previously suppressed person. They would not aim at helping her find the strength to implement new values in her life. Instead they would see Selma as a sick individual needing relief from her suffering and help in readjusting to the same old reality.

Post-Traumatic Stress Disorder

Post-traumatic stress disorder (PTSD) is one of the most useful diagnoses in psychiatry because it actually describes a real-life response to extreme stress. Individuals suffering from PTSD suffer from a persistent reexperiencing of the trauma (through nightmares, flashbacks, restimulation by similar events), a great need to avoid anything remotely resembling the stress, and signs of "increased arousal" (insomnia, irritability, difficulty concentrating, fearfulness, physical signs of anxiety).[3] Individuals suffering from PTSD often feel guilt and shame, but anxiety is frequently the dominant emotion.

Sometimes PTSD can show up years after the trauma—for example, as a response to child abuse. A new event in the individual's life, such as getting married or having a baby, may restimulate the stress reaction from childhood, often without the individual recalling the earlier traumatic event. Some experts believe that childhood sexual abuse *always* leads to PTSD in adulthood.

PTSD is a natural reaction to extremely threatening circumstances of almost any kind, from child abuse to adult rape, as well as experiences of disaster, such as wars, airplane or automobile accidents, and earthquakes. It can be precipitated by one trauma, such as being assaulted or seeing a friend badly injured, or by prolonged exposure to stress, such as physical beatings, repeated abandonments as a child, or prolonged legal conflict as an adult. Many Vietnam vets and nearly all hostages suffer from PTSD.[4] In my experience as a medical expert and a patients' rights advocate I have found that many former psychiatric patients—especially those who have been incarcerated, drugged, and shocked—frequently suffer from PTSD.

PTSD can be relatively short-lived or it can persist for months or years. It's often helpful to relive the trauma with an experienced, caring guide. Sometimes discovering the connection to earlier, similar traumatic events in childhood can be helpful. Sharing with people who have undergone similar experiences can be very useful, especially in overcoming feelings of humiliation following experiences like incest, rape, or involuntary psychiatric hospitalization and shock treatment.

Former psychiatric inmates or patients are especially likely to feel isolated and ashamed when psychiatrists tell them that they are wrong in perceiving themselves as injured by drugs or shock. My books and speeches often are cited by these former patients as helping them overcome their sense of being "abnormal" for feeling so injured by their psychiatric experiences.

Giving psychoactive drugs to people with PTSD can compound their difficulties with concentration and focusing attention.

Drug and Alcohol Addiction

Addictions to drugs, alcohol, nicotine, or food—as well as to work, exercise, sex, and other compulsive activities—are often attributed to underlying anxiety; but they also can be attempts to handle almost any overwhelming emotion, including guilt, shame, anxiety, and anger.*

Alcohol is by far the most common culprit, and public educational efforts have aimed at awakening society to the toll alcohol abuse takes in death through accidents and disease, broken lives, and dysfunctional families. Because addictions can become so invasive and destructive to the entire existence of the individual, it is often useful to seek help from support groups, such as Alcoholics Anonymous (AA). Individuals may

---

*The dangers of addiction and withdrawal in association with the use of sedative drugs, such as alcohol, are discussed chapter 11.

need guidance and moral support in rebuilding their family, social, and professional lives, as well as in establishing more viable values (see chapter 16). The use of alternative means for relaxing, such as self-hypnosis or guided imagery, can be helpful, as can active engagement in health and fitness programs and spiritual approaches of various kinds.

It is also frequently possible to help alcoholics and other addicts through individual psychotherapy and family therapy without the benefit of additional programs; but I believe it is important to offer an ethically oriented psychotherapy—one that encourages self-determination, taking responsibility for the consequences of one's actions, developing new social activities, and living by more fulfilling psychospiritual values (see chapter 16).

Genetic and Biological Theories of Alcoholism

While chronic abuse of alcohol results in many physical ailments, evidence for a biological *cause* is too flimsy to require review, and most textbooks of psychiatry make little or no attempt to argue for it.[5]

The proposed genetic basis of alcoholism also is insubstantial and has been critiqued elsewhere.[6] It is, however, worth noticing that another much-publicized claim for a proven genetic cause in psychiatry recently fell by the wayside. On April 18, 1990, the *Washington Post* headlined GENETIC TIE TO ALCOHOLISM REPORTEDLY DISCOVERED. ABERRANT GENE IS FOUND IN MOST CASES STUDIED. The study from the University of Texas Health Science Center in San Antonio, published in the *Journal of the American Medical Association,* [7] claims to prove the existence of a gene in alcoholics related to one of the dopamine neurotransmitter receptors. Media pronouncements by the investigators gave the impression that it makes neurophysiological sense to relate dopamine receptor malfunction to alcoholism. There were discussions of how dopamine mediates "pleasure." However, as we already have seen, dopamine neurotransmission plays a major role throughout the higher brain (the limbic system and frontal lobes), influencing all intellectual and emotional function, and therefore an abnormality in it probably would produce lobotomy effects or gross mental deterioration (see chapters 3 and 4). Thus I suspected from the start that the Texas findings were flawed; it simply didn't make sense for such a gross defect to produce such a specific problem as alcohol abuse.

As it turned out, within months the study was overturned by one from the National Institute on Alcohol Abuse and Alcoholism.[8] The chief investigator, Annabel Bolos, concludes that the new study "does not support a widespread or consistent association between the receptor gene and alcoholism."⁹

Pitfalls in Alcoholism Treatment

In regard to treatment there are several menacing trends. Psychiatric hospitals and detoxification units are increasingly utilizing AA programs and even forcing involuntary patients to attend AA meetings. This, I believe, undermines the whole spirit of AA as a voluntary organization. Second, psychiatrists and addiction programs in hospitals are pushing the idea that alcoholism is a genetic and biochemical disorder,* and this again undermines AA, especially the principles of ethical autonomy and personal responsibility on which its Twelve Steps are based. These steps include moral principles, such as "Admitted to God, to ourselves, and to another human being the exact nature of our wrongs" and "Made a list of all persons we had harmed, and became willing to make amends to them all." Yet nowadays, publications supporting the disease concept of alcoholism are routinely available at AA meetings, and members mistakenly identify the disease concept with basic AA principles.†

Perhaps most dangerous of all, some clinics and detoxification units encourage families to organize encounters or "interventions" with their relatives in order to force them into treatment. It's one thing for a loving family to confront a member about getting help. That may or may not be ethical and useful, depending on the circumstances. But it's a threat to civil liberties when hospitals or psychiatrists foster these coercive approaches, especially when they also wield the power of involuntary treatment.

Except for short-term help in withdrawing from addictive substances,‡

---

*For example, Suburban Hospital of Bethesda, Maryland, in the November 27, 1987, *Washington Post* has a large advertisement with the headline MOST PEOPLE DON'T KNOW ALCOHOLISM IS A BIOLOGICAL, HEREDITARY DISEASE THAT'S TREATABLE. Smaller print reaffirms, "The fact is that alcoholism is a biological, hereditary disease that affects one of ten Americans who drink."

†While the basic AA literature refers to alcoholism as an "allergy" on a very rare occasion, it is meant as a metaphor intended to discourage even a taste of alcohol. There is no attempt to give evidence or to argue that alcoholism is a physical disease. Indeed, nowhere in original AA literature, such as the primary source *Alcoholics Anonymous* (New York: Alcoholics Anonymous World Services, 1976), is there an actual discussion suggesting that alcoholism is biological or genetic, and the Twelve Steps focus exclusively on psychospiritual problems and solutions. Unfortunately, many AA members are being taught the language of biopsychiatry in detoxification units and through relatively new books popular among AA members, and they are making it a part of their everyday language. They end up undermining AA's principles of personal responsibility by declaring themselves to have a "disease."

‡It can be very dangerous and even life-threatening to stop many drugs too abruptly. Withdrawing from various psychiatric drugs is discussed in the pertinent chapters.

the use of drugs in treating addicts is especially to be condemned. Not only is there a danger of cross-addiction to new substances, but the prescription of drugs encourages the addict's worst tendencies. For these reasons, it makes no more sense to give a heroin addict methadone than it does to give gin to a vodka addict.

Addictions in many respects can be considered compulsions.

Obsessions and Compulsions

Obsessions and compulsions focus our attention on persistent thoughts or ritualized activities rather than on our underlying painful feelings. In this they are similar to phobias, in which the person becomes wholly focused on one specific fear.* While these experiences can become totally debilitating, they may seem less overwhelming to the individual than the panic attacks suffered by Alice, the chronic anxiety experienced by Melissa, or the extreme depersonalization endured by Selma. Focusing on specific thoughts, activities, or fears can become an escape from more overwhelming feelings of anxiety, guilt, or shame. We saw, for example, how Alice initially felt enormous dread but quickly focused her attention on the fear of vomiting. This enabled her to avoid frequent attacks of the more awful fear of personal annihilation.

The woman obsessed with the thought of killing her child may be running from her conflicts about being a mother, her feelings of entrapment within the marriage, her wish to pursue other careers. Guilt won't let her think about a better life for herself at the apparent expense of her husband or her children. The man obsessed over whether he will be late for every meeting may be covering up his frustration and outrage at being so submissive to the demands made on him in the corporate world. Shame over his "unmanly" feelings keeps him from looking at them.

Tony, a young man whose father is a famous surgeon, becomes immobilized by an obsession over which medical school to attend. He's been accepted into several, and selecting one becomes a nightmarish life-and-death struggle. His therapist suggests, "People don't usually become paralyzed over positive choices. Is there some reason you might not want to attend *any*

---

* Usually lumped with the anxiety disorders in modern psychiatric diagnosis, obsessions and compulsions are instead complex attempts to deal with myriad combinations of emotions, including anxiety, guilt, and shame. Obsessions are fixed or persistent thoughts, impulses, or images that usually start out as alien intrusions and eventually seem to take over our minds. Compulsions are actions, often ritualistic and repetitive, that come to dominate our conduct. They usually are driven by obsessive thoughts. Thus we usually speak of obsessive-compulsive behavior. For convenience I may speak of "disorders," but I wish to avoid any suggestion that these are "medical" problems.

medical school?" And the young man blurts out, "My father would disown me!"

Choosing to go to medical school has become the pivotal issue of autonomy in Tony's young life, and he doesn't feel able to handle it. The thought of making a decision raises a hornet's nest of emotional conflicts, including fear of failure, dread of competing with his father, outrage at feeling forced to follow in his father's footsteps, guilt over disappointing his father, and shame over pursuing his own more modest ambitions. The threat of medical school is heightened by the pressure his parents put on him to be "perfect" when he was still a small child. Being a perfect high school and college student seemed attainable, and Tony got straight A's. Being a perfect doctor seems wholly beyond his reach. He thinks he'll be lucky to make a passing grade.

Tony benefited from a patient, long-term therapy that helped him learn to make his own independent choices. In a sense he had to be debriefed from his childhood indoctrination into blind rule following and then introduced to more autonomous, independent principles of living.

Why do obsessive and compulsive individuals tend to be so hard to help? People must have a very rigid outlook on life in order to succumb to repetitive, alien thoughts and to perform endless rituals like handwashing or checking the gas stove again and again. They must be hiding from enormously painful, suppressed feelings in order to drink themselves and their families to destruction. Inquiries into their childhood experiences are likely to be rejected as irrelevant, when in reality they are overwhelmingly painful. The task of psychotherapy or any form of emotional healing may require loosening up controls, exploring emotions, seeking new insights, and pursuing new and better goals. All of that may seem beyond reach to the person who already is sacrificing his or her rationality to avoid facing painful feelings.

People who become enmeshed in obsessions and compulsions sometimes prefer more behavioral forms of therapy that are in themselves obsessive-compulsive, such as substituting "good thoughts" for their bad ones, and being led step by step to change their routines and rituals. Sometimes they seek out therapists who will take over their lives for them. Unfortunately, their personalities can make them easy prey for authoritarian, pseudoscientific approaches. They are likely to grasp at the idea that they suffer from biochemical imbalances and need drugs, and they may fall victim to the psychosurgeons who are taking a renewed interest in operating on them (see chapter 11).

Phobias

Milton was in his early twenties when he came to see me only a few weeks after developing a cancer phobia. After extensive testing for cancer, his physicians had concluded that he needed psychiatric treatment, and reluctantly he came for help. "How can you help me? Isn't everyone afraid of getting cancer? And how do you know I don't have it? The doctors could have missed the early stages."

Milton was new in town. He had taken a job at a bank after college graduation, hoping for specialized training and transfer to the Swiss office. Language and international finance were his interests. Instead he found himself stuck in Washington, D.C. His wife, too, was very disappointed, and she was having trouble making friends or finding a job. For Milton, life seemed at a premature dead end. Then he developed a dreadful fear that he had leukemia.

In the first session Milton recalled something that had wholly escaped his memory. His grandfather had died of leukemia when Milton was a child, and no one had tried to comfort the little boy or to help him understand what had happened. Then he told me about something even more obviously connected to his phobia. Two years earlier Milton's brother had developed a serious yet often curable form of cancer; but the family had been unable to discuss it. Milton had no idea if his brother was expected to survive.

I explained to Milton that his phobia probably was rooted in his family members' experiences with cancer, especially their unwillingness to face their fears about it, and in his own current sense of having reached a "dead end." I suggested that he contact his brother to discuss his health with him and that he consider more vigorous efforts to set his career on the desired course.

By the next session Milton had talked with his mother and father and with his brother. Everyone was relieved to break the silence. It turned out that his brother had a 90-percent chance of complete recovery and was grateful to have Milton showing an interest in him. Milton also had confronted his boss about languishing in Washington, D.C., and to his surprise found out that his boss was wholly unaware of Milton's dissatisfaction with the job placement.

Milton's cancer phobia was gone after the second session and he terminated therapy. A year later he called to say that he was being transferred to Europe and that he was doing fine.

It is unusual to help someone so easily with a phobia. Rarely do psychotherapists get to work with the problem within a matter of weeks after it first rears up. By the time help is sought, most phobias are deeply entrenched and the connections to the person's life are buried out of sight. Phobias share much with obsessions and compulsions. The capacity to focus on one unreasonable fear with enduring intensity is the mark of a mind driven to shift attention away from other, more threatening, passions and problems.

Almost anything or any experience can become the object of phobic fear. The most common phobias focus on being in high places, going outdoors, being trapped in a small or confining space, driving in cars or flying in airplanes, getting diseases like AIDS or cancer or heart disease, and being bitten by animals, such as snakes, bats, or dogs. Eating disorders often involve phobias as well, especially the fear of being overweight.

It's often difficult to help phobic individuals for the same reasons it's hard to help people with obsessions and compulsions. People so driven to displace their emotions in overtly irrational ways are strongly motivated not to face those emotions.

Sometimes great headway can be made with phobias, even when they are long-standing.

Jim was seeing his therapist for other problems when he decided to spend some time dealing with his fear of heights. His therapist encouraged him over several sessions to keep scanning his childhood for times and places that he felt the kind of panic that he now feels in high places.

Eventually Jim recalled a momentous day when he was seven years old. He'd been walking in the woods with his father and his older brother when they came upon a fire observation tower used by the forest rangers. They climbed to the open platform near the top, where his brother began to horse around, feigning to push Jim toward the edge. Jim's father, who never felt much affinity for him, began to ridicule the little boy's fearfulness while his brother went on tormenting him.

In a flash, young Jim's outrage and fear boiled to the surface. His older brother was now perched precariously on the railing and Jim, for an instant, imagined shoving him off. His father would kill him for that—hurl him right off the ledge. He would go flying through the air, screaming in terror, and then die, crushed at the foot of the tower. Little Jim became paralyzed, trapped by his own fear and rage and his terror of the two much larger males. He lay down trembling and clinging to the floor and eventually was dragged screaming down the tower by his irate father. Ever since then, Jim had experienced dreadful fear anywhere near a precipice. If he also happened to feel angry at the time, the fear would paralyze him.

After reexperiencing the episode on the tower, Jim's phobic fear was much reduced. He never would become a mountain climber, but he could handle most of the challenges that previously overwhelmed him. The exploration of the phobia also led him to a better understanding of the rejection, intimidation, and hatred directed at him as a child. In my experience as a therapist, the fear of facing these more threatening insights into the past keeps the phobia in place. The phobia is a kind of mental utility hole cover over an abyss of childhood experiences.

Women and Agoraphobia

Agoraphobia, the fear of going outdoors, is among the most common incapacitating phobias. It occurs by far more frequently in women. It sometimes begins as a panic attack and can manifest itself in many ways, from specific fears of going on public transportation or shopping in food markets to a generalized fear of leaving the house. Often the woman can negotiate these threats, but only in the presence of a spouse or friend. She becomes very dependent and, in the extreme, may stop feeling safe at home alone. This almost happened to Alice (see pages 220–21).

Why are the vast majority of agoraphobics women? Could it be that women have been taught that it's too dangerous to go outside, to meet strangers, to deal with the threatening realities of city life? Could it be that most women find their lives in part controlled by the fear of being abused within their own homes and raped on the streets? Could it be that women, when they do go shopping for food and clothes, may resent their domestic activities? Could it be that being away from home base is both a real threat and a forbidden challenge for many women? In many ways the agoraphobic woman is a caricature of the feminine role (see chapter 14).

Psychiatrist Robert Seidenberg and attorney Karen DeCrow, authors of *Women Who Marry Houses: Panic and Protest in Agoraphobia* (1983), place agoraphobia in its historical perspective as a women's issue. The title of their introduction, "The Streets Still Belong to Men," communicates the thrust of their book. I was especially touched by the chapter "Emily Dickinson: A Woman Who Chose to Stay Home," in which they describe how a creative woman in Emily's era had no place in the society. She had to be a shut-in to be creative.

Seidenberg and DeCrow analyze agoraphobia as both a fear of the social reality created by men and a protest against it. They excoriate therapists who ignore the meaning of being a woman in society and who further abuse these women with behavioral and medical treatments.

When I recommended *Women Who Marry Houses* to a local psychiatrist who runs an agoraphobia clinic she reacted with scorn. "Women *suffer* from agoraphobia," she declared. "It's awful to treat them like their problems are political, or feminist, or whatever." For too many psychiatrists, the fact of suffering redefines a problem as medical rather than psychological, social, or political. The oppression of women, racism, poverty—many social and economic phenomena—contribute enormously to human suffering. We do not discredit human suffering when we examine underlying societal causes. Instead we help the individual find a better perspective on her suffering. When the "agoraphobic" woman discovers that she is being victimized by the age-old oppression of women, she can find solace and understanding in feminist principles (see chapter 14), seek comfort and support from other enlightened women, and rid herself of the mistaken notion that she suffers from a disease. She can begin to overcome her fears through self-empowerment rather than through biochemical theories and drugs.

Women Who Marry Houses has not been read much by psychiatrists. I haven't found it cited in any textbook discussions of agoraphobia. Marketing experts have suggested to Seidenberg and DeCrow that men don't read books with the word *women* in the title, although they may buy them as presents for their wives or girlfriends. Perhaps men are phobic about titles with the word *women* in them. If so, I suspect that the phobia is not biochemical in origin.

Eating Disorders: Anorexia and Bulimia

Anorexia is self-induced starvation. The anorectic rejects food and almost always expresses an intense desire to be as skinny as possible. Anorexia typically is classified as a compulsion but sometimes is labeled a "fat phobia." Anorectic people see fat bulging from their bodies where only taut skin remains. The obsession with losing weight occurs in varying degrees, from almost every young girl's feeling that she's too fat to an all-consuming way of life that ends in death from starvation.

Bulimia, which sometimes occurs along with anorexia, involves bingeing and purging; but the bulimic is not necessarily underweight. The individual will eat, sometimes in great excess, and then compulsively attempt to undo the "damage," typically by vomiting, taking laxatives, or exercising. It, too, can lead to death, especially from metabolic imbalances and cardiac arrest.

The prevalence of these two eating disorders has doubled or tripled in the last two decades, and according to *DSM-III-R*, 90 to 95 percent of sufferers are women. The age of onset is almost always between early adolescence and early adulthood. Male anorexia has been described increasingly in recent years[10] and is probably a copycat response to a phenomenon that is almost wholly female in origin. Rates of bingeing and purging are extraordinary among populations of educated young women, ranging from 13 to 67 percent in surveys of college students.[11]

Psychotherapy, including family therapy, and self-help groups can be effective; but like most severely obsessive people, those suffering from eating disorders can be difficult to help.

Nowadays biopsychiatrists attempt to make drugs, usually antidepressants, the standard therapy. They also try to conjure up biochemical causes; but there's no meaningful evidence to back them up, and it seems fruitless and misleading to seek genetic and biochemical explanations for a problem that has appeared so recently in a social context that would seem to make it almost inevitable.

Both anorexia and bulimia are caricatures of the values imposed on modern young women. Neither "disease" was sufficiently prevalent to gain the attention of psychiatry until the last few decades. Anorexia and bulimia made their appearance simultaneously with the model Twiggy and with the escalating cultural emphasis on skinniness as the standard for the female figure. The preoccupation with being thin has been compounded by the increasingly ambivalent values placed on womanhood itself. The "ideal" young woman is expected to embody within herself an infinite number of conflicted roles, among them sexually alluring female, helpless female, perfect mother, indefatigable housewife, social secretary, helpmate, unisex Peter Pan, companion in recreational athletics, and, finally, professional and wage earner.

It is no wonder that women with eating disorders so often seem utterly lacking in self-esteem. The goals they strive for are unattainable and yet they blame themselves for the failure to achieve them. The extraordinarily high rates of bingeing and purging among college women confirms that the problem is endemic to the culture.

Many young women who suffer from eating disorders are highly motivated, extremely intelligent people who do try to make themselves into everything that could possibly be expected of them—and without help from anyone else. The great majority are from the white middle and upper class and, according to author Hilde Bruch,[12] their mothers typically are high achievers who have been frustrated in attaining their own desired goals in life. Both parents tend to be overly concerned with physical appearance. They tend to have idealized images of their children and to have difficulty being sensitive to their real needs. But it is unfair to lay all of the blame at the feet of parents in a society that places such impossibly conflicting demands on young girls.

Young women with eating disorders can be seen as unconscious and unheralded martyrs to the confused values within our society. Like agoraphobics, their plight is incomprehensible without feminist insights into the situation of modern women. They also can be understood as youngsters suffering from problems within their individual families, often including too high expectations with too little support. Their suffering frequently is intense, from the underlying painful feelings that drive their compulsions and from the physical debilitation and shame associated with their eating disorders.

Because people with eating disorders often are difficult to help, biopsychiatry is gaining influence. It would be far better if therapists were united in rejecting biochemical theories and toxic drugs, in encouraging the young women to face the cultural values and family conflicts that have driven them to such compulsive excesses, in offering them the unconditional love that they so desperately need, and in insisting that the parents of these youngsters join in the process of personal transformation and recovery. In the long run it also would help if more of these therapists addressed women's issues within the society itself.

As we now turn to exploring in more depth psychiatry's impact on children and women, we will find that modern psychiatry remains fiercely insulated from anything that threatens its assumptions. The sexual victimization of women and children, for example, has become a national scandal. Yet psychiatrists continually fail to connect it with the patients they see in their offices from day to day. Child after child, woman after woman, appears before them with all the stigmata of abuse—only to be further abused with medical diagnoses and physical treatments, such as the ones we will look at in the next chapters.

Chapter 11

Suppressing the Passion of Anxiety Overwhelm with Drugs: The Minor Tranquilizers, Including Xanax, Valium, BuSpar, Ativan, and Halcion, and the Antidepressant Anafranil

The next gene to be identified for a psychiatric illness may be for panic disorder, Dr. James C. Ballenger said at a symposium for members of Congress and their staffs.
—Clinical Psychiatry News, *November 1988*

Just as the 1980s was the decade in which those suffering from various forms of depression were identified and treated, so, [NIMH director Lewis] Judd and other specialists hope, the 1990s will be the era when the recognition and treatment of anxiety disorders predominate. Judd recently announced that NIMH will launch a national education and prevention campaign, which, he says, "will be pointed toward early identification and diagnosis."
—Washington Post Health, *May 22, 1990*

From the U.S. Congress to the American public, psychiatry's marketing strategy for the 1990s aims at people who feel anxious. It has become an axiom within modern economics that advertising actually *creates* consumer needs. By targeting people suffering from anxiety, psychiatry should be able to generate an unlimited demand for its drugs. Prescriptions for one class of these drugs, the benzodiazepines, already are estimated at nearly one hundred million a year in the United States, for a cost of about $500 million.[1] Some estimates place the total cost at $800 million or more.

240

This chapter will give special attention to two minor* tranquilizers that have drawn considerable publicity. One is BuSpar (buspirone), whose potentially damaging effects have been largely ignored, even in the psychiatric literature. The other is Xanax (alprazolam), one of the most intensively marketed and yet dangerous drugs in psychiatry. Then chapter 15 will focus on the political campaign that made Xanax so successful.

Unlike most of the drugs discussed in this book, the minor tranquilizers are highly sought after. Even without doctors pushing them, people would want them. Indeed, they are actively sold illegally on the street. This is not surprising, since people often resort to taking anything that promises even temporary relief from anxiety. Millions drink alcohol, smoke cigarettes, and use marijuana, opiates, and other street drugs. Others eat excessively, exercise compulsively, work to exhaustion, watch TV endlessly, escape into books, relentlessly pursue sex, and overindulge any number of otherwise harmless habits in an attempt to escape their tensions and apprehensions. In chapter 10 we saw that obsessions, compulsions, and phobias also can be seen as efforts to control anxiety. Overall, psychiatric interventions play a relatively minor role in humanity's never-ending struggle to deal with anxiety.

The Minor Tranquilizers and Other Sedative-Hypnotics

Among psychiatric medications for the treatment of anxiety, the most commonly used are the minor tranquilizers, starting in 1957 with the introduction of Librium (chlordiazepoxide). In the 1970s the minor tranquilizer Valium (diazepam) topped the charts as the most widely prescribed drug in America, to be replaced by Xanax in 1986. Most of the minor tranquilizers belong to the group called benzodiazepines and are closely related chemically to Librium, Valium, and Xanax. They differ mostly in their duration of action and in the dosage required to achieve the same effect. *They have nearly identical clinical effects.*[2]

The benzodiazepine minor tranquilizers include Xanax, Valium, Librium, Tranxene (clorazepate), Paxipam (halazepam), Centrax or Verstran (prazepam), Klonopin (formerly Clonopin) (clonazepam), Dalmane (flurazepam), Serax (oxazepam), Ativan (lorazepam), Restoril (temazepam), and Halcion (triazolam).

An older minor tranquilizer is Miltown or Equanil (meprobamate).

---

*The drugs are called "minor" tranquilizers to distinguish them from "major" tranquilizers, but nowadays the latter are called neuroleptics or antipsychotics. While the minor tranquilizers might now simply be called tranquilizers, that term itself is somewhat misleading. Basically, they are sedatives.

Other minor tranquilizers are chemically antihistamines, such as Atarax or Vistaril (hydroxyzine).

Sleeping medications also have tranquilizing effects. These include Doriden (glutethimide), Noludar (methyprylon), Placidyl (ethchlorvynol), and Noctec, Somnos, or Beta-Chlor (chloral hydrate), and the various barbiturates, including Seconal (secobarbital), Luminal (phenobarbital), Butibel (butabarbital), Amytal (amobarbital), Nembutal (pentobarbital), and Tuinal (amobarbital and secobarbital).

All of these drugs have the potential for abuse and addiction. Since all have a calming or sedative effect, people addicted to these "downers" use many of them interchangeably, depending on what is available, often mixing them with alcohol. The minor tranquilizers and alcohol make a very dangerous, frequently lethal, combination.

BuSpar, the most recent addition to the minor tranquilizers, is being promoted as nonsedative, nonaddictive, and relatively safe.

The Most Widely Used Psychiatric Drugs

According to FDA data reported by Carlene Baum and her associates in the February 1988 *Medical Care*, there was a dramatic decline in the use of minor tranquilizers and other antianxiety drugs, from a peak of 103 million prescriptions in 1975 to 67 million in 1981 in the United States. There are no complete totals available for recent years, but the APA's task force report, *Benzodiazepine Dependence, Toxicity and Abuse* (1990), estimates that annual prescriptions for benzodiazepines have leveled off since the mid-1980s at about 61 million.

The minor tranquilizers, now led by Xanax, remain by far the most commonly prescribed psychiatric medications. In some countries, such as France, the use of these agents continues to escalate.

Most minor tranquilizer prescriptions—65 percent—were for women in 1984. However, women predominate in all psychiatric drug categories. Thirty-five percent of all patients were sixty years of age or older.

Are the Minor Tranquilizers Something New?

Because of the popularity surrounding the minor tranquilizers, we tend to think that they represent something very new and radically different among drugs; but I recall my medical school professor of psychopharmacology reminding us in 1960 that the sedative attributes of minor tranquilizers differ little from those of the barbiturates, such as phenobarbital. He said, however, that he hesitated to tell this to practicing physicians, because their faith in drugs helped their patients benefit from them. Like most biopsychiatrists, he raised no concerns about encouraging people to have more faith in a pill than in themselves.

Even before the barbiturates, there were sedative and hypnotic drugs, many of which are still in use today. People used them, sometimes got short-term relief from them, and sometimes became addicted to them. Chloral hydrate (Noctec) and paraldehyde (Paral) are among them. Earlier, the highly toxic bromides had their day. And before them, opiates were freely dispensed in private practice and in mental hospitals.

Alcohol Competes with Minor Tranquilizers

To divest the minor tranquilizers of their medical mystique we need only recall that alcohol was prescribed for generations by doctors as a sedative for anxious patients. As recently as 1943, Torald Sollmann's classic text *A Manual of Psychopharmacology* professed:

A certain amount of alcohol, varying for individuals, may be taken occasionally or even daily without demonstrable permanently injurious effects. The relaxation, the easing of strain, of maladjustments, of excessive self-consciousness, of excessive inhibitions, indeed the euphoria, may sometimes be beneficial. . . . (P. 718)

Sollmann goes on to warn about the disadvantages and dangers of alcohol use, but then he reassures the reader:

On the other hand, the moderate use of alcohol is often blamed for shortened duration of life and for various physical injuries, without adequate data, or on the basis of effects that are produced only by very large quantities. (P. 718)

Obviously many people still consider alcohol the tranquilizer of choice, but I am not arguing that doctors should prescribe whiskey or gin. I don't think they should. Nor do I think they should so cavalierly prescribe the other sedative or tranquilizing drugs. I want to emphasize that there is nothing unique or medically sacrosanct about the current drugs commonly prescribed for anxiety. The drugs possess a number of dangerous qualities, many of them similar to the properties of alcohol.

Sedative-Hypnotics and Central Nervous System Depression

All of the commonly used minor tranquilizers—with the possible exception of BuSpar—are central nervous system depressants very similar to alcohol and barbiturates in their clinical effects. Along with alcohol and barbiturates, they are classified as sedative-hypnotics,[3] meaning that they produce relaxation (sedation) at lower doses and sleep (hypnosis) and eventually coma at higher ones. It is important to grasp the principle that minor tranquilizers are central nervous system depressants—and, in particular, sedative-hypnotics—because this classification removes the mystery surrounding these "tranquilizers." The so-called antianxiety effect is merely an early stage of central nervous system depression—sedation.[4] The basic clinical effect on the mind cannot be distinguished from alcohol or barbiturates.

It should be emphasized again that all minor tranquilizers combine with each other or with other central nervous system depressants—such as barbiturates, antidepressants, neuroleptics, lithium, and alcohol—with a potentially fatal result. While they can be lethal when taken alone, they are especially dangerous in combination with these other drugs. A large percentage of drug-related emergency room visits involve minor tranquilizers.

All of the minor tranquilizers impair mental alertness and physical coordination and can dangerously compromise mechanical performance, such as automobile driving.

At low doses the minor tranquilizers are sufficiently potent to impact noticeably on the brain waves on routine EEGs, especially in the frontal lobe region. However, they do not typically have the lobotomizing impact epitomized by the neuroleptics.

Addiction, Tolerance, and Withdrawal Symptoms

All hypnotic-sedatives, including the minor tranquilizers, are habit-forming and addictive and can produce withdrawal symptoms or an abstinence syndrome when they are stopped. In the extreme, the abstinence syndrome can cause life-threatening neurological reactions, including fever, psychosis, and seizures. Less severe withdrawal symptoms include increased heart rate and lowered blood pressure; shakiness; loss of appetite; muscle cramps; impairment of memory, concentration, and orientation; abnormal sounds in the ears and blurred vision; and insomnia, agitation, anxiety, panic, and derealization. Obvious withdrawal symptoms typically last two to four weeks. Subtle ones can last months.

Consistent with the principle that the minor tranquilizers differ little in their clinical effect from other sedatives, the Xanax write-up in the 1991 *PDR* acknowledges that withdrawal symptoms are "similar in character to those noted with barbiturates and alcohol."

Studies of Xanax (see ahead) show that *most* patients develop withdrawal symptoms during routine treatment lasting only eight weeks. Tolerance, or the need for increasing doses to achieve the same psychoactive effect, is the underlying physical mechanism of addiction. Within two to four weeks, tolerance can develop to the sedative effect of minor tranquilizers taken at night for sleep.[5] This again warns against the use of these drugs for more than a few days at a time.

The short-acting benzodiazepines can produce especially severe withdrawal symptoms, because the drug is cleared from the body at a relatively rapid rate. These include Xanax, Halcion, Ativan, Restoril, and Serax.* However, according to expert Louis Fabre in a February 1991 interview with me, tightness of binding to receptors is probably more indicative of addictive potential, and the most tightly binding are Xanax, Halcion, Ativan, and Klonopin.

Individuals who take only one pill daily for sleep or anxiety are not exempt from withdrawal problems. In my private practice during the last few years I have worked with several people who were unable to stop taking a once-a-day standard dose of Xanax, Ativan, Klonopin, or other minor tranquilizers. In each case, the attempt to stop the medication led to a disturbing degree of anxiety or insomnia within twenty-four hours. The problem seemed to be caused by rebound anxiety or rebound insomnia (see ahead).

In a personal communication in late December 1990, internist John Steinberg confirmed that patients taking one Xanax tablet each day for several weeks can become addicted. Steinberg is medical director of the Chemical Dependency Program at the Greater Baltimore Medical Center and president of the Maryland Society of Addiction Medicine. He points to research that Xanax and other short-acting benzodiazepines can cause a reactive hyperactivity of the receptors that they block. The hyperactive receptors then require one or more doses of Xanax each day or they produce anxiety and emotional discomfort. Steinberg calls the impact of Xanax "a fundamental change in the homeostasis of the brain." After the patient stops taking the Xanax, according to Steinberg, it takes the brain *six to eighteen months* to recover. Xanax patients should be warned, he says, that it can take a long time to get over painful withdrawal symptoms. Since doctors frequently don't realize this, they, too, are likely

---

*A drug-by-drug breakdown of half-lives can be found in the 1989 *Comprehensive Textbook of Psychiatry*.

to be confused and to continue the drug in the hope of "treating" the patient's drug-induced anxiety and tension.

Many detoxification beds are occupied by patients addicted to minor tranquilizers and even more by those who are cross-addicted with alcohol and other drugs. Steinberg says that Xanax is "by far and away" the worst offender and that it definitely causes addiction without being mixed with other sedatives.

Steinberg estimates that one in ten patients receiving Xanax will become addicted.* Based on an estimated fifteen million people receiving Xanax each year in the United States, Steinberg concludes that *1.5 million Xanax addicts are produced each year.*

Rebound Anxiety and Insomnia

Rebound anxiety is one of the common reactions to withdrawal or to dose reduction of a minor tranquilizer.[6] As with most psychiatric drugs, the use of the medication eventually causes an increase of the very symptoms that the drug is supposed to ameliorate, and thus rebound anxiety can lead to a false diagnosis of chronic anxiety disorder. As noted in the American Psychiatric Press *Textbook of Psychiatry*, long-term treatment can be erroneously maintained or reinstated when drug-induced rebound anxiety occurs. Addiction is the ultimate outcome.

Some experts, such as John Steinberg, disagree with my assertion that there is no difference between a tranquilizing and a sedative effect. They suspect that in addition to the obvious sedation, minor tranquilizers probably also produce a specific inhibition of anxiety. If true, this means that they also cause a specific rebound anxiety as the blocked receptors become hyperactive.

Rebound insomnia also results from taking most sleeping medications, because the brain reacts against the central nervous system (CNS) depressant effects by becoming more aroused or alert. Medications for sleep generally should not be taken for more than a day or two at a time.

---

*Steinberg does not use the term *addiction* loosely. By addiction he means that the patient periodically loses control of his or her drug intake and has a pattern of compulsive use, despite adverse consequences. If Steinberg were merely speaking of habituation, or difficulty stopping the use of the drug, his estimates would be much higher. He considers Xanax "very easily habituating" and observes that people are especially susceptible to the initial "euphoria or disinhibiting effect" that it has in common with alcohol.

Addiction Can Go Unnoticed

Seriously addicted patients may show no outward signs to their family or physicians until accidentally removed from the medication—for example, following surgery or during a medical emergency. Their withdrawal symptoms may then be wholly misinterpreted as an aspect of some other disorder or as a psychological problem. Marked withdrawal symptoms, including persistent rebound anxiety, can begin as much as five to seven days after stopping the medication and can last up to a month.

Paradoxical Reactions

The minor tranquilizers can produce paradoxical reactions—acute agitation, confusion, disorientation, anxiety, and aggression—especially in children, adults with brain disease, and the elderly. The Xanax report in the 1991 *PDR* states, "As with all benzodiazepines, paradoxical reactions such as stimulation, agitation, rage, increased muscle spasticity, sleep disturbances, hallucinations and other adverse behavioral effects may occur in rare instances and in a random fashion."

In nursing homes the medications may seem to help the insomnia of an elderly patient for a night or two, only to produce generalized brain dysfunction as the medication accumulates in the system. The agitated patient may then be mistakenly overdosed with further medication, perhaps a neuroleptic. According to Robert Hales and Stuart Yudofsky's *Textbook of Neuropsychiatry* (1987), the "routine" prescription of these medications in nursing homes and hospitals "should be avoided," especially for anything but brief periods of insomnia related to a particularly difficult or stressful situation.

As in response to alcohol, some people more readily lose their self-control and become violent when taking minor tranquilizers. There are frequent references to this in the literature, including cases of murder under the influence of minor tranquilizers. Partly because of this disinhibiting effect, the drugs cannot be used effectively for purposes of controlling behavior within institutions.

Halcion has been especially implicated in causing aggressive and suicidal behavior, as well as delirium, hallucinations, and seizures.

Memory Dysfunction from Minor Tranquilizers

Recently there has been much-publicized concern about Halcion producing amnesia for events prior to the taking of the drug. However, this has long been an unheralded problem with minor tranquilizers in general. Years ago I recall noticing that patients who mixed alcohol with Valium the night before a psychotherapy session sometimes would have severe black-out spells and could not recall much of the prior evening. It is well known that the intravenous infusion of benzodiazepines, such as Valium or Ativan, typically produces a similar amnesia for the several hours surrounding the infusion. While this may be a benefit in forgetting the painful effects of surgery, it becomes a potentially serious problem in the routine use of the minor tranquilizers for anxiety or sleep disorders and can interfere with psychotherapy, studying, learning anything new, or recalling previously retained memories.[7]

Long-Term Effects on Mental Function from the Minor Tranquilizers

Despite the obvious need for concern, few studies have attempted to measure the impact of long-term minor tranquilizer usage on overall mental function. Susan Golombok and her colleagues from the Institute of Psychiatry in London published "Cognitive Impairment in Long-Term Benzodiazepine Users" in the 1988 *Psychological Medicine*. Using a variety of neuropsychological tests to evaluate the impact of minor tranquilizers on cognitive function in patients who were administered the medication for at least one year, they found chronic impairment in measures of visual-spatial ability and attention span.

Golombok and her coworkers were unable to follow up with tests after drug termination. However, these findings of chronic brain dysfunction raise a serious concern about possible permanency. The investigators comment:

It is impossible to determine how long it is safe for a patient to continue to take benzodiazepines, or at what dose, before cognitive ability will begin to deteriorate. Nevertheless, it is clear from the inspection of our data that taking a low dose for a short time has little effect, while a high intake is almost always certainly harmful. (P. 371)

The test results indicate that "these patients are not functioning well in everyday life," while they remain unaware of their impairment:

This is in line with clinical evidence that patients who withdraw from their medication often report improved concentration and increased sensory appreciation and that only after withdrawal do they realize that they have been functioning below par. . . . It appears, therefore, that not only are long-term benzodiazepine users at risk of dependence, but that cognitive impairment also represents a very real hazard. (P. 373)

It cannot be overemphasized that brain-disabling treatments render patients less able to evaluate their own dysfunction. The Golombok study is exceedingly important from the viewpoint of the patient who wishes to avoid brain dysfunction and from the viewpoint of the ethical physician who wishes to avoid causing it in his or her patients. *

If doctors wish to prescribe minor tranquilizers or if patients want to take them, it would be prudent to follow the advice of *The New Harvard Guide to Psychiatry* (1988): "The main usefulness of the antianxiety agents is in general medicine in the *short-term treatment* of relatively transient forms of anxiety, fear, and tension" (p. 524).

Brain Shrinkage from Long-Term Minor Tranquilizer Use

An even more terrifying specter haunts the long-term use of minor tranquilizers—the possibility of brain atrophy. Although rarely mentioned in establishment books or reviews, in their letter to the editor in the July 1989 *Archives of General Psychiatry*, Isaac Marks and his ten colleagues summarize the as yet brief literature: "The cerebral ventricular enlargement reported in patients with anxiety/panic disorders who were long-term benzodiazepine users could be due to the disorder or to other factors rather than to the drugs, but wisdom advises caution" (p. 669). In fact, the cerebral ventricular enlargement—the equivalent of atrophy of the brain—is most likely due to the drugs. C. Schmauss and J-C. Kreig in "Enlargement of Cerebrospinal Fluid Spaces in Long-Term Benzodiazepine Abusers" in the 1987 *Biological Medicine* found that "our data suggest that the increase in the VBRs [ventricular enlargement] is dose-dependent on long-term BDZ [benzodiazepine] medication" (p. 873).

I mentioned the studies on brain atrophy to one expert who replied that although he had not heard of them, he was not surprised. "The minor tranquilizers are like alcohol," he observed, "and alcohol when used long-term causes brain shrinkage." He asked to remain anonymous for fear of offending other drug experts.

---

*While insufficiently stressing the problem of memory loss, a discussion and bibliography is presented in the APA task force report, *Benzodiazepine Dependence, Toxicity, and Abuse* (Washington, D.C.: American Psychiatric Association, 1990).

BuSpar—the Latest Miracle Tranquilizer

While the 1989 *Treatments of Psychiatric Disorders* by the APA task force notes that the clinical advantages of BuSpar have not been proven, BuSpar has become the latest fad tranquilizer.

BuSpar, unlike the other minor tranquilizers, is said to have a relatively low potential for abuse, addiction, and withdrawal symptoms. It is slow to take effect, often requiring weeks, and produces a lesser frequency of nervousness, restlessness, headache, and dizziness. That's the "book" on BuSpar, but there are reasons to be skeptical, and even concerned, about its use.

BuSpar, unlike other minor tranquilizers, affects the dopamine receptors, blocking their activity. The possibility of tardive dyskinesia—that untreatable and usually permanent neurological disorder—immediately comes to mind. As discussed in chapter 4, suppression of dopamine activity by neuroleptics frequently causes permanent dopamine hyperreactivity, resulting in tardive dyskinesia. While the mode of dopamine inhibition by BuSpar differs from that of the neuroleptics, the impact is sufficiently similar to raise red flags.

Even the manufacturer, Mead Johnson, shows concern about the drug's impact on dopamine receptors and warns in the 1990 *PDR* about the possible danger of neurological reactions similar to those caused by the neuroleptics, specifically including tardive dyskinesia. Cases of tardive dyskinesia from BuSpar have not yet been reported; but remember, it took twenty years before doctors and pharmaceutical firms recognized neuroleptic-induced tardive dyskinesia. Mead Johnson itself states: "Generally, long-term sequelae of any drug's use can be identified only after several years of marketing."

With a rare exception,[8] the psychiatric establishment isn't showing any concern. I found no mention of the possibility of permanent neurological problems from BuSpar in the relevant section of most of the recently published psychiatric textbooks.

Despite the fact that all minor tranquilizers have been implicated in abuse and addiction, the most current textbooks of psychiatry dismiss or fail to mention this possibility in regard to BuSpar. Yet it is common knowledge in the profession that apparently nonaddictive medications have turned out to be addictive soon after hitting the market and the streets. Darvon, for example, was widely marketed as a harmless analgesic and later turned out to be addictive. Indeed, initially the minor tranquilizers Valium and Librium were promoted as relatively safe in regard to potential abuse, until the FDA, despite legal resistance from Hoffmann-La Roche, placed curbs on them.*

Xanax—Approved for Panic Disorder

The news was announced in 1990 in headlines in Upjohn's eight-page gaudy color advertisements in psychiatric journals: XANAX: THE FIRST AND ONLY MEDICATION INDICATED FOR PANIC DISORDER.[9] Panic disorder (see chapter 10) was officially classified as a distinct psychiatric entity for the first time in 1980 by the APA's *Diagnostic and Statistical Manual*. The recent FDA approval of Xanax as the one and only treatment for this popular diagnosis will catapult the drug to even greater domination of the market.

Yet what is there to distinguish Xanax from the rest of the benzodiazepines? We've already found that there's little or no difference among these drugs in regard to their clinical impact.[10] The same is true in regard to side effects—except that Xanax is short-acting and more tightly bound to its receptors, and therefore, as already discussed, more likely to cause severe withdrawal symptoms and addiction.

Xanax is one of the more dangerous minor tranquilizers. Joe Graedon and Teresa Graedon warn about Xanax in their October 1989 syndicated column "The People's Pharmacy":

Xanax, one of the most commonly prescribed medications in the country, has been associated with confusion, paranoia, depression, hostility and forgetfulness while a person is taking it. Sudden withdrawal from such antianxiety agents can be living hell for some people. We have received letters from readers reporting nerves "jumping," muscle twitching, feelings of disorientation, fear, insomnia, anxiety, agitation and even seizure.[11]

Death from Xanax in combination with alcohol or other sedatives has been a special problem, as reported by Chad Carlton in 1990 in the *Lexington Herald-Leader*: "A commonly prescribed tranquilizer, introduced nearly a decade ago as a safer alternative to Valium, has become increasingly linked to overdose deaths, addiction and street-drug sales in Central Kentucky."[12] It had played a role in ten deaths in a six-month period in Lexington alone. "Doctors are handing it out like candy," says

*See Victor Cohen, "U.S. Curbs Valium, Librium," *Washington Post*, January 31, 1975; and "Justice Department to Control Librium, Valium," *Psychiatric News*, September 19, 1973.

Mark Hyatt, chief of psychiatry at the local Veterans Affairs Medical Center.

The Xanax Studies

On reading Upjohn's eight-page advertisements in psychiatric journals about its FDA studies,*[13] I was struck by something odd. At the top left of one page is a statement that drug evaluations were made at "weeks 1, 2, 3, 4, 6, and 8 of therapy." This gave the immediate impression that Xanax must have been proven effective at eight weeks. But the chart beneath this statement records only the first four weeks. Nowhere in the advertisement is there any discussion of the results after the full eight weeks. Then, at the bottom of the page, there is this explanation: "Because of the high rate of placebo dropouts, week 4 (the last evaluation point where the majority of patients remained in the placebo treatment group) was considered the study 'end point' for efficacy analyses."

In other words, Upjohn was counting only the first four weeks of the study and discarding the final results at eight weeks. Why would Upjohn want to do this?

I was shocked at what I found when I studied the original research report. By the end of the eight weeks, the sugar-pill patients were doing about as well as the drug patients. Indeed, the placebo patients were far better off, because they did not suffer the severe withdrawal and rebound reactions, including an increase in anxiety and in phobic responses, plus *a 350 percent greater number of panic attacks.*

In an unusually negative reaction to a highly touted study, an international group of eleven psychiatrists and psychologists, led by Isaac M. Marks from the Institute of Psychiatry in London, wrote a two-page letter in the July 1989 *Archives of General Psychiatry* criticizing and largely dismissing the Xanax study. They point out that "at the last week after taper [drug withdrawal], patients receiving alprazolam were in a *worse* state than patients receiving placebo, in terms of panic (350% worse, in table 1 of the article by Pecknold et al.), phobias and Hamilton anxiety (other measures were not reported)."

In summary, the FDA Xanax study really shows that most patients were better off if they had never taken the drug. None of this is obvious in reading the actual study by James C. Ballenger and his colleagues.[14] In the introductory abstract, no mention is made of Xanax's effect be-

---

*Studies for official FDA approval are supervised by the FDA, but they are paid for and carried out by the pharmaceutical firm with investigators of its own choosing. See chapter 15 for some of the implications of this arrangement.

yond four weeks. And yet the abstract describes the drug as an unqualified success.

Faced with their own negative results, the Xanax investigators came up with statistical manipulations to show how the data really *should have*—but didn't—come out at eight weeks; but apparently they were embarrassed by these efforts, and they limited the summary and conclusion of their report to data from the first four weeks. As noted, the drug company, with whom they were working closely, followed suit.

In their lengthy critique of the study in the *Archives of General Psychiatry*, Marks and his colleagues point out that a few weeks of relief is hardly worth the consequences of withdrawal and worsening symptoms, especially when the patients had been suffering from anxiety problems for an average of nearly nine years.

Furthermore, they point out that any hoped-for benefit must be balanced against known and unknown dangers of long-term use, including the possibility (see ahead) of brain shrinkage from chronic benzodiazepine use.

Marks and his colleagues summarize, "The unqualified conclusions about efficacy based solely on short-term partial gains in a chronic condition seems biased and arguable."

More Problems with the Xanax Study

As discussed in chapter 8, most people think that FDA drug trials extend for many months or years rather than a few weeks. According to Ballenger and his colleagues, most psychiatrists were giving Xanax for a period of three months to a year before tapering or discontinuing it. Yet Upjohn itself limited its data analysis on efficacy to a mere four weeks. It merits reemphasis: FDA approval does not mean that the drug has been tested with controlled studies for anywhere near the length of time that it typically is prescribed by doctors.

The size of the sample is also a problem, especially in regard to testing for negative side effects. While most people think that FDA-approved drugs have been tested on thousands or tens of thousands of patients, the actual sample size is described in Upjohn advertisements as "more than 500 patients." In fact, only 226 patients took Xanax for the length of the main study.[15] That is hardly a sufficient number to test for relatively infrequent but potentially serious side effects. For example, a side effect that causes death in 0.5 percent of drug patients could easily escape showing up in such a small sample, but it would kill five thousand of the first one million people to take the drug. And, of course, a side effect that doesn't appear until after eight weeks would be missed completely.

Xanax's addictive effects became a serious problem even during short, eight-week trials. J. C. Pecknold and his associates found that even a gradual four-week period of withdrawal did not prevent a "worsening of symptoms" and that "some, in fact most, patients experienced relapse."[16] Thirty-five percent of the patients had "mild to moderate" withdrawal symptoms. Thus after only two months of treatment, a large percentage of the patients were becoming addicted to the drug.

The warning given by Upjohn for Xanax in the 1991 *PDR* states: "If benzodiazepines are used in large doses and/or for extended periods of time, they may produce habituation and emotional and physical dependence." However, the data actually indicate that physical dependence very frequently develops *without* "large doses" and *before* "extended" periods of treatment.* Furthermore, there is no hint in the *PDR* that Xanax is *especially* addictive.

Writing in *The New Harvard Guide to Psychiatry*, George Vaillant indicates that the public is unaware of the addictive qualities of minor tranquilizers, including Xanax: "Contrary to popular belief, physical dependence on diazepam (Valium), chlordiazepoxide (Librium) and especially alprazolam (Xanax) does occur" (p. 711). Because the public is relatively ignorant of the problem and because Xanax is "especially" likely to addict, Upjohn should have made the danger as emphatically clear as possible.

Pecknold and his colleagues recommend that treatment with Xanax be *routinely extended for six months*, to be followed by very slow withdrawal. This adds up to a minimum period of treatment approaching one year. In short, the authors recommend many months of treatment for a drug whose beneficial effect over a placebo was shown to decline to nothing at eight weeks! Furthermore, as Pecknold and associates admit, the increased length of treatment could be expected to worsen the addiction and withdrawal problems. A genuine concern for the patients should have led these investigators to the *opposite* recommendation: that in order to avoid withdrawal and addiction, the drug should be used for *very short* periods of time (such as a few days) or not at all.

Xanax as Alcohol in a Pill

The similarity between Xanax and any other addictive sedative, including alcohol, was verified in the FDA studies.† Russell Noyes, Jr., and his

---

*Also see the discussion of addiction, tolerance, and withdrawal symptoms earlier in the chapter.
† Also see the discussion earlier in the chapter concerning the similarity between the symptoms of alcohol withdrawal and those of minor tranquilizer withdrawal.

associates report that 61.7 percent of the subjects suffered from sedation during the first week and that by the last week 38.7 percent were still aware of the effect.[17] At some time during the treatment, 77 percent reported "at least mild sedation."[18] Clinical experience with alcoholism and drug addiction, as well as the Golombok study of minor tranquilizers, indicates that people taking sedatives tend to deny their drug-induced sedation. People who are sedated often do not appreciate that they are thinking more slowly, getting muddled, forgetting things, slurring their words, or losing their coordination. As almost everyone has noticed at parties where people get "drunk," or from TV and radio ads encouraging us to take the car keys away from our inebriated friends, denial of impairment is *typical* of people experiencing sedation. It is virtually certain that the patients on Xanax were far more sedated than they reported.

In addition to sedation, other "drunken" symptoms were commonly reported by the patients, including ataxia (muscular incoordination), fatigue, slurred speech, and amnesia.

One wonders how the drug would have compared to alcohol, rather than to an inactive placebo,* in its "beneficial" and its toxic side effects.

In another study, after only six days' use, Xanax was found to cause sufficient memory problems to potentially impair educational learning.[19] The investigators warned against taking Xanax before school examinations.

How did Xanax get such an edge on the other benzodiazepines, first by taking the lead in the market and then by becoming the first drug approved for panic disorder? Apparently not on the basis of scientific studies, which show that Xanax is ineffective beyond four weeks, frequently produces sedation and mental dysfunction, and often causes withdrawal problems. In chapter 15 we shall examine how Upjohn's financial support of the psychiatric profession may have influenced the drug's acceptance.

Is There Any "Therapeutic Role" for the Minor Tranquilizers?

Don't people have a right to escape anxiety at times? To use shortcuts if necessary, including sedative drugs? Yes, they surely do. But should doctors encourage this approach to life? I don't think so, except under the most limited circumstances. Because people cannot obtain minor tranquilizers without a doctor's prescription, I don't fault physicians who occasionally prescribe them to help patients get through a difficult few

---

*For a discussion of the need for active or enhanced placebo, see chapter 8.

days or to get a good night's sleep; but their usefulness for more than a few days is highly questionable. Even the prodrug literature has not been able to show a beneficial impact beyond a few weeks, when tolerance and withdrawal symptoms develop.

Minor tranquilizers, like any sedative, can be harmful in the long run not only because they are habit-forming and addictive, but because they cover up anxiety by suppressing the capacity of the brain to generate feelings. The brain, as usual, tries to overcome the suppression and reacts in ways we cannot begin to predict or fully comprehend. As we have seen, drug-induced rebound anxiety is one common effect.

The drugged individual with a suppressed and confused anxiety signal system lives under a considerable handicap. At the least, feelings are pushed down, and with that, self-awareness is muted. More seriously, as the brain reacts against the drug, natural anxiety responses are muted but abnormal rebound anxiety reactions begin to flare up.

What about people who are so overwhelmed by anxiety that they cannot cope at all?

The doctor who offers medication is likely to reinforce the patient's feelings of helplessness. If psychotherapy is being attempted, the drug-induced insensitivity to self can inhibit progress. When a patient has an acute anxiety attack in the midst of a psychotherapy session, for example, it's prime time for understanding the problem and showing the patient various ways to handle it.

Without drugs, severely anxious patients often can be helped rather quickly to overcome the worst of their anguish (see chapter 10). Over a longer period they can learn new approaches to living relatively free of anxiety.

But success in psychotherapy is not guaranteed. Failure may result from a faulty delivery of therapy or from a poorly motivated client, or from a bad "chemistry" between client and therapist. Whatever the cause of the failure, what about drugs as an alternative?

I would rather urge a client to try another therapist, or several other therapists, as well as other approaches, such as group therapy, self-help groups, self-help books, self-hypnosis, relaxation techniques, deep massage, or meditation and other spiritual exercises, rather than to turn to drugs.

Improvement while on drugs is rarely a psychologically clean affair; the improvement almost always leaves an aftermath of persistent personal helplessness. The individual is unable to say with confidence, "I overcame my anxiety and I know how I did it." There is always the lingering suspicion that "the drugs did it."

Even prescribing medications on an occasional basis can interfere with and undermine the real work of psychotherapy.

After a session, a client called me in the evening to request a telephone prescription for a few minor tranquilizers.

"What's up?" I asked.

"Sorry to bother you, Peter. I can't sleep. I just want something to sleep for a few nights."

"How come you didn't bring it up in the session today?" I asked.

"Hey, Doc, you were hardly listening to me today. You seemed in another world yourself."

In an instant I knew he was right. I'd received distressing news by telephone moments before his session, and without realizing it at the time, I hadn't shaken off the effect.

"Thanks for telling me," I said. "If you can come in tomorrow morning, I'll give you a free session to make up for it."

"It's a deal. And forget the drugs. Good-night."

If I had readily acquiesced to the request for a prescription, the patient's real feelings never would have surfaced. Giving drugs runs the risk of distracting from the work of psychotherapy, not only for the client but for the therapist.

Scientific Studies of Efficacy

By now, I hope, the reader will approach the question of "scientific studies" in psychiatry with a large measure of skepticism, and even cynicism. In regard to the minor tranquilizers, there are some blanket endorsements, such as this one from the American Psychiatric Press's *Textbook of Psychiatry*: "The efficacy of the benzodiazepines in the treatment of anxiety, including the symptoms of worry, psychic anxiety, and somatic symptoms (gastrointestinal and cardiovascular), has been clearly and repeatedly demonstrated in many well-controlled studies" (p. 810). On the other hand, there is a detailed review of the literature by Ronald Lipman in Seymour Fisher and Roger Greenberg's *The Limits of Biological Treatments for Psychological Distress* (1989). Lipman finds that, except for the very short-term treatment of generalized anxiety, there is little evidence for the efficacy of these medications. Most reviews suggest that use should be short term and that long-term use is generally dangerous and unwarranted.

Like a growing number of professionals, Lipman actually finds the tricyclic antidepressants to be of somewhat more value than the minor tranquilizers in treating a number of manifestations of anxiety. As already expressed, I have little confidence and much concern about the antidepressants; but after so many years of professionals pushing the minor tranquilizers for anxiety, it is darkly comical to see them turn in frustration to the antidepressants instead.

Authority and Helplessness

That the drugs encourage helplessness and dependency on the physician seems apparent. In *The New Harvard Guide to Psychiatry*, two of the nation's leading psychopharmacologists, Ross Baldessarini and Jonathan Cole, make these observations:

Favorable patient response to antianxiety agents has been associated with lack of psychological sophistication and inability to express unhappiness verbally in terms of intrapsychic or interpersonal conflict; a favorable response also tends to occur in patients with passive and almost magical expectations of the physician. An enthusiastic, charismatic presentation of the medication and its sedative effects by the physician also seems to help. (P. 524)

When drugs are of questionable efficacy and possess serious drawbacks, such as the potential for addiction, one must wonder whether informed consent is incompatible with an "enthusiastic, charismatic presentation."

Anafranil

The antidepressant Anafranil (clomipramine) was approved by the FDA for use in obsessive-compulsive behavior in January 1990. Except for the addition of a chloride radical, this drug is identical in chemical structure to the old-fashioned tricyclic antidepressant Tofranil. It has received a great deal of media hype, including TV specials. Lipman's review indicates that it is of marginal value. Moreover, a 1987 study by W. O. Montiero and others in the *British Journal of Psychiatry* shows a very high rate of interference with orgasm. It can cause a variety of side effects, including dry mouth, sedation, difficulty urinating, weight gain, dizziness, seizures, as well as others that are typical of tricyclic antidepressants (see chapter 8).

Beta Blockers

The use of beta blockers is routine in certain cardiovascular diseases, but it is more speculative in the treatment of anxiety, based largely on the inhibition of the cardiovascular symptoms associated with anxiety, especially increased heart rate and palpitations. These medications also can have a sedativelike effect, dampening emotional responsiveness. My patients who have withdrawn from them sometimes feel considerably more clearheaded. Beta blockers are known to cause depression and, rarely, hallucinations, and may combine adversely with other drugs, including lithium. They can cause memory impairment.

Beta blockers—beta-adrenergic blocking agents—include propranolol (Inderal, Detensol, Novopranol), nadolol (Corgard), metoprolol (Lopressor, Betaloc), oxprenolol (Trasicor), timolol (Blocadren) and acebutolol (Sectral).

The Biology of Anxiety

The biological basis for anxiety overwhelm is so flimsy that one recent textbook, *The New Harvard Guide to Psychiatry*, gives it only a paragraph and labels the exclusively biological approach "an extreme theoretical position that fails to take psychological facts into account." The American Psychiatric Press *Textbook of Psychiatry* does discuss various biological hypotheses as "promising," but it endorses none in particular. The 1989 *Comprehensive Textbook of Psychiatry* makes clear that the data are preliminary, conclusions are tentative, and no biological cause for anxiety has been determined. Each textbook devotes much more space to psychological explanations. Nonetheless, biopsychiatrists have staked out a biology of anxiety in the popular press and mass market books.

On April 28, 1990, NIMH director Lewis Judd told the Southern California Psychiatric Society that anxiety is now known to be a genetic and biological disorder.

Inspired by NIMH, a flurry of newspaper and TV feature stories in recent years have reported that infusions of lactic acid produce anxiety in panic-prone individuals, presumably suggesting a similar mechanism within the body. One national TV news exposé show displayed no skepticism whatsoever when a lactate infusion experiment showed a woman having a panic attack on cue.

Infusions of lactic acid sometimes can produce heart palpitations and probably other feelings of uneasiness, similar to those during an anxiety attack, leading an individual to feel *as if* he or she is getting anxious; but there is no evidence that the production of lactate in the body has anything to do with causing anxiety.

When I wrote a review and analysis entitled "The Psychophysiology of Anxiety," published in the December 1964 *Journal of Nervous and*

*Mental Disease,** I pointed out that even an infusion of adrenaline by itself cannot produce anxiety. People who *fear anxiety* may develop anxiety in response to infusions of adrenaline, while people who do not fear anxiety will observe merely that their hearts are pounding or that their hands are trembling. Large doses of adrenaline, injected into asthmatic patients during medical emergencies, typically produce relief of anxiety, because the patient anticipates or experiences relief of the asthma attack. In the lactate experiments, the panic-prone individuals probably reacted with anxiety to the experimental situation and to cardiac symptoms produced by the lactate. Perhaps they also were fulfilling the expectations of the experimenters in front of the TV cameras.

The Biology of Obsessions and Compulsions

As already described, obsessions and compulsions usually are classified among anxiety disorders, although they can occur in response to guilt and shame as well.

Judith Rapoport, chief of child psychiatry at NIMH and the author of *The Boy Who Wouldn't Stop Washing* (1989), strongly supports the biological viewpoint. In an interview in the March 13, 1989, *People* magazine Rapoport says of obsessive-compulsive disorder (OCD), "It is like a short circuit in the brain. . . ." There are, of course, no short circuits in the brain. Its "circuitry" cannot be compared to house wiring.

In the March 1989 *Scientific American* Rapoport argues that obsessions and compulsions are caused by a defect in the basal ganglia and frontal lobes. By now the words *frontal lobe* and *basal ganglia* may be familiar to the reader (chapter 4). Rapoport would have contributed equally to our knowledge had she said, "I believe the *brain* has something to do with the mind and therefore with obsessions and compulsions."

In her book *The Boy Who Wouldn't Stop Washing*, Rapoport suggests that Anafranil has been found effective in treating some obsessive-compulsive behavior—a conclusion we have already seen challenged. Since Anafranil affects serotonin metabolism, Rapoport further suggests that serotonin is involved in the biology of obsessions and compulsions.

---

*These theoretical formulations on the psychophysiology of anxiety, developed in medical school and published shortly thereafter, have been recently confirmed by David Barlow in *Anxiety and Its Disorders* (New York: Guilford Press, 1988). He states, "Breggin's general impressions are receiving substantial experimental support, as described below in some detail" (p. 116), and Breggin's "psychobiological model, now over 20 years old, still accommodates the laboratory provocation data to a degree that no unidimensional psychological or biological model can attain" (p. 157; see also p. 152). Barlow does note that details have to be modified in keeping with new data. Also see Peter Breggin, "The Sedative-like Effect of Adrenaline," *Archives of General Psychiatry* 12: 255–59, 1965.

But brain cells using serotonin are found in all regions of the brain, especially in the emotion-regulating limbic system and frontal lobes. Of course, serotonin is involved in the obsessive-compulsive process. It's involved in *every mental and emotional process* (see the discussion of Prozac in chapter 8).

Besides, as already discussed, it's impossible to reason backward from a drug *effect* to a brain *defect*. Psychoactive drugs, from alcohol to neuroleptics, exert their impact on normal brain function. Their calming or suppressive effects on emotions have nothing to do with any prior brain abnormality.

Studies that show abnormalities on brain scans in people diagnosed as obsessive-compulsive suffer from all of the problems discussed in regard to schizophrenia (see chapter 4). Most of the patients are severely emotionally handicapped, often with severe depression, and therefore have been treated with a variety of drugs, including antidepressants and neuroleptics.[20] It is most likely that findings of pathology, often located in the striatum, are the result of antidepressant or neuroleptic treatment, or of polydrug therapy with a variety of agents.

Reviving the Menace of Psychosurgery

Speaking of lobotomy, Rapoport says in her book, "I have yet to send a patient for such treatment, but the success of these operations fascinates me because the procedures sever connections in parts of the brain that our brain-imaging studies find abnormal in OCD. This is another clue to the biology of this sickness" (*The Boy Who Wouldn't Stop Washing*, p. 16).* Of course, it's no clue at all; lobotomy is a nonspecific blunting operation (see chapter 3). It also was used on "schizophrenic" people, depressed people, violent people, sexually aggressive criminals, people with chronic pain, alcoholics, and dying cancer patients. And it will blunt animals as well as people.

At the APA's annual meeting, reported in the July 1989 *Clinical Psychiatric News*, Rapoport again raised the possibility of psychosurgery. Going directly to the public in her *People* magazine interview, she describes a man who was lobotomized in 1960:

The procedure is far less common today and would only be considered if every other possible treatment had failed. It cured his OCD, but unfortunately, because the surgery was not as sophisticated 20 years ago as it is

---

* Rapoport also discusses lobotomy on pp. 8–9.

now, he suffered personality changes and began pinching young women and urinating in the street.

So the chief of child psychiatry at NIMH, in professional and public forums, is lending credence to lobotomy, albeit only if "every other possible treatment had failed." That's how lobotomy has always been promoted; but since there are so many "failures" in psychiatry, there will be no shortage of victims available for lobotomy. As documented in chapter 3, her remark that the brain-mutilating surgery is relatively safe nowadays is simply not true.

The promotion of psychosurgery for obsessive-compulsive disorders seems to be taking hold. It rears up in some textbooks and most recently in the April 1990 *Harvard Medical School Health Letter*. Michael Jenike, director of the Obsessive-Compulsive Disorder Clinic and Research Unit at the Massachusetts General Hospital, speaks highly of psychosurgery, specifically an operation called cingulotomy, which electrically melts nerve connections to the frontal lobes. He says, "There is a growing body of evidence that these people will benefit from a precisely localized brain surgery." He does not hint at the inevitable damage to the brain and mind.

I have followed the cingulotomy operations performed at the Massachusetts General Hospital for twenty years.*[21] Indeed, the main surgeon, H. T. Ballantine, recently retired after performing hundreds of them, mostly on women. He did not limit himself to so-called obsessive-compulsives, but even operated on a patient with chronic back pain. There is nothing new about these operations, and they have always been reported in the literature by the surgeons as virtually harmless. Psychosurgeon Ballantine actually claims that his operations had no effect on the mind, adverse or otherwise. As if talking about a subtle intervention that did not coagulate brain tissue with hot electrodes, he opines that the operation corrected biochemical imbalances.

I have now interviewed and studied the records of five of Ballantine's psychosurgery patients as well as patients operated on by other surgeons. All of the patients have lobotomy syndromes, with disabling degrees of mental dysfunction. Of Ballantine's patients, the four who can speak are very bitter about what was done to them. Since the operation, the one who no longer can speak has displayed fear of every doctor who comes

---

* My international campaign in the 1970s to stop lobotomy and other forms of psychosurgery is described, albeit from a negative viewpoint, in Rael Jean Isaac and Virginia Armat, *Madness in the Streets* (New York: Free Press, 1990). I have not written extensively about my reform work, but Isaac and Armat, while attempting to defend lobotomy and to portray my efforts in a negative light, devote a chapter to my success in stopping most of the psychiatric surgery performed in the United States.

near her. She was reduced to a state of severe, chronic mental deterioration (dementia) following the psychosurgery.

I am concerned about so many recent public remarks in favor of psychosurgery by high-ranking psychiatrists. It seems aimed at laying the groundwork for resuming psychosurgery in full force at NIMH, Harvard, and elsewhere. This would reverse the accomplishments of the past decade, which brought most psychosurgery in the country to a halt.

Children and Their Parents

Rapoport's radical biological theories will appeal to those who cannot bear to face their own self-destructive mental processes. Her views also will appeal to some parents who don't wish to believe that they have had anything to do with their offsprings' problems. In her book, Rapoport announces with emphasis a "great piece of news" for parents and sufferers alike: "*It May Not Be Your Fault That You Or Your Child Has Obsessive-Compulsive Disorder!*" (p. 39). This is great news only if you'd rather not take *any* personal responsibility for your own problems or those of your children.

In the next two chapters we shall see how far psychiatry has gone in blaming child-victims for their own problems while exonerating parents, schools, and other authorities. Unfortunately, Rapoport's views are part of an overall NIMH strategy that aligns itself with the parents and custodians rather than with the patients themselves, who are often in conflict with their parents and custodians. It is very dangerous when physicians fail to ally themselves with their patients, and it is even more dangerous when they ally themselves with the parents of mental patients. Too often these parents are angry and frustrated with their offspring.

Obsessions and Compulsions in Brain-Damaged People

There is a relationship between brain disease and increased obsessions and compulsions, but it's the opposite of the one suggested by contemporary biopsychiatrists. Since the early work of Kurt Goldstein (for example, *Human Nature*, published in 1944), clinicians have observed that patients develop obsessive-compulsive tendencies after they have been brain-damaged by war injuries, auto accidents, and psychiatric treatments, such as lobotomy. I also have seen it happen after electroshock. Faced with increased helplessness in dealing with the world, the brain-injured person attempts to control inner anxiety and the outer environment alike with repetitive rituals. Everything must be put in the right place, no routines may be changed, plans must be reviewed again and again, simple ideas must be repeated over and over, reassurance about irrational worries will be asked for endlessly.

It's unlikely that the obsessive-compulsive behavior is directly caused by the injury. More likely it is a psychological defense aimed at increasing the individual's sense of security in the face of reduced mental function. This is confirmed by the fact that heavy reliance on obsessions and compulsions can be seen at both ends of the age spectrum, in childhood and in old age. A small child getting ready for bed often needs a fixed ritual with no deviations in order to handle bedtime without too much anxiety or insomnia. Many young children go through periods of time when everything in their room must be in its proper place before going to bed. Similarly, the elderly become more set in their routines and more focused on controlling small details of their daily activities: when and what they eat, when they go to the bathroom, when they visit with people, what they watch on TV or read, when they go to bed, how they arrange their possessions. Often their communications become compulsively repetitive.

In the normal childhood, there's no reason to believe that brain damage or malfunction plays any role in the frequent tendency toward obsessions and compulsions. In old age, the loss of mental acuity and other physical infirmities affecting the mind and the body increase the individual's sense of helplessness and dependence, encouraging reliance on obsessions and compulsions to give a semblance of control over one's life.

Obsessions and compulsions also are apt to occur or to worsen at times of severe stress. People subjected to constant stress, such as athletes, are notorious for their rituals. So are soldiers at the front. In ordinary life, obsessive-compulsive problems rear up when a frightening decision is at hand, such as choosing a new career direction or deciding to get married.

Genetic Studies

Despite all the hopes for finding a genetic basis of anxiety disorders, none has been demonstrated. A remarkable headline in the December 4, 1987, *Psychiatric Times* reads GENETIC FINDINGS. The story begins with the statement, "A study in the November *Archives of General Psychiatry* offers preliminary evidence that panic disorder may be caused by a gene on chromosome 16." Toward the end of the brief report it is admitted that the finding was "not statistically significant," but that the investigators believe that more research is warranted. Donald Goodwin, in *Anxiety* (1986), was reduced to pointing to differences in fearfulness among animals and to one unidentified study of identical twins supposedly showing that they have a similar degree of fear of strangers. Some studies do show a familial pattern for certain anxiety problems, but this is not surprising. Psychotherapists typically find that anxious patients have learned their emotional reactions in part, at least, from their parents.

Anxiety sometimes can be *temporarily* alleviated by a variety of sedative drugs, including minor tranquilizers, barbiturates, opiates, alcohol, and perhaps antidepressants. But the effects are short-lived, with little or no evidence for sustained relief, and the hazards are considerable, including addiction, withdrawal reactions, rebound anxiety, mental dysfunction, and lethality.

Even if these drugs were more effective or safer, should physicians prescribe them for the relief of anxiety? Few psychiatrists would keep a pitcher of martinis at hand in the office to ease the anxiety of their patients; yet most are willing to reach into the drawer for a sample of "alcohol in a pill," the minor tranquilizers. Both alcohol and minor tranquilizers accomplish the same thing—a brief escape from intense feelings by suppressing or sedating normal brain function.

It is understandable that some people want to try to handle their problems through psychiatric or recreational drugs, but should doctors endorse this dangerous and self-defeating avenue as a form of medical treatment? As physicians or psychotherapists we should empower our patients to trust themselves and their capacity to triumph over frightening emotions. We should help them overcome anxiety through self-understanding, improved self-control of their minds and actions, more courageous attitudes, and more successful principles of living.

Part IV

Women, Children, the Homeless, and the Psycho- Pharmaceutical Complex

Abandoning Responsibility for Our Children: A Critique of Hyperactivity, Attention Deficit Disorder, Learning Disabilities, Dyslexia, Autism, and Other Diagnoses

Children have more need of models than of critics.
                    —*Joseph Joubert (1754–1822)*

The wildest colts make the best horses.
                    —*Themistocles (524?–460?* B.C.*)*

Considering the joylessness of many schools with their authoritarian structures, it is fair to speculate that hyperactivity may be a "normal" response—indeed, even a healthy reaction—to an intolerable situation.[1]
                    —*J. Larry Brown and Stephen R. Bing (1976)*

It is easy to substitute our will for that of the child by means of suggestion or coercion; but when we have done this we have robbed him of his greatest right, the right to construct his own personality.
                    —*Maria Montessori (1870–1952)*

Nothing measures the quality of a society better than how it treats its children. Nothing predicts the future of a society better than how it nurtures and educates its children. In America today, children as a group are in trouble, and psychiatry is moving in to take over.

The Discarded Child

A 1990 report from the House Select Committee on Children, Youth and Families finds that the "discarded child" population has reached 500,000 and will soon grow to 850,000. These are children who live in detention centers, hospitals, foster homes, and mental health facilities. In many cities children are being born with drug addiction or AIDS, and many newborns are abandoned as "boarder babies" in hospitals. The root causes of discarded children are identified by the House committee as alcohol and drug abuse, homelessness, family breakup, poverty, and child abuse. Notice that none of these identified causes lie within the child in the form of genetic defects or biochemical imbalances.

The Child of Poverty

Driven by increasing poverty among the poorest of the poor and by the decreasing availability of low-cost housing, more and more families have been driven into the streets. It is estimated that up to one-quarter of the homeless are children. According to a 1990 report from the Columbia University National Center for Children in Poverty, five million children under six live in poverty. That's almost one in four children.

Child Abuse and Neglect*

Reported figures on child abuse reveal only the tip of the iceberg. Even so, they are tragic. As summarized by Richard Gelles and Claire Cornell in *Intimate Violence in Families* (1990), 16 percent of children undergo some form of maltreatment each year, including abuse and neglect of a physical, sexual, or emotional nature. During 1987 over two million children were reported to state agencies for suspected neglect and abuse.

The latest survey discloses 2.4 million suspected neglect and abuse cases in 1989.[2] The U.S. Advisory Board on Child Abuse and Neglect declares, "Each year, hundreds of thousands of children are being starved, abandoned, burned and severely beaten, raped and sodomized, berated and belittled," often by members of the family. Child maltreatment is strongly correlated with poverty. It was seven times more likely to occur in families with an income of under $15,000.

* My concerns about these issues have led me to teach a course entitled "Interpersonal Conflict: The Male Abuse of Women and Children" at the Institute for Conflict Analysis and Resolution at George Mason University in Fairfax, Virginia.

Physical violence is rampant. Surveys indicate that about one in ten children is subjected to serious violence each year. Between twelve hundred and five thousand children a year die from abuse.

A recent state-of-the-art survey indicates that 38 percent of women were sexually abused as children. In *Secret Survivors* (1990), E. Sue Blume suggests that the true rates must be even higher, because people tend to repress their childhood memories of sexual abuse and therefore cannot report them to interviewers (see chapter 12). While men report much lower rates, they typically are more ashamed of admitting to sexual victimization. Convicted pederasts often confess to molesting more boys than girls.

Increasing numbers of children live in single-parent homes. Thirteen percent of white and 43 percent of black families are headed by a woman, and one-third live in poverty. Many other children are latchkey kids, with two working parents. Most people concerned with family life in America find that the modern family produces many stresses for its children.

A survey of seventeen thousand parents conducted for the National Center for Health Statistics (1990) found that one in five children have emotional problems largely attributable to the breakup of the two-parent family. The most frequently troubled children are those who "experience parental divorce, were born outside of marriage, or are raised in conflict-filled families or low-income, low-education, single-parent households."[3] They also cite possible contributions from the increasing survival of low-birth-weight babies, environmental contamination, and crack-addicted mothers.

The Schools

During the 1960s the schools of the nation were subjected to scorching criticism from many sources. Social critic Paul Goodman spoke of "compulsory mis-education" and former teacher John Holt asked, "Why can't Johnny read?" In 1967 and 1968, as a full-time consultant in mental health and education at NIMH, I was aware of a widely recognized crisis in education.

Reform never took hold in the schools. More than two decades later, in June 1989 and then in January 1990, reports continue to confirm the escalating failure. The first was issued by the Carnegie Council on Adolescent Development and the second by the Massachusetts Institute of Technology on the problem of minority education. They are in substantial agreement, and I'll focus on the more comprehensive one, the Carnegie report, *Turning Points: Preparing American Youth for the 21st*

Century. It deals with the middle schools, where students entering their adolescence are educated. The council included business leaders, governors, university presidents and deans, school superintendents, and professors from many fields.

The Carnegie Council found that seven million youths, one in four adolescents, are "extremely vulnerable to multiple high-risk behaviors and school failure," and that another seven million are "at moderate risk, but remain a cause for serious concern." It points to dramatic changes and new pressures confronting young people, including sexual promiscuity, drugs, the breakdown of social relationships in the community, and a lack of adult guidance.

The report declares that the schools too often contribute to the problems of the students:

A volatile mismatch exists between the organization and curriculum of middle grade schools and the intellectual and emotional needs of young adolescents. Caught in a vortex of changing demands, the engagement of many youth in learning diminishes, and their rates of alienation, substance abuse, absenteeism, and dropping out of school begin to rise.

Wholly unlike the psychiatric analyses we shall examine, the report is very critical of the schools:

Many large middle grade schools function as mills that contain and process endless streams of students. Within them are masses of anonymous youth. . . . Such settings virtually guarantee that the intellectual and emotional needs of youth will go unmet.

The Carnegie Council makes several recommendations for transforming the schools, among them the creation of small communities of learning within the larger schools, a better core curriculum, greater attention to the students' actual educational needs, the availability of at least one concerned adult to take a special interest in each child, and the involvement of families and communities in education. My concern, however, is not with supporting one or another reform program, but with drawing attention to the society-wide stresses placed on today's children.

Making Trouble for Teachers

Given the sorry state of our schools, it is no surprise that making trouble for teachers is the single most important reason that children get referred for psychological and psychiatric help. The September 1989 *Clinical*

Psychiatry News cites a Duke University study demonstrating that "the amount of trouble that children are causing adults, particularly teachers, appears to be the driving force determining children's referrals to mental health services." It was noted without comment that most of the children referred were "black, male, and poor."

The schools have provided the mental health professions with the entering wedge for turning a large proportion of children into involuntary psychiatric consumers.

Recognizing the Effects of Neglect and Abuse

When I volunteered in nursery schools as a young parent, it was easy to pair up the most disturbed pupils with their parents merely by sizing up the parents as they came to pick up their children. Most children who display serious psychological or social difficulties are having serious problems at home in the form of severe conflicts between the parents or of abuse and neglect. It's usually so obvious that fifth or sixth graders are likely to put it together. "Oh, yeah, Jimmy's parents are getting divorced, that's why he's so weird right now," or "Sure Joanie's freaked out; you should see her parents." But much of the abuse to which children are subjected goes unnoticed outside the family and denied within it.

A variety of popular books vividly make the connection between childhood neglect and abuse and subsequent emotional problems in children and adults. Some that are good reading and easy to obtain are Jane Middleton-Moz's *Children of Trauma* (1989), John Bradshaw's *Healing the Shame that Binds You* (1988), Pia Mellody's *Facing Codependency* (1989), Susan Forward's *Toxic Parents* (1989), and E. Sue Blume's *Secret Survivors* (1990). Alice Miller's *For Your Own Good* (1983) is now a classic, and my own *Psychology of Freedom* (1980) also links abuse to psychological problems in children and adults.

The growing public awareness of the importance of child abuse comes at exactly the moment that biopsychiatry is trying to reverse the trend by fixing the problem within the genetics and biology of the child.

The Psychological Effects on Children of Abuse and Neglect

A growing body of psychological research confirms the obvious—that troubled families raise a high percentage of troubled children, who go on to become troubled adults.[4] In a professional book called *Children of*

Battered Women (1990), Peter Jaffe and his colleagues review scientific studies demonstrating that "physical, emotional, and sexual abuse" produce children who typically get labeled with psychiatric or school-related diagnoses. Cognitive and emotional problems in children are caused not only by direct abuse, but by witnessing violence and by typical "marital discord, separation, and divorce."[5] In *The Creation of Dangerous Violent Criminals* (1989), Lonnie Athens dramatically describes the family and group indoctrination that produces the extreme of "insanity," the dangerous maniac who severely brutalizes other human beings.

A chapter entitled "Physical and Sexual Abuse of Children," by psychiatrist Arthur H. Green in the *Comprehensive Textbook of Psychiatry* (1989), discloses that all commonly diagnosed disorders of childhood can be linked to abuse and neglect. These include not only the traditional diagnoses, such as depression and anxiety, but popular school-related ones, such as attention deficit disorder (ADD), or the newer attention-deficit hyperactivity disorder (ADHD),* and a variety of so-called learning disorders (LD). Green describes in detail how "pathological object relations" (avoidance and withdrawal from people), "poor self-concept and depression," and "impaired impulse control" can result from abuse. Abuse and neglect produces "difficulties in school," such as "cognitive impairment, particularly in the areas of speech and language, combined with limited attention span and hyperactivity." Furthermore he writes, "These children frequently demonstrate specific learning disabilities, such as dyslexia, expressive and receptive language disorders, and perceptual-motor problems." In short, the whole spectrum of so-called psychiatric and psychological disorders in children can be traced to child abuse and neglect, including the latest school-related fad diagnoses.

More startling, Green summarizes research indicating that the brain damage and dysfunction occasionally found in children also are related to child abuse. While the biopsychiatrist latches onto any hint of brain damage in order to point the finger at a defect in the child, someone wishing to help a child should be willing to look to the conduct of the parents and other potential abusers in the child's environment.†

Not only do biopsychiatrists working with children tend to deny these obvious conclusions, so do the other psychiatric contributors to the same *Comprehensive Textbook of Psychiatry*. Chapter after chapter is written about one or another "disorder" in children and adults, without connecting them in any way to childhood experiences of any kind. As if the

---

*The *DSM-III-R* (1987) combines attention deficit disorder with hyperactivity to form one diagnostic category, attention-deficit hyperactivity disorder. The distinction is not critical for this chapter.
†Also see chapter 6 on depression and chapter 14 on women for research substantiating the importance of childhood trauma.

reality behind Green's chapter did not exist, child abuse typically goes unmentioned. Instead, the so-called disorders are linked to unproven but presumed biochemical and genetic defects.

Psychiatry Offers to Fill the Void

The mental health professions, led by psychiatry, have rushed into the void left by the default of the family, the schools, the society, and the government. Recently NIMH announced that 20 percent of children need psychiatric care! In another pronouncement NIMH estimated that by 1990 one million children would be taking the drug Ritalin, an addictive substance used to manage difficult children with various diagnoses. Whether or not NIMH's figures reflect an actual escalation of problems among children, they unquestionably indicate the psychiatric establishment's voracious appetite for children.

In blaming the child-victim, psychiatry takes the pressure off the parents, the family, the schools, and the society. By diagnosing, drugging, and hospitalizing children, psychiatry enforces the worst attitudes toward children in our culture today and exonerates those adult institutions that need reform.

Psychiatry has been joined by factions within behavioral and educational psychology in exonerating the schools and blaming the children. The question asked by John Holt, "Why can't Johnny read?" has been answered, "Because he has a learning disability."

We shall look first at the movement to label children ADD and hyperactive and to drug them. It originated largely out of medicine and psychiatry. Then we shall look at the LD movement, spawned mostly by psychology but now adopted by psychiatry as well.

Andy: A Hyperactive Child

A nationally known psychiatrist affiliated with NIMH already had diagnosed ten-year-old Andy as having attention deficit disorder, indicating that he suffered from an inherent and presumably genetic and biological difficulty in focusing his attention on school work. He had no trouble focusing on video games, sports, and other things that interested him. Because he fidgeted, squirmed, and looked nervous in school, Andy also was diagnosed as hyperactive.

The NIMH expert had prescribed Ritalin for Andy. Andy's mother, aghast at the idea of medicating her child, had come to me for a second opinion.

Following a consultation with the parents, they dropped Andy off at my office for us to get acquainted.

"He's like a bull in a china shop," his father warned me as he left. "That kid will break everything you own."

I took my son's cockatiel, Sydney, out of his cage to introduce him to Andy, and abruptly he flew onto Andy's shoulder and began nipping the boy's ear. Sydney is three times the size of a parakeet and when he bites, he can draw blood.

Andy didn't move. With exquisite self-control, he tolerated Sydney's directness in getting acquainted. Following my instructions exactly, Andy then raised his finger to Sydney's chest, endured a few pecks on his knuckle, stroked the bird's belly, and gently lifted him onto his finger.

Outside at the old picnic table Andy explained to me that he got along fine with his mother, except he didn't listen to her very well. He couldn't explain why he gave her such a hard time. He said he didn't think his dad loved him. School was just plain boring. "Gruesome" and "d-u-m-b" was his way of putting it.

Sitting there in the sunshine with this wonderful youngster, the idea of putting toxic drugs into his brain appalled me.

Over the next few months, I rarely asked to see Andy. Already feeling badly about himself, he didn't need the stigma of being "the patient." Instead I worked with his parents. I explained, "Right now, your son isn't feeling loved by his dad, and he's not feeling disciplined by his mom, and he's getting very mixed messages about how to behave. The one message he is getting is that his dad doesn't love him and that he's a problem for everyone."

Dad cried during our fourth session and told me that he did love his son, but he was treating him exactly like his own father had treated him. Dad's vulnerability and honesty was a good sign. Within two months, life at home was much better.

I encouraged the parents to stop trying to enforce a hodgepodge of confusing rules, and instead to focus on only a very few. The main new rule for Andy was simple enough: treat your parents with respect and expect them to treat you in the same manner. This rule imposed discipline on every member of the family, including the parents, who had to learn more dignified and rational ways of communicating their own needs to their children. Previously, fear had ruled everyone, including Andy and his parents. Andy was afraid of his father; Mom and Dad, in turn, were intimidated by Andy's rebelliousness. Respect allowed for the eventual flowering of love.

Andy, remember, had been diagnosed as ADD, meaning that he lacked the ability to focus his attention. The real "attention" problem Andy had was the attention he *wasn't getting* from his father—the good, loving attention and consistent, firm discipline he needed as a normal, energetic child. A better diagnosis for Andy was DADD—dad attention deficit disorder. Mom was also missing out on attention from Dad, causing her to express hostility toward him and to cling too closely to Andy. She was suffering from HADD, husband attention deficit disorder. The couples therapy for Mom and Dad dealt in part with their own childhood experiences and how the extreme abuse they had endured was being replayed in their new family. It's common knowledge among all clinicians who work in the field that most abusive parents were themselves abused as children.

While the improvements at home took a great deal of pressure off Andy, he remained bored at school. Fortunately, his parents had the option of trying another public school, one that was somewhat more child-oriented. As it turned out, his new teacher was a young man.

"I just wanted to warn you," Andy's mom told the new teacher, "the teachers at his other school said he's forgetful. Sometimes he leaves his books home, and if he has to change classes, he's likely to forget his pencils. He means well, but he's too friendly and likes to talk in class."

"Sounds like nothing special to me," the teacher responded. "Just a kid." Andy's "hyperactive" days ended the moment he met his new teacher, a warm, playful man who was willing to provide discipline, when occasionally necessary, in a firm but gentle manner. More relaxed at home and eager to please his new teacher, Andy began to do well in school.

Regina: The Daughter Who Had No Problems

Andy's younger sister Regina had no school problems, no family problems, and no psychiatric problems. The psychiatrist who diagnosed Andy pointed to Regina as proof that Andy's problem was unique to him and due to his genetic defects and biochemical imbalances. "So you see," he had told Andy's parents, "you're not to blame for his problems." I met Regina briefly. She was so shy, she couldn't reach out at all, even to our docile rabbit. She was positively terrified of the cockatiel and wouldn't let me open his cage. Her problems were far more debilitating than her brother Andy's.

Psychiatry has no diagnoses for children who are too conforming, too inhibited, and just plain too good. Shyness has to reach the proportions of autism or schizophrenia before psychiatry will take notice of it. If the child is a girl, even the most morbid inhibitions may go unnoticed.

Hyperactivity: The Invention of a Disease

Hyperactivity, as much as any so-called psychiatric disorder, justifies the axiom that "disease is in the eye of the beholder." Teachers typically initiate the process of labeling children as behavior problems, and as Russell Barkley confirms in *Hyperactive Children: A Handbook for Diagnosis and Treatment* (1981), many teachers believe that a large percentage of their students are aberrant. In one study they labeled 57 percent of the boys and 42 percent of the girls overactive. In another study teachers found that among the boys, 30 percent were overactive, 46 percent disruptive, 49 percent restless, and 43 percent short in attention span.[6]

Hyperactivity (HA) is the most frequent justification for drugging children. The difficult-to-control male child is certainly not a new phenomenon, but attempts to give him a medical diagnosis are the product of modern psychology and psychiatry. At first psychiatrists called hyperactivity a brain disease. When no brain disease could be found, they changed it to "minimal brain disease" (MBD). When no minimal brain disease could be found the profession transformed the concept into "minimal brain dysfunction." When no minimal brain dysfunction could be demonstrated, the label became attention deficit disorder. Now it's just assumed to be a real disease, regardless of the failure to prove it so. Biochemical imbalance is the code word, but there's no more evidence for that than there is for actual brain disease.

The appalling history of these attempts to blame children for the failings of their parents and schools is described in detail by Peter Schrag and Diane Divoky in the *Myth of Hyperactivity* (1975) and Gerald Coles in *The Learning Mystique* (1987). Schrag and Divoky call it "inventing a disease." Even the staid *Principles of Neurology* (1985), by Raymond Adams and Maurice Victor, finds no significant physical basis to "minimal brain dysfunction." In "The Role of Attention Deficit Hyperactivity Disorder in Learning Disabilities" in the March 1991 *Seminars in Neurology*, Gerald S. Golden finds no consistent evidence for an underlying physical or chemical cause.

In her chapter in Seymour Fisher and Roger Greenberg's *The Limits of Biological Treatments for Psychological Distress* (1989), Diane McGuinness refers to ADD as "the emperor's new clothes." She observes, "It is currently fashionable to treat approximately one third of all elementary school boys as an abnormal population because they are fidgety, inattentive, and unamenable to adult control." She concludes, however, that "two decades of research have not provided any support for the validity of ADD" or hyperactivity. Neither clinical studies nor psychological testing has been able to identify such a group. The problem, according to McGuinness, is how to get professionals to give up such a vested interest in the use of this powerful label:

We have invented a disease, given it medical sanction, and now must disown it. The major question is how we go about destroying the monster we have created. It is not easy to do this and still save face, another reason why physicians and many researchers with years of funding and an academic reputation to protect are reluctant to believe the data.

But the Labels Keep Coming

Meanwhile, new labels have been added to describe various learning disorders, such as dyslexia, often supposedly found in association with ADD. Most of the routine problems of growth and development in children are called disorders in the APA's official *Diagnostic and Statistical Manual*.

How many children get stuck with one or another label is not known, but it surely runs into the millions. Mental health authorities indicate that many millions of children—remember the 20 percent estimate from NIMH—*should* be given psychiatric diagnoses. From *DSM-III-R*, I added up the prevalence rates for the various school-related diagnoses. They totaled up to as much as 57 percent of all girls and 64 percent of all boys. Granted, these totals reflect the top estimate for each disorder, and there also would be some overlap among the diagnoses. On the other hand, the totals do not include the traditional psychiatric diagnoses, such as phobias, depression, and autism. I counted only the new, school-related ones, such as language and reading disorders. The totals are so outlandish that nobody on the *DSM-III-R* committee probably bothered to add them up.

In the 1970s the media, Congress, and the public generated a considerable amount of criticism aimed at the diagnosing and drugging of children; but a review of psychiatric textbooks from the time period discloses that the criticism was either dismissed or ignored. We'll find that up to one million children a year are being drugged with Ritalin alone (chapter 13). Tens of thousands of others are being given minor tranquilizers, neuroleptics, antidepressants, and other psychiatric drugs. And the idea persists that there is evidence of a physical basis for childhood problems.

Paul Wender and the Myth of the Child Monster

Then a research psychiatrist at NIMH and a professor at Johns Hopkins, Paul Wender set the standard for the radical biological approach to children. He is the coauthor of relevant chapters in recent textbooks. You may recall from chapter 5 that he was also a key investigator in the ludicrous Danish studies that "proved" schizophrenia genetic on the basis of an increased rate of schizophrenia among half brothers and sisters on the father's side.

In *The Hyperactive Child: A Handbook for Parents* (1973), Wender announces that five million children suffer from hyperactivity. Although Wender calls hyperactivity a disease, he admits that "many of the symptoms are present in all children to some degree at some particular time." It's a continuum, and the hyperactive child has an "excessive degree."

An excess of what? Energy is the answer. They are "active and restless," they "stood and walked at an early age," and they get into all kinds of trouble because of their energetic inquisitiveness. So begins the disease pattern.

In a sequel nearly fifteen years later, *The Hyperactive Child, Adolescent, and Adult* (1987), Wender inflates his estimate to include up to 10 percent of all children among the diseased. The child labeled ADD and hyperactive is now seen as a miscreant born into a mostly flawless world, which he then goes on to despoil. This is no exaggeration of Wender's view; he compares the child to the awesome giant ape King Kong:

As these infants become toddlers, many of them are bundles of energy. The parents frequently report that after an active and restless infancy, the child stood and walked at an early age, and then, like an infant King Kong, burst the bars of his crib and marched forth to destroy the house. He was always on the go, always getting into everything, always touching (and hence, usually by mistake, breaking) every object in sight. When unwatched for a moment he somehow got to the top of the refrigerator and appeared in the middle of the street. In a twinkling, pots and pans were whisked from cupboards, ashtrays knocked off tables, and lamps overturned. (P. 10)

Parents who love their children are likely to chortle as they envision them in that description—until they realize that Wender means to drug them.

The Problem of Obedience

In his earlier work, Wender is very clear about the crux of the problem in dealing with hyperactive youngsters, their failure to comply with requests and prohibitions. The central problem is obedience—but obedience to what? Wender acknowledges that "much of any school experience *is* boring, tedious, repetitious," and that parents who visit the modern school often wonder how children could pay attention under such regimented conditions. The conflict between the child and the school comes up one more time when Wender declares, "A child who cannot force himself to complete tedious, disagreeable school tasks will have trouble in mastering reading, spelling, and arithmetic" (p. 37). Apparently these observations on the oppressiveness of the schools were too much of an embarrassment to his biopsychiatric ideology. They are edited out of the later edition.

Wender also observes that many of these children do fine outside of school, so that medication does not have to be prescribed for "weekends, holidays, and vacations."

Wender recognizes that the families of these children are often very disturbed, but he doesn't see this as causing the child's problem. Instead, "family disturbances are often the result and not the cause of the child's problem." In Wender's world, the people with the power and authority —the parents and the schools—are the victims, while the children, who have neither power nor authority, are the perpetrators. Contemporary psychiatric literature has turned psychosocial wisdom and knowledge on its head, and increasingly the child is blamed for problems in the family, schools, and society.

Wender is a strong advocate of drugs, but he admits that children "never like the medication." After drug treatment, the children "generally become calmer and less active, develop a longer span of attention, become less stubborn, and are easier to manage." In his 1987 book he advocates medication for most ADD and hyperactive children.

While Wender is a radical biopsychiatrist, he is a leader in the field of ADD and hyperactivity, and even moderates follow the same basic themes.[7]

Research on ADD

Reviews by Gerald Coles in *The Learning Mystique* (1987) and Diane McGuinness in Fisher and Greenberg's *The Limits of Biological Treatments for Psychological Distress* (1989) show that research does not confirm the existence of an ADD syndrome. For example, in the October 1984 *Exceptional Children*, Lisa Fleisher and her colleagues find that the ADD syndrome lacks supportive evidence and should be clinically discarded. In the February 1985 issue of the same journal, S. Jay Samuels and Nancy Miller find no differences in attention span between normal children and those with school problems. They do find that all children focus their attention better in small classes with more teacher involvement. Common sense suggests that some children have more difficulty focusing their attention in school than do others. The natural exuberance and imagination of many children make them "drift off" while sitting in a classroom. I've talked to highly successful professional adults who confess to daydreaming the moment they sit down in their kids' elementary school classrooms on parents' night. For other children drifting off can be a sign of post-traumatic stress disorder due to neglect, beatings, or sexual abuse.

Other kids are under too much stress at home to focus their attention

281

properly. Or they come from economically and socially impoverished homes where there's little help in learning how to focus their attention. Daniel Hallahan and his team report in the April 1978 *Journal of Learning Disabilities* that these children lack a sense of "locus of control." They don't believe in their own ability to control their environment, so they don't pay attention to it. To these children, "Positive and negative events happen because of luck, fate, involvement of other persons, or as 'just one of those things.' " This has been designated "learned helplessness" by other researchers. In my *The Psychology of Freedom* it is called psychological helplessness and the failure to be self-determining. It's a psychosocial problem.

Why Boys?

The vast majority of children who get labeled ADD or hyperactive are boys. Russell Barkley cites estimates as high as nine boys for every one girl but favors the ratio of six to one. The reasons for the disproportionate number of boys are not difficult to ascertain. Boys are brought up to express more of their activity, aggressiveness, independence, and defiance; they therefore run into more conflict with harried, inadequate, or absentee parents and with boring, understaffed schools. Boys learn their aggressiveness from their male peers, from school sports, from the TV and movies—from everywhere in the culture.

Conversely, girls are carefully taught to be more submissive, to pay more attention to the requirements of other people, and to keep themselves under good control. In school this translates into "paying attention."

As Andy's story dramatized, so-called hyperactive children are often at war with the world while their fathers sit on the sidelines. In addition to love, they need attention, a firm hand, and a stimulating environment. These *normal* needs can be read between the lines of the diagnostic descriptions in the *DSM-III-R*: "Signs of the disorder may be minimal or absent when the person is receiving frequent reinforcement or very strict control, or in a novel setting or a one-to-one situation (e.g., being examined in a clinician's office, or interacting with a video game)." Notice that these children are so hungry for attention that their symptoms sometimes do not show up when being examined one-to-one in the clinician's office! Attention deficit disorder reflects our own unwillingness to give enough attention to our children.

On the other hand, children like Andy's sister Regina are crippled precisely because they can so regularly conform to the demands of school.

Mary Ann's Learning Disorder

Thus far we've been critiquing ADD and hyperactivity. Nowadays learning disorders (LD) are diagnosed more frequently than either of these, although often a child gets labeled both ADD and LD. LD children are supposed to have difficulties caused by neurological and genetic factors rather than by normal differences among children or by failures on the part of the family and the educational system.

Fifth grader Mary Ann was very talented and a strong achiever—in all of the areas her school didn't value very highly, such as art, music, dancing, and socializing. At home with her friends, it was a snap for her to organize a show that delighted children and adults alike. She was a social ball of fire who lit up any room fortunate enough to contain her.

Mary Ann's mother hoped that Mary Ann would buckle down to more serious studies. As a struggling single parent working as a secretary, she wanted more for her daughter's future. And so when Mary Ann got behind in math homework, her mother grew frightened. This, in turn, paralyzed Mary Ann with anxiety.

Mary Ann's teacher, responding to the child's "math anxiety" as well as to Mom's anxiety, decided to refer Mary Ann to the learning disability team. They diagnosed Mary Ann as an "LD child," exactly as they did every referral that year. Then they met with Mary Ann's mom and explained that the problem was beyond parental help because Mary Ann had a "different wiring in her brain."

Mom didn't know that in order to continue getting funds for the school's LD program, the school required several more recruits before the end of the year.

Mary Ann was introduced into a special LD program. Some of it resembled old-fashioned remedial math, and some involved fancy audio-visual equipment with video games. She didn't especially improve in math, but her teacher and her mother thought she was more relaxed about it.

No one discussed Mary Ann's feelings about being labeled an LD child until many years later, when she sought psychotherapy during college. She wanted to go to medical school but feared "How can I be a doctor when my own wires are crossed?" Despite the best of efforts from her therapist, Mary Ann continued to believe that she was defective. Even a book that claimed that Einstein had also been LD didn't bolster her self-esteem. She dropped out of her premed courses.

The LD Movement Springs From the Ashes of Reform

LD is a diagnosis generated not by research or even by clinical experience, but by a parents movement. Unable to confront the failure of the public schools, the difficulties in their own families, or the lack of motivation or aptitude within their children, parents began searching for another explanation for the lack of success of their children in school.

As described by Gerald Coles in *The Learning Mystique,* a combined parent-professional movement burgeoned around the theme of a new class of defective children. Enthusiastic national conventions were held. It soon snowballed with religious fervor across the nation. A whole new professional discipline was born, with its own training programs and degrees. Dyslexia, the LD version of being a slow reader, became a familiar term. By 1985 nearly two million schoolchildren were diagnosed as LD.

The LD movement offered a special twist that served the esteem of parents. The presumed "neurological disability" wasn't stigmatized as a psychiatric disorder or even a disease. It typically was seen as limited to a special problem, such as reading or math, and sometimes to a more narrow defect, such as word reversal.

LD became a financial boondoggle. Behavioral psychology thrived on a whole new subspecialty with unlimited involuntary clients. The schools also benefited. With little funding for remedial education and no funds for genuine school reform, LD programs could tap state and federal mental health coffers.

Does Dyslexia Exist?

All children have learning problems, or they wouldn't need help from teachers—they would simply learn on their own. Learning, for all of us, is a difficult process. So there's an endless number of problems associated with learning. But are there learning disabilities—based on presumed genetic and neurological deficits—that can be clinically described, diagnosed on testing, and treated with special techniques?

As it turns out, the answer is no. There are no known neurological deficits, no known genetic traits, no consistent clinical descriptions, no specific diagnostic testing, and no reliable techniques of treatment.

Gerald Coles's review makes clear that there is no known physical basis for learning disorders: "After decades of research, it has still not been demonstrated that disabling neurological dysfunctions exist in more than a minuscule number of these children" (p. xii). For example, "The truth is that reversal errors by both normal and disabled readers can more consistently be explained by lack of adequate instruction than by any organic deficiencies" (p. 30). They also can be explained by the different rates at which individuals mature. Michael Rutter reviews "Syndromes Attributed to 'Minimal Brain Dysfunction' in Childhood" in the January

1982 *Archives of General Psychiatry*. While he finds the neurological and genetic hypotheses interesting and worth pursuing, he admits that there is no substantial evidence to support them. LD children rarely are found to suffer from any demonstrable brain disorder; and when brain damage can be found in children, it does not consistently produce any specific learning disabilities.

As described in *Casarett and Douell's Toxicology* (1986), poisons such as lead can produce generalized brain dysfunction at relatively low blood levels in children, resulting in a variety of unpredictable symptoms. Physical abuse, such as violently shaking an infant, can cause closed-head injury and also produce generalized brain dysfunction. But real-life threats like these rarely get checked for in children who get labeled LD. Too often there's a rush to make the convenient diagnosis rather than to get at the true cause, whether it is psychosocial or medical.

Word Reversal

Do specific learning disabilities exist? For example, what about word reversal? The observation that some children reverse words and letters has especially gripped the imagination of the public when it comes to believing there must be something to the LD concept. Not only is word and letter reversal simply a normal part of the struggle to learn to read, it rarely plays any role in chronic reading problems. As he reported in 1973 in the journal *Perceptual and Motor Skills* (36:895–98), F. William Black compared one hundred normal readers and one hundred poor readers in regard to word and letter reversal. Word reversal was infrequent in both groups and there was no difference between the two. He concluded it was not a useful concept.

In the April 1977 volume of *Exceptional Children*, Sandra Moyer and Phyllis Newcomer come to similar conclusions. Word reversal is not a neurological or perceptual deficit, but simply a problem of learning "directionality," something that can be taught "with proper instruction, even to 4 and 5 year olds."

An Empty Label

In the 1982 *Journal of School Psychology*, Bob Algozzinc, James Ysseldyke, and Mark Shinn found that the LD label added up to no more than the gross observation that a child wasn't achieving as high as his or her potential suggested. LD is a "sophisticated term for underachievement." They conclude that "the fear that LD may be anything the diagnostician wants it to be appears justified" (p. 305).

In short, LD is a label of convenience for schoolteachers, educational psychologists, and some parents; but it does not correspond to any existing phenomenon within the minds or brains of children. As we heard Diane McGuinness aptly conclude in regard to ADD, "The major question is how we go about destroying the monster we have created."

Little Help From the LD Programs

Nor do the special LD training programs demonstrate any usefulness beyond the usual help afforded by individual attention and remedial education. There's no evidence that LD kids benefit in the long run. Mary Poplin published a lengthy review entitled "Reductionism from the Medical Model to the Classroom: The Past, Present and Future of Learning Disabilities" in the 1985 journal *Research Communications in Psychology, Psychiatry and Behavior.* She observes, "Today there is little agreement among psychologists or educators regarding the definition, diagnostic criteria, or education . . . of learning disabilities" (p. 38). Traditional psychologists use one treatment approach, behaviorists another, and cognitive psychologists still another. Educators from differing backgrounds will promote different approaches as well. Poplin debunks the most basic LD approach, its emphasis on finding specific learning errors: "Errors are a substantial part of learning. . . . Rather than designing errorless learning environments, holistic teachers design environments where errors are natural and go unpunished" (pp. 65–66). Contrary to much of the LD thrust, it's important not to stress the errors a child makes. Errors come and go; the child needs a good, positive learning environment and more individual attention.

Depression

Children get labeled with the old, familiar adult diagnoses, too.

In its May 4, 1987, cover story, *Newsweek* promotes the latest psychiatric estimates that approximately 6 to 7 percent of adolescents and 2 percent of younger children are depressed, including about 400,000 children age seven to twelve. Again notice the enormous numbers that add up to big business for psychiatry, as well as for pediatrics and psychology. Growing numbers of doctors are described as prescribing antidepressants for children instead of talk therapy.

Newsweek quotes a noted biopsychiatrist who compares depression in children to a "bodily infection" and who initiates treatment with drugs. He gave antidepressants to a little boy, David, whose "bad feelings" happened to coincide with witnessing his pregnant mother fall down a flight of stairs and break her ankle.

Studies of families of depressed children indicate a high rate of psychological problems among the parents, especially depression in mothers and alcoholism in fathers, according to "Childhood Mood Disorder Tied to Parental Mental Ill" in the August 1988 *Clinical Psychiatry News*. By the time people become adults, the childhood antecedents of their hopeless, despairing feelings may require excavation. In children they are always lying as large as life right on the surface. Biopsychiatrists must blind themselves in order to make believe that childhood depression is anything but a response to real-life conditions.

Schizophrenia

To diagnose children as schizophrenic is to fix them in psychiatric formaldehyde. A preadolescent child can become acutely disturbed—hallucinating monsters and other eerie sights while awake and contemplating suicide—directly as a result of situational stress, such as a divorce or the loss of a parent. One seven-year-old girl recovered in days from such apparent madness when her divorced parents stopped quarreling over her and improved their own relationship. In keeping with my own clinical experience, Sotiris Kotsopoulos and colleagues in the May/June 1987 *Journal of the American Academy of Child and Adolescent Psychiatry* found that many hallucinating children were reacting to upsetting family crises in which they were receiving little emotional support. Most did well with psychosocial interventions without medication.

Autism

Responding to a PR blitz from biopsychiatry and from parents of autistic children, represented by the Autism Society of America, the media have been promoting the idea that autism is now a known physical disorder, that parents have no role in creating the problem, and, further, that no one in the profession believes anything else. None of these assertions is true. The evidence for a physical basis for autism is as flimsy as the evidence in regard to other psychiatric disorders; and as R. Peter Hobson documents in a review of psychological theories of autism in the July 1990 *American Journal of Orthopsychiatry*, the psychosocial viewpoint has not yet expired. It is unfortunate that the Autism Society of America has lent its weight, successfully, to creating a false public image of autism research. *

The autistic child tends to treat people as if they are objects, with no love or affinity for them. He or she may literally bump into a human being without acknowledging the individual's existence. "Like furniture" is the common analogy for how the autistic child treats people. Typically they learn speech later than expected, and often they do not learn to talk at all. While many test low in IQ, this is due primarily to the language problems. Like Dustin Hoffman's movie character in *Rain Man*, they may be gifted in mathematics, music, or other nonsocial, nonlanguage areas. For unknown reasons, the great majority (three or four to one) are males. Regardless of their theoretical bias, nearly all of the experts agree that the primary problem lies in the realm of "reciprocal relationships."

The pioneering work of Leo Kanner, described in his 1948 textbook *Child Psychiatry*, first defined autism as a distinct syndrome of early childhood withdrawal. Kanner views autism as a psychological disorder resulting from parental upbringing, especially the failure of the parents to connect emotionally to offspring in the early years of life.

In her book *Autism* (1988) psychologist Laura Schreibman describes how parents initially consider them "good babies" because they make no demands: "Indeed, the children not only do not actively seek cuddling, hugging and kissing, but may, in fact, actively resist the affectionate overtures of others" (p. 15). When picked up, their mothers report, the children frequently become "rigid, like a wooden doll, or flaccid, like a rag doll." Overall, "there is a definite lack of attachment to others and a failure to bond with parents" (p. 14).

Schreibman, while not espousing a psychosocial cause for autism, tells the story of a child who was always resistive and rebellious when the mother tried to bottle-feed her. Then the mother developed a severe cold and tried to protect her child from the infection by propping the bottle up on a pillow. The child fed without problems from this artificial mother but again immediately became resistant when the real mom tried to feed her again. Observes Schreibman, "It was apparent that the child was most content when not in contact with the mother" (p. 15). Examples

---

* Unlike NAMI, the largest parent group, the Autism Society of America (ASA) is very concerned about the excessive use of psychiatric drugs. Its leadership is aware that drugs reinforce the isolation and withdrawal of autistic children and adults. In 1990, for example, they invited me to address their national convention on the dangers of psychiatric drugs. Nonetheless, like NAMI, they are adamantly opposed to any hint of a psychosocial explanation for the problems of their children. Their leaders boasted at the conference about how ASA single-handedly made professionals feel "guilty" about "blaming parents." They explained how, in a brief five-year period, they had politically engineered the PR transformation of autism from a psychosocial to a biological disorder. Their efforts are a dramatic illustration of the politics of psychiatric diagnosis—in this case, in the service of exonerating parents.

of this desire not to be in contact with the mother, according to Schreibman, are commonplace and the literature "abounds" with them.

At a legislative hearing on autism where I was testifying, one mother recently retold how her child's "biological disorder" made him shrink away from her and wipe his face in disgust when she pressed kisses on him. Her frantic, nonverbal child was disrupting the hearing while the mother, ignoring his existence, was focused exclusively on declaiming her plight to the legislators.

It is difficult to learn about the inner experience of autistic children because they speak little or not at all. But it is common to see autisticlike patients in psychotherapy who can, with patience and encouragement, communicate about their feelings and experiences. They display shyness, a fear and resentment of close contact with people, and a tendency to withdraw. They report similar feelings in childhood, including isolation from parents and siblings and a tendency to be preoccupied with objects, such as the furniture in their rooms, designs in the wallpaper, or lamps and other objects around the house. Their early childhood memories may literally have more to do with their chairs, beds, and household appliances than with their family. Their parents showed them little warmth or attention and typically continue to be remote as adults. Family photographs from childhood show little or no touching or emotional relating with their parents. The lesson seems to be that some children treated as objects will relate to other people as if they are objects, too.

The Biology of Autism

Although a few of these children and adults do have various brain disorders, including epilepsy, no consistent neurological symptoms or patterns of brain dysfunction have been identified. Perhaps there is an increased rate of autism among brain-damaged children; but this would not prove that the damage caused the autism. Autism, like depression and like obsessive-compulsive disorders, may sometimes develop as a psychological reaction to brain dysfunction and the social isolation it can impose on the child. On occasion brain impairment may make it harder for children to relate to their parents or harder for their parents to feel love for them. However, these are conjectures, as are any attempts to connect autism with brain dysfunction.

Many autism researchers and the American Society for Autism, the parents organization, rally around any suggestion that autism is genetic and physical in origin. There was great media celebration when investigators at the Children's Hospital Research Center in San Diego, led by Eric Courchesne, reported finding abnormal areas in the cerebellum of fourteen of eighteen autistic individuals by using brain-imaging techniques. One national news magazine carried the story without a hint of skepticism and estimated that 350,000 Americans suffer from the newly proven brain disorder.

Courchesne's report appears in the May 26, 1988, issue of the *New England Journal of Medicine*, trumpeting in the opening line of its abstract, "Autism is a neurological disorder. . . ." Unconscionably, there is no mention of the *drugs* these autistic people had been exposed to during their lifetimes, when in all likelihood, most or all had been treated with large doses of neuroleptics and other toxic agents.*

A few months after publishing the study, Courchesne himself admitted that no one had corroborated his findings of cerebellar atrophy and that the results were possibly of minimal significance. In an interview published in the winter 1988 issue of *The Advocate*, the magazine of the Autism Society of America, he said of cerebellar atrophy in autism, "We don't know if it's going to be 5% that show it or 50% or 80%." Nonetheless, the public knows only of his highly publicized study with its premature claims.

The "Biomedical Update" feature of the *Autism Research Review International* (vol. 1, no. 4, 1987) lists no fewer than four recent studies implicating differing physical factors, all unrelated to one another, as causes of autism. It also cites a study implicating the season of the year in which the child is born. Biopsychiatry marches on, but rarely are any two strides in step. Often they trip over each other.

In the fall 1987 issue of the *Clinical Psychologist*, Victor Sanua of St. John's University describes the dominance of biological mythology in current autism research circles and laments how manuscripts are rejected by journals in America simply because they don't confirm the prevailing ideology. In Europe, he observes, minds are somewhat more open and papers criticizing the biological model are more likely to get published. In this report, and in others he has published, Sanua debunks research claims for a biological basis for autism with analyses of specific studies, much as I have done for schizophrenia, depression, and manic-depression in this book. His work is must reading for anyone concerned with the area.[8]

Meanwhile, it's hard for me to grasp how a biochemical defect could specifically drive a child to withdraw from other people and to treat them wholly without love or affinity, while sometimes maintaining a normal intelligence or even special intellectual gifts. On the other hand, it's very easy for me to see how an inherently intelligent child, treated as an object, would learn to treat others in the same fashion.

---

*Compare this to the same oversight in the same journal in regard to brain atrophy in a twin study of schizophrenics treated with neuroleptics (chapter 5).

Even among experts who believe in a physical cause of autism there is general agreement that human services, such as education and rehabilitation training, are the best approach. Psychiatrist Lorna Wing is founder of the National Society for Autistic Children in Great Britain and author of a 1982 booklet entitled *Children Apart*. Wing declares that "there is as yet no medical treatment" for autism and "there is no medication which can help the underlying handicap," including social withdrawal and language problems. She sees a limited application for behavioral training but cautions that "human beings, even handicapped ones, are not machines."

While there is a familial tendency for autism, it is relatively slight. Only 2 percent of autistic children have autistic siblings. There are no adequate genetic studies in the field.

In *The Advocate* (Winter 1988) drug expert Magda Campbell states, "We do not believe drugs should be prescribed to control children's behaviors." She warns about tardive dyskinesia from neuroleptics and a worsening of behavioral and mental problems from Ritalin. She sees a limited use of medications to make some children more amenable to the all-important, indispensable psychosocial and educational help. Nonetheless, in many institutions around the world people diagnosed as autistic are warehoused and subdued with psychiatric drugs. Even Campbell herself seems more prodrug when writing for doctors, rather than for parents, as in her chapter in the APA's *Treatments of Psychiatric Disorders* (1989).

In children, as in adults, there is no evidence that any of the common psychological or psychiatric disorders have a genetic or biological component. The typical school-related diagnoses—attention deficit disorder and learning disorder, as well as so-called hyperactivity, depression, autism, and schizophrenia—tend to cover up the abuse, neglect, miscommunication, and family conflict that drive children into despair and failure.

Psychiatric labeling inflicts additional humiliation and injury on already damaged children. It can rob them of all self-esteem, shatter their identity among their peers, and relegate them to inferior status in the eyes of parents and teachers. Often the stigma remains for a lifetime. David Simmonds points out that children cannot resist the labeling process, and he suggests, "A child's rights may indeed include the right not to be a scapegoat. . . . Psychiatric labels have not proved to be assets to individuals in their future endeavors."[9] In the subtitle to his essay, Simmonds poignantly captures the child's plight: "Daddy, why do I have to be the crazy one?"

291

While diagnosing and labeling is injurious, most children can be helped relatively easily by interventions aimed not at the child but at the family and the school. Even some severely disturbed autistic children can be helped toward an improved life with caring educational interventions, especially when they involve the parents and help them to relate better to their children.

Adults, not children, have the power, and therefore they have both the responsibility and the satisfaction of improving the lives of the children in their care. Because children are so in need of love, discipline, and guidance from adults, the parents of unhappy, frustrated, and even despairing children can almost always be sure of helping their children improve the quality of their lives. If the adults who plan and run our schools also were willing and able to do their part, many other so-called childhood disorders would never surface. Those that remained would be largely due to broader societal factors, such as poverty, male supremacy, and racism, as well as parents who for one reason or another cannot learn to adequately raise their children.

Clearly, however, the efforts of individual adults will not always suffice. The single working parent can do his or her best, but society also needs to do something to relieve the parent's plight. Similarly, overburdened principals and teachers need the support of educational reform.

Too often it seems easier to diagnose and blame the children, and too often the mental health professions encourage that seemingly easier solution. And as harmful as psychiatric labeling is for children, it frequently is but the first involuntary step along a still more disastrous path. We turn now to the wholesale drugging and escalating incarceration of children.

Suppressing the Passion of Children with Hospitalization and with Drugs, Such as Ritalin and Mellaril

If a child has an attention disorder, then he has a chemical problem and needs Ritalin as much as a diabetic needs insulin.[1]
—*Pediatrician Martin Baren (1988)*

As a society, we are ready to put people in jail for smoking a single marijuana joint, but we seem strangely uninterested in setting limits on legal speed [for example, Ritalin]. The reasons are pretty clear. We believe in drugs. If they can be viewed as medicine.[2]
—*Carole Wade Offir (1974)*

The practice of drugging children has no sound basis in law, medicine, or social policy. As such, it represents an ominous step along the Orwellian continuum of social control through psychotechnology.[3]
—*Physician Larry Brown (1975)*

An estimated 180,000 to 300,000 young people a year are locked up in private psychiatric hospitals, and the numbers are increasing rapidly. Over one million more children are being prescribed drugs to control their behavior in school and at home. Carving out this largely involuntary consumer group has vastly increased the income, power, and influence of modern psychiatry. It has also greatly increased the psychiatric menace to children.

On Being a Child in Insane Places

His mom and dad had been divorced for six years when ten-year-old Sammy decided he wanted to live with his father; but Mom had custody and refused to let him go. When Sammy tried to run away, she brought him to a psychiatrist at a famous California hospital, who hospitalized him.

From Sammy's viewpoint, he'd been "locked up in the loony bin" by his mom and "her psychiatrist." He was stuck on the ward with youngsters who were "dope heads" and "criminal types." He saw one boy hallucinating and another popping street drugs. "I'm gonna learn to be a real thug in here," he tried to jest with his father on the phone.

Used to saying what he thought with his dad, Sammy made the mistake of "talking back" to one of the doctors. He was told that patients had to "earn" their liberties and was reduced to the lowest disciplinary level—no visitors, no books, no radio, "no nothing," as he later told his dad. In retaliation, Sammy refused to talk with his doctor. That created a spiraling cycle of psychiatric control.

The hospital psychiatrist agreed with Sammy's mom that Dad was stirring up trouble, and he prohibited the father from phoning or visiting. With the mother's agreement, he started Sammy on an antidepressant to control the "depression" that was causing him to "resist" treatment.

By the time his dad obtained a lawyer, Sammy's insurance had run out and he was discharged anyway. But armed with hospital records to confirm that Dad was "uncooperative with Sammy's psychiatric treatment," Mom got a court order prohibiting any contact between father and son. Cut off from his father and drugged, Sammy concluded that his dad didn't love him anymore.

Humiliation and Powerlessness

The power psychiatry has over people becomes nearly total once an individual is hospitalized. Children, under these circumstances, are wholly at the mercy of the psychiatrist, who may even override parental wishes through his authority, outright intimidation, or the courts. Also, some overwhelmed, frustrated, or embittered parents will go along with or even instigate extreme forms of psychiatric control. And sometimes parents may act out of selfishness. One hospital plan administrator recently told me about three sets of parents who hospitalized their children at the same time—and then took a European vacation together.

Psychiatric hospitalization is at the least a humiliating experience for most patients. In a January 19, 1973, article in *Science* entitled "On Being Sane in Insane Places," psychologist D. L. Rosenhan reports on an experiment in which adult "pseudopatient" volunteers had themselves admitted to mental hospitals, including some of the best in their respective communities. None of the staff knew that these adults were "normal volunteers" participating in a research project. Indeed, Rosenhan didn't even tell the hospital administrations what was going on. The fake patients universally felt humiliated by an "overwhelming sense of powerlessness" on the wards:

Powerlessness was evident everywhere. The patient is deprived of many of his legal rights by dint of his psychiatric commitment. He is shorn of credibility by virtue of his psychiatric label. His freedom of movement is restricted. He cannot initiate contact with the staff, but may only respond to such overtures as they make. Personal privacy is minimal. Patient quarters and possessions can be entered and examined by any staff member, for whatever reason. . . . His personal hygiene and waste evacuation are often monitored. The water closets have no doors.

At times, depersonalization reached such proportions that pseudopatients had the sense that they were invisible, or at least unworthy of account.

As bad as mental hospitals are for adults, they can be much worse for children. Since the rights of children are easier to ignore or rationalize away, the control tends to be more arbitrary and more complete. Typically there is a tier system of privileges, similar to those used in behaviorally oriented prisons for the criminally insane or in institutions for the developmentally disabled. Every privilege, from listening to a radio to eating candy or visiting with a friend, will be codified and assigned a level. The child's degree of freedom will depend on his conduct—that is, how conforming he is.

It is exceptionally hard for a child to resist feeling spiritually crushed, abandoned, and worthless under such conditions. With a less formed sense of self than an adult has, a child is less able to resist the shame attached to being diagnosed and labeled a "mental patient." Children also may find it much harder to conform to institutional life. They are naturally energetic, rambunctious, at times strident, often noisy, and resistant to control. If a boy doesn't conform, he is considered "ill" and can be subjected to physical restraints, solitary confinement, and toxic drugs.

A teenager was visiting her friend in a mental hospital. While they were giggling together in the privacy of her friend's room, a nurse stuck her head in and warned them, "Laughing too loud is not allowed." The young patient instantly grew solemn.

A mental hospital is almost never a "haven" in which a child can gain a needed respite from overburdened, desperate, feuding, or abusive parents. Psychiatry is not oriented around defending children and promoting their needs and rights. That would put the doctors and hospitals into conflict with the parents who are paying the bills.

The Financial Waste

Psychiatric hospitalization for a child can cost $800 a day or more. That adds up to $24,000 for one month. That kind of money could provide tuition for four years at many private primary and secondary schools or fund a personal social worker for a year full time.* And if the aim is to create havens for children, the cost of a month's hospitalization could instead provide $2,000 per month *for a year* to fund a less costly nonmedical and educational environment. But none of those solutions would put megabucks into the psychiatric coffers.

A Bustling Industry; An Unlimited Supply

Why the recent burgeoning of psychiatric hospitalization for children? Drastic cutbacks in insurance funding for outpatient psychotherapy have decimated private practice for psychiatrists. This has been exacerbated by competition from social workers, counselors, family therapists, and psychologists, including many women who charge less for psychotherapy and frequently offer more meaningful, caring services. Meanwhile, many adults resist psychiatric hospitalization, with its loss of freedom and stigmatization, but children are given no choice.

Also, most psychiatrists have little or no training in family crisis intervention or conflict resolution and are ill equipped to advise parents on how to raise their children. Naturally they turn to methods they understand: hospitalization and medication.

Financial pressures within the general medical delivery system have motivated chains of hospitals and individual facilities to increase their psychiatric beds. The utilization of medical and surgical beds has come under federal and insurance carrier scrutiny. The cost and length of stay often are carefully monitored. This is not as yet happening extensively in psychiatry. In addition, medical and surgical beds have a huge overhead compared to psychiatric beds. Finally, the utilization of medical beds is constrained by the reality of how many people need or want them. The supply of medical patients has a limit. By contrast, if parents can be convinced to send "difficult" or "problem" children and teenagers into hospitals, the supply is infinitely expandable.

Parents, too, have financial motives for resorting to hospitalization.

---

*Communities are beginning to take advantage of the financial savings in providing intensive home care instead of institutionalization. Several organizations now offer alternatives to hospitalization in the form of daily home visits for several months to help families regain their social or economic equilibrium and to help individual members with specific problems (see chapter 16). Meanwhile, some hospitals charge double the figures cited here.

The insurance coverage is much better than for outpatient therapy, while there's no insurance coverage at all for educational tutoring, private schools, intensive in-home care, and similar nonmedical interventions more to the advantage of the family and the child.

High-Pressure Advertising

Hospitals now bypass the customary source of referral, local physicians, by reaching directly to parents through advertising on radio, on television, and in the newspapers. Many of these facilities are part of national chains with huge funds available for advertising and with access to cooperation from major medical centers.

Charter Hospitals have been especially vigorous in their ad campaigns. For its "grand opening" on Saturday, June 24, 1989, Charter Hospital of Sioux Falls—"a community resource, providing programs for people with emotional problems and chemical dependencies"—acted more like a new car franchise than a new hospital. In advertising its grand opening it offered "Charter Teddy Bears" to the first five hundred children, plus "refreshments, balloons, face painting," and "picture[s] taken with Charter Chum." The excited youngster also could meet a Minnesota Vikings football linebacker and "take home a signed autograph."

A glossy one-page handout from the same hospital offers a sixteen-bed "Child/Pre-Teen Program" for children ages four through twelve. At the top of its list of "Problem Areas Treated" are "Hyperactivity," "Dangerous or Disruptive Behavior," and "Emotional and Anxiety Problems." "Family Crisis" is listed as another treatment problem.

Two-thirds of the hospital's beds—forty out of sixty—were set up in advance for individuals age seventeen and younger. Is it any wonder that increasing numbers of Sioux Falls children are now being psychiatrically hospitalized?

In an article entitled "Teen-Agers End up in Psychiatric Hospitals in Alarming Numbers," in the February 3, 1989, *Wall Street Journal*, James Schiffman describes how Charter Redlands Hospital in California "started giving entry blanks for a raffle to employees who helped to get patients admitted. The grand prize was a Caribbean cruise. The contest was canceled after a patient-rights advocate complained."

Charter recently bought thirty minutes of prime time television in Atlanta to broadcast a "documentary" purporting to tell the story of troubled teens and how hospitals are helping them. According to the *Wall Street Journal* report, the TV story presents chilling statistics on teen suicide, interspersed with testimonials from teenagers, while displaying Charter hospital telephone numbers on the screen.

While hospitals in the Charter chain are dressed up to look more like condos than psychiatric facilities, Schiffman points out that "once inside an institution like this, a young person is in for full-blown psychiatric treatment." He describes an eleven-year-old boy tied down to a bed in four-point restraint in a windowless seclusion room. The boy, a victim of sexual abuse, had banged his head and tried to bite his shoulder, according to the hospital. High-priced psychiatric care doesn't necessarily mean individual care. It can mean the same old resort to restraints and isolation.

Schiffman reports that hospital chains—such as Charter Medical Corporation, Hospital Corporation of America, and National Medical Enterprises—"plan to build at least 45 more psychiatric hospitals in the next three years."

Hospitals find psychiatric beds much more remunerative than medical beds. In 1989 the *Doctor's People,* a consumer newsletter founded by pediatrician Robert Mendelsohn, ran a brief report under the title "Teens Big Business for Psychiatrists." It observed,

Adolescence has long been regarded as a troubled time. It was almost universally expected that adolescents would rebel, and that with maturity would come socially-accepted behavior. But today, adolescence is fast becoming a condition in need of treatment. In recent years, as hospitals found themselves with high vacancy rates—often higher than 50%—it became financially attractive to convert empty beds to profitable psychiatric beds.

The process of conversion continues. A February 3, 1990, report in the *Washington Post* by Lynne Duke describes how one local hospital, swamped by indigent patients, "is seeking government approval to swap scores of medical/surgical beds for high-revenue psychiatric beds." The hospital hoped to keep from closing down by transforming medical beds to psychiatric beds.

In response to the need to keep psychiatric beds filled, one Boston psychiatrist, who specializes in adolescence, set up a business to facilitate the placement of patients in empty beds. A glossy advertising brochure asks, "Is A High Occupancy Rate for Your Hospital's Psychiatric Beds a Priority?" The ad material notes that "the availability of beds at any institution waxes and wanes throughout the year" and that the computerized service "provides a way to fill beds when hospitals need them filled. . . ." The service also provides "an effective marketing tool to expand hospital market territory and visibility."

When Profit Is the Primary Motive

An exposé by Dave Parks in the October 1, 1989, *Birmingham News* describes how "Millions of Federal Medicaid dollars are fueling a national welfare system in which thousands of delinquent, abused and neglected children are being inappropriately sent to expensive, private psychiatric hospitals. . . ." Ira Schwartz, director of the Center for the Study of Youth Policy at the University of Michigan, told Parks that Medicaid covered $425 a day. "It's a way to fill empty beds. It's become a very significant money-making issue for hospitals." Noting that hospitals were converting empty medical beds to psychiatric beds, Schwartz explains, "Kids can be admitted for really vague diagnostic disorders" without due process to protect their rights. Schwartz estimates that about 300,000 children are sent to private psychiatric facilities each year. Figures reported by the industry are nearer to 180,000.*

The Profession Takes Notice

In an unusual move, the nation's three main psychiatric newspapers, quoting several psychiatrists, came out in 1989 with criticisms of the excessive hospitalization of children and adolescents.

Clinical Psychiatry News, a newspaper sent to all U.S. psychiatrists, rarely publishes stories that blemish the image of the profession, but a report in the April 1989 issue begins: "The growing use of psychiatric hospitals to treat children and adolescents is drawing criticism from some psychiatrists. . . ." Several psychiatrists speak critically of practices such as giving bonuses to physicians who refer patients for hospitalization and using theatrical TV advertising to pressure guilt-ridden, stressed parents into hospitalizing their children.

In the July 7, 1989, issue of *Psychiatric News*, the official newspaper of the American Psychiatric Association, a past president of the APA is quoted as saying that "most of the criticism is justified." Lawrence Hartmann, chair of an APA committee on children and adolescents, condemned "shortsighted profiteering" by some private for-profit hospitals.

In an opinion piece aptly entitled "Psychiatry's Time Bomb" in the November 1987 *Psychiatric Times*, physician Adam Blatner sounds warnings about the greed factor in hospitalizing youngsters. He is critical of both the hospital chains and individual practitioners:

---

*In the *Wall Street Journal* article by James Schiffman, Ira Schwartz was quoted as saying, "The primary motive of hospitals is profit and because of the competitive atmosphere they're in, I think the pressure causes their objectivity and, at times, ethical considerations to go right out the window."

The proliferation of private psychiatric hospitals in the last few years represents a socio-economic trend which poses a major threat to the psychiatric profession. It generates a significant pressure for admitting patients and keeping them in the hospital, a pressure which distorts criteria for the indications for such costly treatments. It is only a matter of time until the public, consumer groups, and organizations of third-party payers become aware of this situation.

Blatner questions the ethics of incarcerating youngsters at the demand of their parents. He laments that financial considerations may lead psychiatrists to "collaborate with the stated helplessness of parents in coping with a difficult youngster," leading to the unjust locking up of their children.

Despite such critical remarks, organized psychiatry has shown no inclination to do anything about these abuses of children. As in other issues raised in this book, pressure will have to come from outside psychiatry.*

Medicating Youngsters in Hospitals and Institutions

Many hospitalized and institutionalized young people are given the same drugs as adults receive. Among the most frequently used are the neuroleptics, such as Thorazine, Mellaril, and Haldol. Increasingly, however, a wide variety of agents have been used for emotional and social control, including antidepressants, sedatives, beta blockers, and anticonvulsants. Thus far there has been no outcry over the medicating of children and adolescents in general in psychiatric hospitals and other institutions, in part because no consumer group adequately represents their interests. NAMI pushes drugs the way the NRA promotes guns, but fortunately, the parents of developmentally disabled and autistic children have often criticized the resort to medication for control.

Medicating the Developmentally Disabled

Children and adults with developmental retardation are an especially vulnerable group frequently subjected to neuroleptic treatment. For example, a survey by the Ohio Legal Rights Service in 1987 of eleven facilities found that the percentages of patients on neuroleptics ranged from 18 percent to 70 percent. Five of the eleven facilities prescribed

---

*This conviction led me to write an op-ed piece, "The Scapegoating of American Children," in the Wall Street Journal, November 7, 1989. It deals with hospitalization, diagnosis, and drugs.

neuroleptics for more than 50 percent of their inmates. A large percentage of developmentally disabled patients also are given a variety of sedatives, including anticonvulsant drugs in the absence of epileptic disease.

Medications frequently are used when persons with retardation try the patience or test the limited ability or time of their caretakers. Almost any problem can lead to drugging, from bedwetting to uncooperativeness, hyperactivity, and aggression. Most often drugs are used to subdue them. The frequent results, documented in chapter 4, are tardive dyskinesia, tardive akathisia, tardive psychosis, tardive dementia, and suppression of maturation. Often the medication causes a deterioration in the limited cognitive abilities and self-care skills of the developmentally disabled individual.

As described in chapter 4, a particularly nasty cycle develops when hyperactivity in the individual is treated with a neuroleptic. In half or more of patients, neuroleptic treatment results in akathisia with an anxiety or discomfort that drives the individual into motion. If the akathisia is mistaken for the original hyperactivity, then the medication is increased. Eventually the drug-induced akathisia can become irreversible, in the form of tardive akathisia, and the hapless individual is tortured for life.

Worsening Retardation Among the Retarded

In *The Psychiatric Uses of Seclusion and Restraint* (1984) Timothy Kuehnel and Katherine Slama observe that "antipsychotic medications decrease the rate of learning in some developmentally disabled clients, an effect that must be considered especially unfortunate in a population whose principal shared characteristic is slowness to learn." Attempts to use educational and behavioral approaches can be impeded by the blunting effects of the drugs. The worsening of behavior in drugged patients also may be due to "a more general result of the discomfort of neuroleptic drugs' neuromuscular effects, such as akathisia, muscle tension, and dystonias, or of the sedative 'snowed' effect, which may reduce a client's positive response to learning cues."[4]

Tardive Dyskinesia in Children

Tardive dyskinesia—the largely irreversible and wholly untreatable neurological disorder that causes involuntary bodily movements—is among the greatest threats to children treated with neuroleptics. As described in chapter 4, the profession initially discounted the threat of tardive dyskinesia to children; but children often suffer from especially disabling forms

of the disease, including dystonias of the trunk or limbs that are painful
and can make it difficult for the child to stand or walk.

Again as mentioned earlier, C. Thomas Gualtieri and his colleagues
confirm the bad news when they published "Tardive Dyskinesia in Young
Mentally Retarded Individuals" in the April 1986 *Archives of General
Psychiatry*. They report a tardive dyskinesia rate of 34 percent among
institutionalized children and young people and declare, "One may conclude that TD, including severe and persistent TD, represents a substantial hazard to young retarded people treated with neuroleptic drugs."

Nine of thirty-eight patients developed new negative behaviors during
drug withdrawal—behaviors that had not been listed as reasons for ini-
tiating treatment. These included "agitation, hyperactivity, screaming,
self-injurious behavior, aggression, destructiveness, and insomnia."
Gualtieri and his group attribute these symptoms to damage produced by
the drugs. In addition, institutionalization itself can drastically worsen a
child's condition.

Writing in *Tardive Dyskinesia: Biological Mechanisms and Clinical
Aspects* (1988), Gualtieri and L. Jarrett Barnhill also warn that neuroleptics cause lack of energy, painful emotions, motor impairment, and
cognitive dysfunction and tend to " 'blunt' the personality of treated
patients." They further warn about the danger of dementia—generalized
deterioration of the brain and mind—from long-term neuroleptic treatment (see chapter 4).

John Singer, from the pediatrics and neurology departments of the
Johns Hopkins University School of Medicine, has issued a warning
entitled "Tardive Dyskinesia: A Concern for the Pediatrician" in the April
1986 issue of *Pediatrics*. He states, "Based on the recognition that all
currently available antipsychotic drugs, regardless of potency or type, are
capable of inducing tardive dyskinesia, the use of these medications
should be restricted. Whenever possible, other therapies should be considered." He also calls for the informed consent of both the patient and
parents.

Failing to Warn Families

In a September 1985 report in the *Annals of Neurology* by Faye Silverstein
and Michael Johnston entitled "Risks of Neuroleptic Drugs in Children
with Neurological Disorders," 410 pediatric neurologists were surveyed
concerning what they told families about the "risks" of neuroleptics. The
largest portion of pediatric neurologists wholly failed to warn families
about tardive dyskinesia, while only a small fraction of them acknowledged the actual rate.

In *The Hyperactive Child, Adolescent and Adult* (1987), Paul Wender, one of the nation's most influential biopsychiatrists, concludes his discussion of neuroleptic side effects with this extraordinarily misleading paragraph: "Although these side effects do occur in some children, they are infrequent. It is necessary to be aware of them, but not necessary to be very concerned about them" (p. 71). A physician prescribing the medications on the basis of Wender's viewpoint may end up committing malpractice. A family acting on Wender's viewpoint would have been grossly misled.

Medicating Autistic Children

Many parents of autistic children fear and resist the drugging of their children. In the *Pen Sac Newsletter and Journal*, sponsored by the parents of autistic children, Constance Torisky writes with understandable maternal outrage about "Street Drugs vs. Prescription Drugs":

All the publicity and recent posturing about teaching the youth of America to say "no" to drugs has delivered a very painful and outrageous message to parents who have spent years trying to say "no" FOR their handicapped child. The message is that OUR CHILDREN DO NOT COUNT. They are less than perfect, therefore it is perfectly O.K. to damage their brains, distort their bodies, and permanently alter their psyche with strong chemical tranquilizers, AGAINST THEIR WILL, and the will of their parents, because THEY DON'T COUNT. . . . This double standard presupposes that the mentally handicapped or mentally ill child simply cannot "make it", so it is O.K to zap him with enough chemical control to wipe out his muscle control, his desire to learn, his sensitivity to the world around him, and his very sense of who he is, just to cover up a few objectionable behaviors, and make things easier for the families or institutional personnel around him.

Ritalin: An Iatrogenic Drug Epidemic

The most commonly prescribed drugs for children are the psychostimulants, especially Ritalin (methylphenidate). Ritalin is commonly given to children diagnosed as ADD or hyperactive while attending public schools. It also is dispensed to quiet children in institutions. And Ritalin usage is escalating. The FDA was forced to double its proposed ceiling on the production of Ritalin, according to William Schmidt's "Sales of Drug Are Soaring for Treatment of Hyperactivity," in the May 5, 1987, *New York Times*.

Estimates on the use of Ritalin usually exceed 500,000 children a year in the United States, and reach as high as a million. In "Medical News and Perspectives," in the May 6, 1988, *Journal of the American Medical Association*, Virginia Cowart estimates the 1988 total at 800,000 children. The title, "The Ritalin Controversy: What Made This Drug's Opponents Hyperactive?" facetiously dismisses concerns about the problem. A January 16, 1989, *Time* magazine report puts the figure for Ritalin-treated children at 750,000 and cites NIMH predictions of one million by the early 1990s. *Time* also cites an NIMH estimate that one in ten boys suffers from hyperactivity. From this and other more inflated claims (see chapter 12) it is possible to envision the eventual Ritalin drugging of an even larger percentage of America's male children.*

Although there are some differences among them, the psychostimulants can be discussed as a group. Dexedrine (dextroamphetamine), produced by Smith Kline and French, accounts for a small share of the market, as does the stimulant Cylert (pemoline). The lion's share goes to Ritalin, a product of CIBA.

The Effects of Ritalin on the Brain and Mind of Children

The actual impact of stimulants on the brain and mind of children are poorly understood and, despite administering the drug to millions of youngsters in the past several years, psychiatry shows little interest in the question. In none of the many standard and even specialized textbooks I consulted could I find any interest in how children *feel* when taking stimulants. The subjective experience of the child is ignored. It is as if we are putting coins (instead of pills) into one end of a black box (instead of a child) and getting an output at the other end. What happens *inside the box* is of no concern; all we care about is the behavioral end product. This disregard for the person's subjective response is due in part to the dual stigmatization of the patients: not only are they "mental patients," they are children. That they are involuntary patients makes it all the easier, and in some ways necessary,† to ignore their feelings.

Indeed, one of the few references I could find to the child's subjective experience of Ritalin was one voiced by Paul Wender, who observes in *The Hyperactive Child* (1973) that "they never like the medication." In

---

*To a great extent, widespread Ritalin use is an American phenomenon. On a recent trip to Scandinavia I found little evidence of drugging children. In their more child-oriented schools and culture, it was considered abhorrent. But there was fear that Scandinavian psychiatrists would try to "catch up" with their American counterparts.

†We rarely want to know the real feelings of people we are coercing or abusing. I discuss this in *The Psychology of Freedom* (1980) and in the forthcoming *Beyond Conflict*.

the American Psychiatric Press's *Textbook of Psychiatry*, Mina Dulcan observes that children report feeling "funny" on the drug.*

The youngsters I have talked to have felt that Ritalin put them "out of touch" and made them "feel weird," blunting their feelings and subduing them.

In adults we know that stimulants energize and cause a hyperalert feeling, not unlike drinking a lot of coffee, but more so. In increasing doses they create agitation, an artificial high, psychotic euphoria or mania, and, finally, convulsions. In large enough doses they would have the same effect on children of any age. But those who prescribe the drug are certainly not aiming at producing a high in already "hyper" children. When the child in the classroom sits still, stops fussing, and becomes more obedient—the desired drug effect has been achieved. And children on Ritalin often do look as if they are taking a "downer" rather than an "upper." They are emotionally suppressed or flattened.†

Children do seem to react differently to uppers and downers compared to adults. For example, phenobarbital, a reliable sedative for adults, is not generally used to quiet children, because it tends to excite them.[5] These confusing results in children are rarely mentioned anymore in psychiatric textbooks, which simply recommend the drug because it "works."

The idea that Ritalin or other stimulants correct biochemical imbalances in the brain of hyperactive children, although promoted by Wender and others,‡ is false on two counts. First, there is no known biochemical imbalance in these children, and second, it generally is accepted that Ritalin has the same effect on all individuals, regardless of their psychiatric diagnosis or behavior.[6]

Frequently listed as side effects are sadness or depression, social withdrawal, flattened emotions, and loss of energy.[7] Consistent with the brain-disabling principle of biopsychiatric treatment (chapter 3), I believe that these subduing effects are not side effects but the *primary "therapeutic effect,"* rendering the child less troublesome and easier to manage.

Other negative effects of Ritalin include growth suppression (both height and weight), tics, skin rashes, nausea, headache, stomachache, and psychosis.[8]

Abnormal movements, such as tics and spasms, sometimes develop.

---

* In fact, there is little evidence for an improvement in attention span, and as we shall see, prolonged use tends to disrupt attention span.
† Frequently the clinical effect is mixed, quieting the child during the day but causing insomnia at night, or producing up-and-down cycles. Also, Ritalin can make a child more irritable rather than calmer.
‡ See quote from Martin Baren at the head of the chapter.

Many cases of full-blown Tourette's syndrome are reported, characterized by both facial and vocal tics. Sometimes these neurological disorders do not subside after termination of treatment, and tragically, neuroleptics may be prescribed to control them, increasing the risk of further neurological disorders. Pemoline frequently is associated with involuntary movements at commonly used doses. Parents should be warned about this risk and experts should recommend stopping the drugs as soon as any abnormal movements are noted.

While there is some growth rebound when Ritalin is stopped, the degree of growth recovery is not known. Although little concern is shown in the literature, it seems unlikely that the negative impact on the body is limited to the loss of a few inches or pounds. Such a gross effect likely would be associated with more subtle and difficult-to-ascertain developmental abnormalities. The cause of the growth inhibition is unclear, but it is not due to loss of appetite alone.

The stimulants also produce a chronically elevated heart rate and blood pressure in many children. The long-term impact of chronically revving up the cardiovascular system is unknown.

Cocaine in Disguise?

Some drug advocates claim that the psychostimulants do not cause addiction in the doses typically prescribed to children. Meanwhile, we do know that stimulants are highly addictive and often abused as illegal drugs, called speed and uppers. The Drug Enforcement Administration (DEA) puts Ritalin and other psychostimulants in Class II, along with morphine, barbiturates, and other prescription drugs that have a high potential for addiction or abuse. *Goodman and Gilman's The Pharmacological Basis of Therapeutics* (1985) points out that Ritalin is "structurally related to amphetamine" and says simply, "Its pharmacological properties are essentially the same as those of the amphetamines" (p. 586). It considers Ritalin among the highly addictive drugs.

The APA's *DSM-III-R* (1987) has special categories for abuse and dependence involving amphetamine and "amphetamine-like" drugs, specifically including Dexedrine and Ritalin. The pattern of abuse for Ritalin and related medications is described as "very similar to those of Cocaine Dependence and Abuse." The *DSM-III-R* then observes, "Controlled studies have shown that experienced users are unable to distinguish amphetamine from cocaine."

Ironically, the *DSM-III-R* description of Ritalin abuse exactly parallels the enforced "treatment" of children:

Chronic daily, or almost daily, use may be at high or low doses. Use may be throughout the course of the day or be restricted to certain hours, e.g., only during the working hours or only during the evening. In this pattern there are usually no wide fluctuations in the amount of amphetamine used on successive occasions, but there is often a general increase in doses over time.

Yet this is the pattern imposed by physicians on as many as one million children annually.[9]

Causing Inattention, Memory Problems, and Hyperactivity with Ritalin

It seems to have escaped Ritalin advocates that long-term use tends to create the very same problems that Ritalin is supposed to combat— "attentional disturbances" and "memory problems" as well as "irritability" and hyperactivity.[10] When children are prescribed Ritalin for years because they continue to have problems focusing their attention, the disorder itself may be due to the Ritalin. A vicious circle is generated, with drug-induced inattention causing the doctor to prescribe more medication, all the while blaming the problem on a defect within the child.

As Ritalin treatment is continued, its calming or subduing effects can diminish, requiring increased medication. It can become more and more difficult to prevent rebound hyperactivity, talkativeness, and other signs of euphoria.* This drug rebound effect is easily confused with the child's original hyperactivity, again causing the doctor to mistakenly continue or to increase the medication. We have seen similar patterns with the use of neuroleptics, minor tranquilizers, and antidepressants.

As with any addictive drug, withdrawal from psychostimulants, even in routine use, can be very difficult. Again we are educated by the official *DSM-III-R*, which has a special category for withdrawal reactions caused by amphetamine and amphetaminelike drugs, including cocaine and Ritalin. After "several days or longer" of medication, withdrawal from the drug can produce depression, anxiety, and irritability as well as sleep problems, fatigue, and agitation. The individual may become suicidal in response to the depression. Again, no distinction is made between children and adults.

---

*The 1990 *PDR* has a special box on "Drug Dependence" for Ritalin, including warnings that drug withdrawal can be accompanied by "severe depression" and hyperactivity.

Ritalin as a Street Drug

In the 1960s and early 1970s an epidemic of psychostimulant abuse spread over America and a number of other industrial nations. In response the National Institute of Drug Abuse, a branch of the U.S. Department of Health, Education and Welfare, published a large compendium of 150 studies dealing with the abuse of amphetamines and related drugs, including Ritalin, making clear the seriousness of the then-rising epidemic and the government's concern about stemming it.[11] Yet estimates of the size of that epidemic of drug abuse do not approach the highwater mark of up to one million children now taking Ritalin.

One study in the compendium, authored by P. H. Connell and reprinted from the 1966 *Journal of the American Medical Association*, states that the regular ingestion of only two or three tablets a day constitutes abuse and that the self-abuser "would certainly be better off without them." This limited use of the medication, described as abuse, is exceeded frequently in the routine treatment of children.

Ethical Implications

Despite these warnings, little or nothing is said about addiction and withdrawal problems by the profession in its textbooks, popular books, and media statements.

Why would a profession's ethics consider a pattern of abuse a serious epidemic disease, except when it is called a "treatment" for children? Why would it describe serious withdrawal symptoms after only a few days of self-abuse with a drug, but dismiss the same potentially bad outcome when prescribing the same drug for years at a time to children?

Brain Damage From Ritalin?

There is reason to be concerned about brain tissue shrinkage as a result of long-term Ritalin therapy, similar to that associated with neuroleptic treatment. A 1986 study by Henry Nasrallah and his colleagues of "Cortical Atrophy in Young Adults with a History of Hyperactivity," published in *Psychiatric Research*, found the brain pathology in more than half of twenty-four young adults. Since all of the patients had been treated with psychostimulants, "cortical atrophy may be a long-term adverse effect of this treatment" (p. 245). One study is suggestive rather than conclusive, but there remains a cause for concern. It bears repeating that the use of any potent psychoactive drugs is not good for the brain.

Drug Combinations

Combining antidepressants and psychostimulants increases the risk of cardiovascular catastrophes, seizures, sedation, euphoria, and psychosis. Withdrawal from the combination can cause a severe reaction that includes confusion, emotional instability, agitation, and aggression. Combining neuroleptics with Ritalin causes a much-increased risk of sedation, stupor, and emotional flattening as well as adding the withdrawal problems associated with neuroleptics.

Moral and Psychological Harm From Giving and Taking Ritalin

In the American Psychiatric Press *Textbook of Psychiatry* (1988), Mina Dulcan summarizes some of the harmful psychosocial effects on children who are given Ritalin:

. . . indirect and inadvertent cognitive and social consequences, such as lower self esteem and self efficacy; attribution by child, parents, and teachers of both success and failure to external causes, rather than the child's effort; stigmatization by peers; and dependence by parents and teachers on medication rather than making needed changes in the environment. (P. 993)

The "stigmatization by peers" is worth underscoring. Often children are ridiculed and rejected by their peers as a result of taking psychiatric drugs, in contrast to taking illegal drugs, which may have a certain glamor or status associated with them. Being a "mental patient" who needs "medication" is anything but a status symbol among the young.

A recent unpublished report confirms that taking Ritalin badly affects a child's self-esteem as well as the attitudes of parents, teachers, and doctors. The study, "Why Johnny Can't Sit Still: Kids' Ideas on Why They Take Stimulants," was conducted by physicians Peter Jensen, Michael Bain, and Allen Josephson. Jensen is an experienced researcher from the Division of Neuropsychiatry at Walter Reed. Using interviews, child psychiatric rating scales, and a projective test entitled "Draw a Person Taking the Pill," the authors systematically evaluated twenty children given Ritalin by their primary care physicians.

Many of the children thought they were taking the pill to "control them" because they were "bad." They often attributed their conduct to outside forces, such as eating sugar or not taking their pill, rather than to themselves. The researchers conclude that taking the drugs produced (1) "defective superego formation" manifested by "disowning responsibility for their provocation behavior"; (2) "impaired self-esteem development"; (3) "lack of resolution of critical family events which preceded the emergence of the child's hyperactive behavior" and (4) displacement of "family difficulties onto the child."

Jensen and his colleagues warn that the use of stimulant medication "has significant effects on the psychological development of the child" and distracts parents, teachers, and doctors from solving important problems in the child's environment.

Does Ritalin Help?

While psychostimulants can blunt a child sufficiently to make him more amenable to control in a classroom or at home, at least for a few weeks, there is little or no evidence of any beneficial long-term effect on academic or psychosocial life. Surprisingly, this rather negative conclusion is confirmed in standard textbooks. As Dulcan observes in the American Psychiatric Press *Textbook of Psychiatry*, "Stimulants have not yet been demonstrated to have long-term therapeutic effects. . . ." Furthermore, "it is clear that medication alone is not sufficient treatment" (p. 990).

In addition, the *PDR* and other sources make clear that the long-term negative effects of taking Ritalin have not been evaluated. The 1990 *PDR* specifically warns that "sufficient data on safety and efficacy of long-term use of Ritalin in children are not yet available." Statements such as these are hair-raising in view of the frequency with which children are subjected to long-term Ritalin treatment.

There is general agreement, even among advocates, that Ritalin never should be given to a child as the primary or sole treatment. Psychosocial interventions are also required in the school and home.

James H. Satterfield, executive director of the National Center for Hyperactive Children in Encino, California, coauthored a follow-up study of medicated children in the 1987 *Journal of the American Academy of Child and Adolescent Psychiatry*. The inclusion of counseling for both the child and his parents in the treatment program resulted in fewer arrests and lower rates of institutionalization. Drugs alone produced no long-term beneficial effects on school performance or socialization. Satterfield sees psychotherapy as the chief modality, with the medication required in the short run to help some children settle down for therapy. What about psychotherapy alone? Sadly, the Satterfield study didn't give any children counseling by itself.

In evaluating the impact of Ritalin, the importance of the placebo effect must be taken into account. As the American Psychiatric Press *Textbook of Psychiatry* points out, while as many as 75 percent of children are rated improved during the initial treatment (and subduing) phase with Ritalin, 40 percent of placebo or nondrug controls are rated similarly. This suggests that placebo may account for more than 50 percent of the supposed Ritalin effect.

McGuinness's review chapter in *The Limits of Biological Treatments for Psychological Distress* (1989) confirms that there is no convincing evidence that the medications help learning or attention problems. While Ritalin sometimes can reduce "fidgety behavior," it does so in all children regardless of any diagnosis. Beyond temporarily calming children, says McGuinness, "the data consistently fail to support any benefits from stimulant medication." She also warns that "stimulant medication is a drastic invasion of the body and nervous system," with potentially adverse effects that we cannot anticipate.

McGuinness concludes by calling for the abandonment of diagnoses such as ADD and hyperactivity as well as the mass medicating of these children.

It may be a painful admission to recognize that one has spent 10 to 20 years studying something that doesn't exist, but when considering the accumulated amount of human suffering, the substitution of medication for otherwise remedial behavior problems, then it is time to stop and think.

In *The Learning Mystique*, Gerald Coles similarly concludes that there is no scientific evidence that Ritalin helps hyperactivity or ADD.

The Ritalin Controversy

Ritalin is advertised heavily by the pharmaceutical company CIBA in psychiatric journals. The irony of pushing psychiatric drugs for children is graphically portrayed on a page of the April 1987 *Clinical Psychiatry News*. Across the top of the page is a headline, AMA INITIATES PROGRAM TO IMPROVE HEALTH OF ADOLESCENTS. The report laments that two-thirds of all high school students have tried an illicit drug before graduation, that one in five smoke cigarettes daily, and that many abuse alcohol. But the report takes up less than half the page. The dominant display on the page, sporting a large picture of a child doing his school work, is an ad for Ritalin entitled "ADD therapy that's easy to live with." Within the ad, a small box of fine print is labeled "Drug Dependence."

In a 1988 letter to me psychologist David Keirsey, the author with Marilyn Bates of the best-seller *Please Understand Me* (1984), excoriates those who prescribe Ritalin for children:

The people who prescribe chemotherapy for inattention and restless action have no idea of how damaging it is. . . . As for mental effects, such as the child coming to see himself as a damaged person, these prescriptors remain quite oblivious. And the claim that these chemically abused children pay more attention to the teacher and learn better remains undocumented, the teachers' reports that they are less restless and more docile hardly constituting evidence of learning. Who wouldn't be docile if spaced out on speed or crashed from sleepless nights from speed? And as for the unavailability of alternative interventions, well, just because physicians are not trained to treat behavior is no reason for them to assume that others aren't.

The drugging of children seems to garner far more public sympathy than the forced drugging of adults. On June 10, 1988, Ted Koppel's "ABC News Nightline" estimated that 800,000 children were taking Ritalin and that its production had doubled in recent years. The subject of the show is nine-year-old Casey Jesson, whose school system told him to take Ritalin as a part of its "educational plan." When Casey's parents protested, the New Hampshire Department of Education upheld the school's decision.

The superintendent of schools appeared on "Nightline" to affirm the school's right to insist on medication. What other alternative did Superintendent Brown offer the parents? "They have the right to withdraw their child from school."

Intimidating parents into drugging their children is a common practice around the United States, especially among the poor and minority groups. There are cases in which schools have obtained Ritalin and given it to children without parental knowledge or permission.

Psychiatry Ignores the Controversy

The controversy surrounding Ritalin has been going on a long time. Two decades ago, on September 29, 1970, the Committee on Government Operations of the U.S. House of Representatives held hearings entitled "Federal Involvement in the Use of Behavior Modification Drugs on Grammar School Children." Already 200,000 to 300,000 children were being drugged, and the subcommittee correctly summarized that eventually the figures would "zoom." The subcommittee noted the irony that "each and every school child is told that 'speed kills,' " while many other children are being forced to take speed in the form of Ritalin. It warned about the effect of this on "our extensive national campaign against drug abuse." It further condemned "a certain glibness about the experimentation on young children in this country, used as guinea pigs." Testimony was received about a pattern of teachers and school administrators intimidating parents into giving Ritalin to their children.

Commenting on the diagnosis of hyperactivity, educator John Holt's presentation told the committee:

We consider it a disease because it makes it difficult to run our schools as we do, like maximum security prisons, for the comfort and the convenience of the teachers and administrators who work in them. . . . Given the fact that some children are more energetic and active than others, might it not be easier, more healthy, and more humane to deal with this fact by giving them more time and scope to make use of and work off their energy? . . . Everyone is taken care of, except, of course, the child himself, who wears a label which to him reads clearly enough "freak," and who is denied from those closest to him, however much sympathy he may get, what he and all children most need—respect, faith, hope, and trust.

Largely outside of psychiatry, the controversy around school-related diagnoses and Ritalin has continued to simmer over the years. As reported in the May 7, 1975, *Psychiatric News*, at the annual meeting of the American Orthopsychiatric Association physician Larry Brown, director of the Massachusetts Advocacy Center, pointed out that drugging children distracted attention away from the faults of the school system. He finds this "blaming of the victim" a "low point in professional ethics" and a political problem as well. He declares, "When drugs are used as a cheap alternative to reform of the schools, then the practice of drugging children must be seen as a political act."

The year 1975 also marked the publication of Peter Schrag and Diane Divoky's pathfinding critique, *The Myth of the Hyperactive Child*, which includes criticism of the growing use of Ritalin. While the public controversy has been heated for more than two decades, psychiatry has remained impervious to it. Most textbooks of psychiatry don't bother to mention the controversy, and the drugging goes on at an escalating rate.

Something other than media exposés will be required to stop this rampant abuse. Pressure must come from the public in the form of legislation and legal actions.

Children: Our Most Vulnerable Citizens

Children are our most vulnerable citizens. More than any other group, they need our love, our interest, our sympathy, and our protection. They also need us to create mutual respect between themselves and us. Out of mutual respect grows the most healthy kind of discipline. Raising children is the most difficult job in the world, requiring a balance of love and respectful limit setting that rarely comes easily to parents and caretakers. Being parents confronts us with our own personal problems, many of which stem from difficulties in our own childhoods that we cannot bear to face. Our preference for the company of adults, our preoccupations with adult concerns, our confusion over how to parent, mismatches of temperament between ourselves and our children, our impatience or tiredness—all of these compound to make parenting and teaching children difficult.

Raising children is probably the easiest job in the world to botch, not only because it is so difficult, but because there's almost no one to hold us accountable. As parents we may at times feel baffled and impotent or even completely helpless; nonetheless, we exercise a degree of power and authority in the home that is unparalleled in the remainder of our lives. We never could lose our temper at the boss, or even at our employees, and get away with it so easily. We never could ignore the needs of our friends with such impunity. Nor could we hit or spank anyone else with whom we came into conflict.

Our difficulty in raising children often is complicated by the stresses of our own adult lives. Many parents, especially single mothers, live in poverty; many families grow up amid racism; and all children and adults suffer from the effects of sexism and male supremacy. Many marriages are torn by conflicts that frighten and confuse the children.

When our children finally go off to school, it is often to a more unsatisfactory situation than the one at home within the family. Typically children are forced to endure long, boring hours in regimented classrooms that give almost no attention to their personal needs or unique attributes. In many schools children are beaten and humiliated as a means of control.

Child abuse and neglect are rampant. Instead of covering up this tragedy with diagnoses, drugs, and hospitals, psychiatry should be leading the society toward a more sympathetic understanding of the plight of children. Given what we've seen in this book, there's no chance that the profession can make such a turnaround in the imaginable future.

An End to the Scapegoating of Children

The schools virtually have given up on educational reform. Children who cannot or will not fit the mold are sent off to mental health professionals, frequently for stupefying and addictive medication. Parents similarly forsake their responsibility for raising their own children by handing them over to mental health specialists, not only injuring their offspring, but depriving themselves of the satisfaction of being good parents. The children are stigmatized and carry within themselves feelings of guilt and shame over problems that are almost wholly beyond their control.

Which way shall we go—toward blaming our children for our own problems, including an epidemic of child abuse, or toward finding better family, educational, and social solutions? Modern psychiatry pushes us in one direction—toward blaming the victim and exonerating the adult authorities. It's the easy way out for all of the adults, including the child abuser; but it's a disaster for the child.

We need a drastic turnabout in which we, as caring adults, retake responsibility for our children. Freeing ourselves from biopsychiatric mythology can become the single most important step in that direction.

Chapter 14

Suppressing the Passion of Women

Your young girls . . . are not happy with their American husbands
because they are not afraid of them. It is natural, even though it is
archaic, for women to want to be afraid when they love.[1]
—*Carl Jung (1912)*

It must be admitted that women have but little sense of justice, and this
is no doubt connected with the preponderance of envy in their mental
life. . . . We also say of women that their social interests are weaker
than those of men, and that their capacity for sublimation of their
instincts is less.[2]
—*Sigmund Freud (1932)*

The three most distinguishing traits of female personality were, in
Freud's view, passivity, masochism, and narcissism. . . . The position of
women in patriarchy is such that they are expected to be passive, to
suffer, and to be sex objects; it is unquestionable that they are, with
varying degrees of success, socialized in such roles.[3]
—*Kate Millett, Sexual Politics (1969)*

In medical psychiatry . . . women appear to be the prime subjects of
shock treatment, psychosurgery, and psychotropic drugs.[4]
—*Elaine Showalter (1985)*

Our anger is real. Our anger at our experiences of oppression as women
and as psychiatric inmates, of being raped, beaten, locked up, drugged,
shocked, is valid and strong. It is not a "symptom" to be drugged or
therapized away. It is, instead, a source of our power, a fuel for our
outrage and our activism. . . . [W]e refuse to calm down and "adjust" to
a "reality" that defines us as inferior.[5]
—*Virginia Raymond et al., "Mental Health
and Violence Against Women" (1982)*

Once upon a sunny morning a man who sat in a breakfast nook looked
up from his scrambled eggs to see a white unicorn with a golden horn
quietly cropping the roses in the garden.

316

So begins misogynist James Thurber's modern fable, "The Unicorn in the Garden." In this brief tale, the husband tells his cynical, controlling wife about seeing the unicorn. She calls him a "booby" and declares, "and I am going to have you put in the booby-hatch." At her behest, a psychiatrist and a policeman come to the house. When the two men arrive, she tells them that her husband has seen a unicorn in the backyard; but thinking her to be the crazy one, they pounce on her and put her in a straitjacket.

When the husband returns from the garden, the psychiatrist and the policeman ask him if he's seen a unicorn. He denies it. Turning the tables on his wife, he declares, "Of course not. . . . The unicorn is a mythical beast." The psychiatrist and the policeman take away his wife, "cursing and screaming, and shut her up in an institution." The husband lives "happily ever after." Thurber's stated moral for the fable is "Don't count your boobies until they are hatched."

The covert message of the fable is how to use authority—in this case, psychiatry—to triumph over one's wife.

"The Unicorn in the Garden" might have been funny, as intended, if it were not true. Men have long been using psychiatry to dominate and oppress their wives.

The Real Situation of the Middle-Aged Woman

Consider the real situation of a middle-aged woman who ends up in a mental hospital.

Instead of being Thurber's aggressive and overwhelmingly dominant woman, Clara is depressed, helpless, and dependent. She is forty-five years old and her children have left the nest. Her lifelong job as mother and homemaker has been terminated.

Before having the children, Clara had wanted to go to college to "become someone"; now she could have a second chance. She thinks about ordering college catalogs but never gets around to it. She can hardly imagine herself going back to college. She has no idea that many colleges have special reentry programs for mature women. She's not sure that her high school courses and grades will qualify her for admission and she's embarrassed to look into it. And has she retained the intelligence to go to school?

"You'll look ridiculous among the college kids," her husband Sam tells her, not noticing her wince. "Getting a bachelor's degree won't get you a decent job. We turn them away all the time at the office. Tuition will be money down the drain when we need to be putting it away. Come on, Clara, I just got through putting four kids through college. Not another one!"

317

Clara's husband is anything but Thurber's caricature of the henpecked, fearful husband. Sam at age forty-five still looks handsome, youthful, vibrant. His gray hair has made him appear more distinguished. He plays tennis three times a week at the club and is fit and trim. One furtive glance at her own body, four children later, and Clara feels it's hopeless for her. TV's "Golden Girls" notwithstanding, she sees only a downhill career for herself as a woman. There's no prize for being a nice middle-aged women. Therein lies the ultimate terror: her husband seems more enamored with his twenty-eight-year-old secretary than with his forty-five-year-old wife.

Unlike Thurber's version of the sensitive male and the insensitive female, it's Clara who is more likely to see the unicorn in the garden. Sam almost never sets foot in the garden. Clara is the poetic soul who got married and started having children—bing, bing, bing, bing; four in a row—instead of pursuing her ambition to teach English and to write. Sam, on the other hand, is a practical, down-to-earth man. Sports and business turn him on. With the children gone, he and Clara have almost nothing in common.

In reaction to her husband's escalating hours away from home, Clara gets more depressed. She becomes difficult, irritable, and sad. She awakens in the middle of the night feeling as if the day will bring her nothing good. She begins to lose weight, which briefly seems like a miracle—until she can't even force herself to eat. She becomes afraid to be alone and has "panic attacks" when her husband goes on trips . . . with his secretary. In the mirror she now looks to herself like a bag of loose skin. Better off dead . . .

Within her husband's hearing, Clara mutters to herself about feeling worthless enough to want to die. She talks about "old horses" and "pastures." When she mentions the possibility of seeing a psychiatrist, Sam agrees to it—as long as he doesn't have to participate and as long as the insurance holds out.

Clara's psychiatrist! We've already met him in so many places in this book. He's the one who's never read a feminist book and maybe not even a psychology book. Clara, who's devoured numerous paperback self-help books, actually knows more modern psychology than her psychiatrist does. But that would never dawn on her. She assumes that the psychiatrist knows more than she does about everything that matters in life.

Almost in passing, the psychiatrist asks her, "How are you getting along with your husband?" Embarrassed to confess the truth about the suspected affair, she mutters, "Fine. Oh, just fine."

The psychiatrist tells Clara she has a "genetic and biological disorder," major depression. To prove it he lists her "physical" symptoms, including weight loss, sleeplessness, and loss of energy. After fifteen minutes in his office he suggests starting her on antidepressants.

Six months later, when none of the drugs have touched Clara's despair, the psychiatrist hospitalizes her for electroshock. Her husband urges her to sign the consent form for the shock treatment . . .

A Vivid Image

The connection between women's issues and shock treatment brings a vivid image to my mind. It's a television documentary in favor of shock therapy. The patient is a beautiful young woman lying passively on her back. She is sedated and then rendered limp by the muscle-paralyzing agent. Two male physicians and two male orderlies or nurses stand solemnly over her prostrate, vulnerable body. The psychiatrist leans over, places the electrodes on her forehead, and her body quivers as the electricity passes through her brain. The men watch as if spellbound. It is as if I am watching a ritual rape and the men, on some level, are experiencing the gratification of it.

Poor Preparation

Being entertained by Thurber's fables as a young teenage boy hardly prepared me for recognizing the actual power imbalance between men and women. When I began my successful antilobotomy campaign in the early 1970s I found that women were lobotomized at least twice as often as men. One Canadian team was lobotomizing only women because they couldn't get permission to do it on the men's ward.[6] Two-thirds of shock patients are women.[7]

Although impressively gruesome, the statistics on shock and lobotomy are merely the reflection of much more fundamental hazards facing women who become enmeshed in modern psychiatry. As Clara's story illustrates, one of the biggest threats to a woman is having her real-life. issues ignored while she is defined as biologically defective.

Causes of Depression in Women

Advocates of shock defend themselves by saying that more women than men get depressed. That doesn't account for the lobotomy imbalance, since lobotomy has rarely been done for depression. Besides, why do women get depressed more often? The biopsychiatrist finds the fault in their female bodies. Few women and fewer feminists would agree.

A recent study from the American Psychological Association, *Women and Depression: Risk Factors and Treatment Issues* (1990),[8] relates increased depression in women to several factors: (1) "avoidant, passive, dependent behavior patterns, pessimistic, negative cognitive styles, and focusing too much on depressed feeling instead of action and mastery strategies"; (2) high rates of sexual abuse in childhood, so that "depressive symptoms may be long-lasting symptoms of 'Post-Traumatic Stress Syndrome' for many women"; (3) the burdens of marriage and childrearing, which fall much more heavily on women; and (4) poverty, in which women and children are vastly overrepresented.

While the report leaves open the possibility that biology may sometimes contribute to depression, the chair of the project, Ellen McGrath, told the *Washington Post*: "The Task Force found that women truly are more depressed than men primarily due to their experience being female in our contemporary culture."*[9] Columnist Judy Mann comments trenchantly on the report:

You don't have to be a psychologist to figure out that a class of people who are underpaid in the workplace, beaten up at home and raped almost routinely on college campuses are going to suffer much more from depression than people who aren't victimized. What is important about the study, however, is that it bears the stamp of authority of the APA and marks the first time it has linked cultural causes to depression in a formal task force report.[10]

Yet how disappointing that psychologists and psychiatrists so often are the last to know what seems obvious to other enlightened observers of human life.

Feminism

Betty Friedan's ground-breaking 1963 book *The Feminine Mystique* remains a good starting point for those uninitiated into the feminist philosophy. I was influenced more personally by Kate Millett's *Sexual Politics*, published six years later.† Millett's critique disillusioned me about some of my favorite male authors and helped enlighten me about my own corresponding chauvinistic values. Millett, who went on to have her own negative encounters with psychiatry, became active as both a feminist and an ex-psychiatric inmate in criticizing the mental health

---

*Representing establishment psychiatry, Alan Leshner, acting director of the federal Alcohol, Drug Abuse and Mental Health Administration, warned against overlooking biological causes. However, there is little evidence to support a genetic or biochemical basis for depression. See chapter 7.

†This is not the place for presenting a complete feminist philosophy. In addition to the books by Friedan and Millett, a good starting point is Marilyn French's *Beyond Power* (1985), which presents a unique and extremely comprehensive view of feminism and a good critique of psychiatry as well. Gerda Lerner's *The Creation of Patriarchy* (1986) offers an academic analysis of the historical development of the subjugation of women.

establishment. Her most recent book, *The Looney-Bin Trip* (1990), is a courageous account of her own abuse at the hands of psychiatry.

It is difficult for most men and many women to appreciate the meaning of feminism. The very word strikes discomfort, if not fear, into the hearts of many. Yet what *is* feminism? It means, as a start, *equality in all things for women*—that women and men should have equal opportunity and equal recognition as human beings. Feminists believe that young women should be able to imagine every possible future and that grown women should have complete recognition and opportunity as human beings. Equality is a matter of dignity as well as equal rights. It means that when a young man looks at a young woman, he looks her in the eye, and with respect; and that when she looks at him, she does so without a hint of diffidence, deference, or shyness.

There is also a more broad critique offered by feminism—the notion that male supremacy has gotten us into much of the trouble that threatens life on this planet, from nuclear war to the defilement of the earth. It suggests that in dominating and abusing women and children and in establishing a social order that suppresses women, men have established the model for how they further abuse one another and the earth itself.*

When a little boy grows up feeling that little girls are inferior to him and that everything "girlish" should be the butt of ridicule, he prepares himself for a role of superiority in other relations as well. And in forsaking all things girlish, he deprives himself of sensitivity, tenderness, caring, affinity, and community.

As Carol Gilligan describes in *In a Different Voice* (1982), women bring a special set of values from their experiences and responsibilities within the family. In place of the power, control, abstract principles of justice, and alienated individualism so commonly valued by men and male theoreticians, women more frequently promote sensitivity to the feelings of others, responsibility for the well-being of others, a desire for solutions that meet the needs of all involved, and a concern for the network of human relationships. Men have tended to place the highest value on autonomy, while for women, maturity is often based more on interdependence and attachment.

---

*In feminist theory the term *patriarchy* is used to designate the institutions and values that sustain male supremacy. "Hierarchical" is the adjective used to describe the fundamental structure of patriarchy—the division of people into superior and inferior and the implementation of power and control over those deemed less worthy. From patriarchy springs not only the degradation of women but of children, racial minorities, religious and ethnic groups, and others labeled inferior. Because patriarchy and hierarchy are inherent within modern culture, feminists do not believe that putting more women into positions of authority will solve the world's problems, although it would be a step in the right direction toward equality. What is needed is a transformation of institutions and values away from power and control and toward treasuring all people and the earth itself.

Thus feminism is something more than a demand for equality of the sexes in everything. It's a hope for new and better values based on liberty *and* love, on individualism *and* valued relationships, on reasoning *and* passionate connection. In the process feminism demands that men look at what their domination hath wrought.

Modern psychiatry, unfortunately, is one of those things that male supremacy hath wrought.

Women and Madness

Psychologist Phyllis Chesler's *Women and Madness*, first published in 1972, set the stage for all future feminist critiques of psychiatry.* Mostly in my own words and embellished with my own interpretations, the following is a summary of some of her main points.

In the nineteenth century women were the primary victims of the asylums of the day and the primary models for madness as studied by psychiatrists. Husbands often dumped unwanted wives into these wretched lockups. In 1860, for example, Elizabeth Packard's husband incarcerated her in a mental hospital because she engaged in "free religious inquiry." She had insisted on teaching in Bible class that human beings are born good, not evil. Deprived of her inheritance, her clothes, and all personal belongings, including writing paper, Packard nonetheless kept a record and kept her wits. She graphically depicted the brutality of the doctors and staff and was the first to compare asylum psychiatry to the Inquisition.

From the beginnings of psychiatry until today, the treatment of patients in mental hospitals has been based on the female role model in the family. Patients are treated as "helpless, dependent, sexless, unreasonable—as 'crazy.' " The hospital experience is even more spiritually debilitating to women than it is to men, because being treated like a woman lies at the root of the female patient's problems in life. Hospitalized women learn that being a mental patient is in many ways similar to being a wife. This disillusionment often drives them to enact the helpless role with still more fervor.

Therapists can take an especially demeaning stance toward their female

---

*It has been supplemented recently by Elaine Showalter, *The Female Malady: Women, Madness and English Culture, 1830–1980* (New York: Pantheon, 1985). Showalter believes that a third revolution in psychiatry has been inspired by feminism and feminist psychology. "Together these have insisted that the cultural connections between 'women' and 'madness' must be dismantled, that 'femininity' must not be defined in terms of male norms, and that we can expect no progress when a male-dominated profession determines the concepts of normality and deviance that women perforce must accept."

patients. According to Chesler, "Clinicians, most of whom are men, all too often treat their patients, most of whom are women, as 'wives' and 'daughters,' rather than as people: treat them as if female misery, by biological definition, exists outside the realm of what is considered human or adult" (p. xxi).

The ideal patient from the male psychotherapist's viewpoint is a young, attractive female with a bachelor's degree. Note that the therapist doesn't want his ideal to have as much education as he has. It would threaten his status. This was so obvious to us as young psychiatrists in training that I recall jokes being made about it.

Mental health professionals have a lower standard for a mature woman than for a mature man. Male psychology is equated with adult maturity. Female psychology is degraded as more childlike.* Since this observation by Chesler, the problem has been found to be pervasive throughout academic disciplines as well, including psychology and philosophy, as shown in Carol Gilligan's *In A Different Voice* and in Marilyn French's *Beyond Power*.

Far more women than men develop "careers" as mental patients, spending substantial portions of their lives on psychiatric drugs, in psychotherapy, or in mental hospitals. Women may seek these psychiatric careers because it's even more painful to be forced into the same humiliating role within the home and because they desperately desire the nurturing they cannot obtain in the family. I would add that women are taught to see themselves as flawed or inferior and that this identity fits in with being a chronic mental patient.

Because women are far more restricted by society in what they can do and how they can behave, women more than men are easily diagnosed as deviant or mentally ill. This socialization begins in early childhood, when "boys will be boys" but girls must be inhibited. Indeed, as social psychiatrist Ruth Peachey has reminded me in personal conversations, it can begin prior to birth. With modern amniocentesis, gender can be determined from cells withdrawn from the amniotic fluid that surrounds the fetus, and then gender distinctions are typically prearranged before the infant sets foot outside the womb. Typically the female is greeted with pink and frills and with more feminine expectations that quickly are communicated through verbal intonation and physical handling.

There are "female diseases" and "male diseases" in psychiatry. Hospitalized women are in the majority in several traditional psychiatric diagnostic categories: psychotic depression, manic-depression, psychoneurosis, and psychophysiological reactions. In categories related to

*One could make a case that men, in their rejection of values more commonly associated with women, are in fact frozen in early adolescence, with its emphasis on competitiveness and its rejection of tenderness, caring, vulnerability, intimate communication, and mutuality.

depression, women are preponderant by a rate of two to one. Still according to Chesler, women are so frequently depressed because of their condition in life, "a continual state of mourning—for what they never had—or had too briefly, and for what they can't have in the present, be it Prince Charming or direct worldly power."

"Suicidal gestures" in women are a ritual sacrifice to their role as women. Madness "is a cry of powerlessness which is mercilessly punished."

A major characteristic of supposedly schizophrenic women who are hospitalized is their refusal or inability to do housework. Drugs are given to women to reinforce their enslavement to the women's role. To this observation of Chesler's I would add that instead of understanding the woman's symptoms as an expression of frustration, outrage, and despair over her place in the family and society, the psychiatrist prescribes spirit-blunting medications that reinforce the status quo in her life.

According to Chesler, feminist political insights into the role of women are more liberating to women than typical psychological self-insights, which tend to blame the victim. As victimologist Emilio C. Viano points out in the introduction to the book he edited, *Crime and Its Victims* (1989), "Serious questions have been raised by some in recent times about the role of psychology, psychiatry, social work, and counseling vis-a-vis the victim" and their tendency to try to make the individual fit the society and its injustices. He suggests that instead of accepting "the existing social order as a given," the psychosocial approach should "support the individual whose problems stem from an unjust social order" and try to reform the social order "to fit the individual." Whether dealing with men or women, the therapist must confront this issue on a daily basis in regard to the oppression of women by society and psychiatry.

Finally, Chesler urges women to band together and to love and support one another in order to gain strength and their rightful place in society.

The Special Threat of Psychiatry to Women

In some ways the problem of women in relation to psychiatry is no different than that of women in regard to most other social institutions. Women are abused and humiliated in psychiatry as they are in any other power structure, from our religious and fraternal institutions to business, academia, and government. While we may wish that psychiatry held itself to a higher standard, it's no surprise that it does not. That psychiatric abuses of women exceed the norm in society derives from the fact that its legal authority is excessive and that its orientation is power and control.

Yet in still other ways, the relationship between psychiatry and women has an especially insidious quality not found in other institutions.

Psychiatry is the institution socially mandated to respond to personal helplessness and failure. The woman who seeks help from psychiatry or who is forced into the psychiatric system often is suffering from exactly those issues that feminism attempts to address—the feminine mystique of helplessness and dependency. On the one hand, she has failed in some important aspect of life, often with easily identifiable women's issues underlying her failures. She may be depressed in part because of conflicts related to being a woman. Or she may be anorexic, bulimic, or agoraphobic, problems we have already addressed as obvious women's issues (see chapter 10). On the other hand, by going to a psychiatrist she is doing what women are trained to do best: she is placing herself in a dependent role, more or less at the mercy of an authority.

Psychiatry, unlike other powerful social institutions, such as corporations, universities, and churches, is typically implemented on a one-to-one basis, placing the woman in an especially precarious position. The individual woman is seeking help, or being forced to seek help, from a single other person of authority, usually a male. She's more vulnerable there than in church, where the minister's power usually is defused by the sheer numbers of parishioners and by the limitations he sets on his sphere of interest and influence. It's not like going to work, where the boss's main interest in her, in most cases, is as one worker among many. In psychiatry, the most important exchanges take place in one-on-one encounters, and the woman's entire life is fair game. Nothing is off limits to the psychiatrist's inquiries and influence.

In the psychiatric hospital setting, where a treatment team is involved, the doctor stands at the top of the pyramid. The psychiatrist, most often male, is the one before whom the patient will have to plead her case for changes in her status or her drugs. Every wish she has, every action she desires to take, is subject to his control. Indeed, the doctor may be so elevated in the hierarchy that he rarely, if ever, visits the patient, instead gaining information from nurses and aides and handing down his orders "from on high," like an invisible deity.*

Beneath the doctor in the hierarchy is the rest of the team of nurses, aides, and social workers. The majority of this team, as in the patriarchal family, are women. At the very bottom is the female patient.

Thus the woman's role in the family is reinforced by the hospital

---

* Attorney Pam Clay tells me that psychiatrists in the California state system complained about new regulations requiring them to explain drug effects to their patients, because this would force them to *talk* with each patient. They were accustomed to supervising treatment and prescribing drugs on the basis of information provided by the nurses and aides.

experience. She's not likely to be discharged feeling inspired with feminist fervor and or brimming over with self-empowerment. Indeed, such attitudes would get labeled "resistant" or "oppositional" in the hospital and earn her more severe restrictions, a larger dose of medication, or electroshock. In rare cases nowadays they even may lead to psychosurgery. I have compared the situation of mental patients to that of battered women.[11] Both the patient and the battered woman are most in danger of being treated violently when they reject being controlled and attempt to leave the hospital or the domestic relationship.

For the woman relating to a psychiatrist, the full panoply and potential fury of male-female relationships comes into play. Her lifelong relationships with authorities—such as her father, husband, teachers, and employer—are evoked. Even if the doctor is a female, her ambitions and training are likely to mimic the authoritarian father or manipulative older brother more than the nurturing mother or sister.

From the psychiatrist's vantage point he is playing the authority role to its fullest, because his patient is a woman, precisely the category of person toward whom he already feels superior.*

The woman in therapy with a male therapist faces a potentially demoralizing situation, especially if the man does not actively promote the empowerment of women. Not only are women's issues important in a general way, but more specifically, some of her acute difficulties probably relate directly to individual men, such as her father or husband. In the psychiatrist, especially the biopsychiatrist, she confronts a caricature of the world according to her father and her husband. All of her doubts about herself are reinforced if this man fails to view her as a person and a peer.

The Male in Therapy

We should not overlook what the male patient faces when he enters into this same male-dominated system. Yes, he is more likely than the woman to find confirmation of his values and identity. If he is confident or successful enough in his own right, he may even feel some comfort from being in a good-old-boy's network. But what inner struggle brought him into therapy?

Often the male entering therapy is struggling with the suppression of the so-called feminine side of himself. He has denied his feelings, his

---

* Psychiatry, growing out of its medical school and hospital heritage, is an especially hierarchical structure in which compliance is expected and enforced in regard to lesser professionals and patients alike.

sense of vulnerability, his loneliness, his need for companionship and tender love. Indeed, he may be so "out of touch" that he has no idea what's going on inside him. When the psychiatrist as human engineer, as caricature of male values, gives him a drug, a good-old-boy communication is cemented between the men. The doctor, in effect, says, "As one guy to another, forget the soft and painful side of yourself."

While men in therapy are likely to be struggling with a suppressed side of themselves that might be called feminine, women may be struggling with what they identify as their suppressed masculinity, especially their assertiveness.

It's no accident that men and women have suppressed aspects of themselves that are thought to belong to the other gender. Our society promotes an extreme polarity between the sexes. Instead of whole people, too often we are halves, people wrenched away from ourselves by the sexual stereotypes. This cleavage is part of why so many people have severe emotional conflicts.

Anyone who has children of both sexes quickly learns how early in life the polarization begins. Despite one's efforts as a parent, the culture succeeds in enforcing a split within the first few years of life. Typically the male will try to be more objective, more rational, more distant from his inner feelings, less vulnerable. The female will be more intimately involved with other children, more emotional, and more in touch with her feelings. She may be less afraid to seem vulnerable. The boys will stop crying and stop holding hands long before the girls do. The girls will learn to stop "acting up" and "getting into trouble" long before the boys do.

While some men adopt a more "feminine" identity and some women take on a more "masculine" one, it remains rare for people to find an optimal balance or wholeness. The man with softer qualities is seen as "effeminate" and the woman with tougher traits is labeled "mannish." It's not easy for anyone to establish and retain an equilibrium in a world that is polarized and dominated by male values.

Biopsychiatry as an Extreme Expression of Male Values

The biological viewpoint deemphasizes to the point of denial the spiritual or psychological self and the important human values inherent in the existence of a subjective thinking, feeling, and decision-making human being. The behavioral viewpoint accomplishes the same thing by analyzing only external actions and by trying to modify them by manipulating rewards or punishments and by constructing new routines or strategies for the individual to follow. To the extreme behaviorist, such as B. F.

Skinner, the subjective, inner human being has no more relevance than for the biological psychiatrist.* Neither the biological nor the behavioral outlook cherishes introspection, personal responsibility, self-expression, or striving for the fulfillment of higher values.

In negating the subjective person, the biobehavioral psychiatrist eradicates the softer feminine side of men and women alike. The objective, scientific, remote masculine overview takes precedence. The phrase *hard science* tells us how essentially masculine the viewpoint is.

A sensitive, aware woman recently described to me a dinner party with the leading lights of the National Institute of Mental Health (NIMH). "They didn't talk about people," she said. "They talked about physical brains all night." Biological and behavioral psychiatry reflect and epitomize most of what is wrong with exaggerated male values.

Looking for Women in the *Archives*

As I took a break from writing that last paragraph, my June 1989 issue of the AMA's *Archives of General Psychiatry* arrived in the mail. Of the eleven "original articles" listed on the cover, not one deals with remotely psychological or personal issues. Two, for example, study cerebral blood flow during anxiety, one analyzes cerebral glucose metabolism in people who developed obsessive-compulsive disorders as children, and another investigates an aspect of hormonal responses in depressed people. A couple of reports demonstrate a behavioral orientation as well, such as one that studies the brain's electrical response to auditory stimuli in schizophrenics and normal people. They aren't talking about people in the *Archives of General Psychiatry* any more than they are at NIMH.

I decided to look up the sex of the authors of the articles as well as the staff of the magazine. When gender was unclear, I called the journal to confirm it.

- Only one out of eleven of the senior authors in this recent issue is a woman.
- Only one out of twenty-three members of the editorial board is a woman.

---

*In *Beyond Freedom and Dignity* (New York: Bantam, 1971), Skinner writes of behaviorism:

The direction of the controlling relation is reversed: a person does not act upon the world, the world acts upon him. (P. 202) . . . An experimental analysis shifts the determination of behavior from autonomous man to the environment—an environment responsible for both the evolution of the species and the repertoire acquired by each member. . . . It is the autonomous inner man who is abolished, and that is a step forward. (P. 205)

- No women are among the ten chief executives, from the executive vice-president on down.
- The managing editor is also a man.

Counting them all up, there are *two women* and *forty-three men* involved in the writing, editorial, and top management functions of this issue of the *Archives of General Psychiatry*.

The *Archives* does hire women—for positions on the less prestigious and more poorly paid publishing staff, where they are in the vast majority. The masthead shows women filling most of the posts as staff assistants, copy editors, art assistants, and proofreaders as well as various production roles. The publishing staff of a magazine has nothing to do with the actual content, which remains the domain of the almost exclusively male side of the magazine.

Our best hope for the future is that history will look back with ridicule at the irrelevance to human life of the biobehavioral research that today preoccupies the male-dominated journals and psychiatric institutions. But suppose instead that this sort of psychiatry eventually gains as much credence in both popular and intellectual circles as the Freudian approach once did? The frequency with which educated people now talk of "biochemical imbalances" and "genetic predispositions" and the almost uncritical acceptance of biopsychiatric pronouncements in the media suggest that we are on our way to a world dominated by these values.

Husbands and Wives in Therapy

Somewhat oversimplifying to illustrate a point, we can compare the contrasting views of men and women who participate in couples psychotherapy. Most of the couples I see in my practice—perhaps nine out of ten—display a female-male stereotype of relating that seems typical for middle- and upper-middle-class white culture. The husband's views of himself and of life are largely interchangeable with those of a typical biopsychiatrist. The wife's views are more like someone the psychiatrist would label mentally ill.

About Feelings

He views himself as relying on reason and tends to suppress or avoid strong feelings. He associates passions with being effeminate, womanish, childish, out of control, or crazy. If he had his way, he wouldn't have any strong feelings, except perhaps anger.

She views herself as struggling with strong feelings that often overcome her rationality. She believes that her feelings are important and that she has a right to them; but she's not confident about it and sometimes wonders if she is too childish or even crazy.

About Communication

He talks about ideas and thoughts and is not comfortable with feelings. Resenting his wife's demands to communicate, he feels as if she is "pulling" on him. He tries to be tolerant. Since she is the one "making all the noise," it's easy for him to identify her as the problem and himself as the innocent bystander.

She displays many feelings and wants to talk about them. She is often openly frustrated and angry when her husband won't respond. She'd do anything to get him to "open up."

About Feelings of Helplessness

He is baffled and put off by feelings of helplessness, denying the feelings in himself and ignoring them in his wife. When she does act helpless, he feels both guilty and confirmed in his male superiority.

She often feels helpless and resents her husband's unwillingness to express or to deal with similar feelings. She wishes she could rely on him when she feels needy.

About Personal Problems

He has a "Mr. Fix It" approach to any problem she brings up and rushes in to find a quick solution with a minimum of effort. He can't understand why his wife wants to "go over the same thing again and again."

She wants to explore problems from varying angles, taking into account a variety of feelings and attitudes, and especially she wants to know her own subjective viewpoint before leaping to a solution.

She feels rejected by his desire to solve a personal issue as soon as she brings it up and he feels put down by her refusal to validate his solutions by accepting them.

About Higher Values

He is uncomfortable with spiritual and romantic concepts or with idealized images of how people can and should relate to each other. He never reads romances or pop psychology books. He's more pragmatic and down-to-earth. He genuinely wonders what people mean by "love." Sex is very important to him, and he believes he could become more loving *if* he were more sexually satisfied by his wife.

She believes in spiritual values, including love, and secretly or openly wants more romance in her life. She doesn't want to have sex without love.*

About Their Lengthy Conflict

After years of marital conflict, he is trying to be stoic, objective, and distant. He has withdrawn into himself.

She feels in severe turmoil, as if coming apart at the seams. She cannot separate herself from the conflict and "takes everything personally."

About Psychotherapy

At least initially, he resents and feels ashamed of seeking help, and attends the first sessions at his wife's insistence. He's embarrassed to think of himself as a patient and may not want to use his health insurance for fear that people at work will find out. He's most comfortable thinking that he's tagging along to help his wife with her problems.

She actively wants help for herself, her husband, and the marriage and wishes her husband had more personal motivation in the same direction. Being a patient seems acceptable to her.

The Biopsychiatrist as a Caricature of Male Values

Now consider what we know of the biopsychiatric viewpoint. It is identical to that of the man in crisis and conflict—the man walled off from himself who has suppressed his own feminine or softer side. The following is a point-by-point comparison.

About Feelings

The biopsychiatrist tries to suppress passions with drugs or shock treatment. A strong expression of anxiety, depression, anger, or the like by

---

* Some feminists see romantic love as a trap for women and believe it has fostered dependency in some women and motivated them to stay in self-injurious relationships. However, my overall experience as a therapist is that men often tend to reject romantic love in their marriages because of the values it tends to call forth: equality, intimacy, passion, caring, and vulnerability. Women often yearn for romantic love because it places a premium on these values. In *The Psychology of Freedom* I discuss how liberty and individuality are often expressed in romantic love. Also see Peter Breggin, "Sex and Love: Sexual Dysfunction as a Spiritual Disorder," in *Sexuality and Medicine, vol. 1: Conceptual Roots*, ed. Earl Shelp (Boston: D. Reidel, 1987).

the patient will bring out the prescription pad or, worse . . . involuntary treatment and electroshock.

About Communication

The biopsychiatrist remains aloof, parries or rejects any attempt on the patient's part to get more personal with him, and doesn't want to spend too much time listening to the patient's feelings. Sessions will tend to be short: fifteen minutes to monitor the drugs may be enough. Eventually, telephone calls for prescription refills may suffice. (The female patient may end up with *two* men in her life whom she can hardly get in touch with at work and whom she never encounters in a personal manner.)

About Personal Helplessness

The biopsychiatrist views personal helplessness as an expression of mental illness, a symptom rather than a feeling in need of exploration.

About Personal Problems

The biopsychiatrist is the "Dr. Fix It" par excellence. Like an auto mechanic, he listens to the noises coming from the patient only long enough to diagnose the problem and to prescribe. Like the frustrated mechanic, he may even "kick the machine" with shock treatment. *

About Higher Values

Issues such as love, romance, and the meaning and purpose of life, are foreign to his work. They are mentioned nowhere in the psychiatric textbooks that he refers to as authoritative.

About Their Lengthy Conflict

The biopsychiatrist isn't focused on resolving conflicts through love, communication, and the fulfillment of basic needs. † He conceptualizes severe

---

* Actually, only a deranged mechanic would do to an auto engine what psychiatrists routinely do to the human brain.

† For the conceptualization of deep-rooted conflict (both personal and political) as emanating from unsatisfied basic needs—such as the need for valued relationships and recognition—see John Burton, *Conflict: Resolution and Prevention* (New York: St. Martin's Press, 1990). Also Peter Breggin, *Beyond Conflict* (tentative) (New York: St. Martin's Press, forthcoming).

conflict as the product of mental illness in one of the participants. If the patient's illness is cured, the family and social conflicts presumably will dissipate.

About Psychotherapy

The "modern" psychiatrist doesn't believe in psychotherapy, except perhaps for very mild problems, the sort that somehow never find their way into his office. He doesn't even know how to do individual psychotherapy (see chapter 1), and he has even less awareness of other alternatives, such as couples and family therapy, self-help groups, the human potential movement, and various religious and spiritual approaches (see chapter 16). From his viewpoint, "talking to a disease" is pointless and even can make it worse.

In sum, there is a close similarity between chauvinistic male values at their most extreme and run-of-the-mill biopsychiatry values. At the same time, there is a similarity between female values and what biopsychiatrists perceive to be mental illness.

The Abuse of Women and Female Children: Prevalence and Aftereffects

Physical and sexual assault of women and children is a staggering phenomenon that only recently has drawn public attention. According to a 1986 report from the U.S. Department of Justice, two million women a year experience a severe beating at the hands of their husbands, and these estimates are generally thought to be low. Many of these women are forced into sex—that is, they are raped by their husbands. Some states still do not recognize rape as a crime if committed by the victim's husband. The physical and sexual abuse of women is so epidemic that in the September/October 1990 issue of *Ms.*, Jane Caputi and Diana E. H. Russell proposed the term *femicide* to characterize it.

A report in the April 16, 1988, *Lancet* by Paul Mullen and his colleagues found a rate of "psychiatric disorder" of 20 percent among women who had been abused as children, compared to 6 percent among those who were not. "These findings indicate that the deleterious effects of abuse can continue to contribute to psychiatric morbidity for many years." Recent studies continue to demonstrate sexual exploitation of female children, usually by men, with disastrous consequences later in life.* E. Sue Blume, in *Secret Survivors: Uncovering Incest and Its Aftereffects in Women* (1990), surveys the literature and reports that older research on the average has reported that 25 percent of American women were molested as children "by someone they knew and trusted," while "newer research, done more carefully and accurately, indicates that as many as 38% of women were molested in childhood." She concludes that the actual number is even higher: "It is my experience that fewer than half of the women who experienced this trauma later remember or identify it as abuse. Therefore it is not unlikely that *more than half of all women* are survivors of childhood sexual trauma" (p. xiv, italics in original).

My experience confirms that the vast majority of women have been sexually abused in childhood. In both my psychotherapy practice and among my friends, recollection of the trauma frequently occurs later in life, often in an attempt to explain seemingly irrational fears that have plagued the individual for a lifetime.

A large proportion of sexual victimization takes place in infancy, often striking two year olds, and thus a great deal of it falls into the mental darkness of childhood amnesia. Even when recalled it may not be reported.

Victims almost always feel ashamed and guilty, even about an experience in which they had no control or responsibility. This shame and guilt, as well as the helplessness bred by exploitation, leads them to repress memories and to withhold facts even when they can be recalled. In psychotherapy, abuse often is casually dismissed, denied, or simply forgotten by the client until the therapist begins to make direct inquiries.

Psychiatry, Women, and the Self-Defeating Personality Disorder

Despite all of this mounting evidence, psychiatry marches off madly in its own aberrant direction—blaming the victim with psychiatric diagnoses

---

*In a book edited by Gail Wyatt and Gloria Powell, *Lasting Effects of Child Sexual Abuse* (Newbury Park, Calif.: Sage Publications, 1988), a team lead by Judith Stein surveys more than three thousand men and women in Los Angeles. Of those women reporting sexual abuse, almost 63.6 percent at some time in their lives met the standards for a psychiatric diagnosis, compared to 29 percent among the nonabused. The authors conclude, "Substance use disorders, major depression, phobia, panic disorder, and antisocial personality also showed elevated prevalence among those abused as children—even when gender, ethnicity, age, and education were controlled . . ." (p. 146). In the same book, Stephanie Peters examines "Child Sexual Abuse and Later Psychological Problems" and finds increased rates of various psychological problems among these women.

and committing further abuse in the form of physical interventions. Indeed, the nonmedical literature has never been richer on the long-term negative effects of childhood victimization within alcoholic, incestuous, and otherwise dysfunctional families, but biopsychiatry barely gives lip service to the influence of the family on adult personality and problems.

The authors of the APA's *DSM-III-R* (1987) originally proposed a relatively new diagnosis, the "self-defeating personality." Concerned that this label would be attached to women without regard to the context of their oppression as children and adults, feminist groups successfully pressured the APA to drop it from the main text of the report. Nonetheless, the diagnosis can be found in "Appendix A: Proposed Diagnostic Categories Needing Further Study." The lengthy write-up acknowledges the origin of the diagnosis in "psychoanalytic views of female sexuality and the implication that a person with the disorder derives unconscious pleasure from suffering." This is a variation on the self-serving male theme, "They really like it."

To its credit, *DSM-III-R* does briefly mention that grown women may become self-defeating in response to maltreatment as children. Under "Predisposing factors" it states, "Having been physically, sexually, or psychologically abused as a child or having been reared in a family in which there was abuse of a spouse may predispose to the development this disorder." *DSM-III-R* considers the self-defeating personality to be one of the most common personality disorders. This makes it especially menacing that some textbooks have given it legitimate status as a diagnosis with no regard for women's issues.*

Criticisms of Psychiatry

Investigators who have blown the whistle on the physical and sexual molestation of women and children usually have been critical of psychiatry's response to these problems.

Erin Pizzey, in *Scream Quietly or the Neighbors Will Hear* (1974), expresses outrage that the female victims end up in mental hospitals far more often than their perpetrator husbands. The victims get diagnosed and hence blamed, and often psychiatrically abused, while the persecutors go free. Typically these women already have been treated for depression

---

The New Harvard Guide to Psychiatry (1988) discusses the self-defeating personality without mentioning the controversy surrounding it, the threatening implications for women, or any relationship between the diagnosis and a history of childhood abuse. The American Psychiatric Press *Textbook of Psychiatry* (1988) mentions some of the controversy but does not connect the diagnosis to harmful treatment in childhood. There's no significant discussion of child abuse in the book.

and suicide attempts before hospitalization. It is not a coincidence that Pizzey's breakthrough book on the abuse of women was also among the first to confront the psychiatric exploitation of these people. The psychiatric approach has tended to cover up the battery and sexual exploitation of women and children; both had to be exposed at once.

Del Martin, author of *Battered Wives* (1981), confirms that battered women often find that psychiatrists want to suppress their complaints and their feelings with massive doses of tranquilizers and even electroshock. But women have no such recourse with their perpetrator husbands:

If a woman tries to have her husband committed to a mental institution because of his violent behavior, however, no one talks about pills to tranquilize him or electric shocks and lobotomies to relieve him of his violent rage. Instead, mental health professionals recommend psychotherapy and say that nothing can be done unless the man comes in voluntarily.

In *Post Traumatic Therapy and Victims of Violence* (1987, edited by Frank Ochberg), Evan Stark and Anne Flitcraft note that wife battering often is compounded by institutional and professional mistreatment of the victims, including "neglect, inappropriate medication, and labeling women who persistently seek help."

In *Secret Survivors* (1990) E. Sue Blume is also critical of the mental health establishment for labeling and treating women inappropriately without regard for the traumatic childhood origins of their problems. Hospitalization, she believes, can become another abuse. Later in her book Blume asserts that schizophrenia, with hallucinations and delusions, can result from childhood sexual assault (p. 85). In chapter 3 we saw that many so-called schizophrenics speak in seemingly irrational metaphors that, when taken seriously, suggest veiled references to child abuse, and that battered women often are labeled schizophrenic.

Psychoanalysis and the Abuse of Children

Both poles of modern psychiatry, the biopsychiatric and the psychoanalytic, have led the way in covering up the victimization of women and female children and in exonerating men in general.

In *Freud: The Assault On Truth* (1984), Jeffrey Masson,[12] former psychoanalyst and former director of the Sigmund Freud Archives, describes how he inadvertently discovered the secret of Freud's collaboration with Victorian society and the medical profession in covering up the sexual abuse of young women and girls. Masson became interested in the evolution of Freud's theory of the Oedipus complex. Briefly, the Oedipus complex designates his cornerstone theory that little children normally or naturally develop a lustful attachment to the parent of the opposite sex, with fear and hostility toward the parent of the same sex. Girls were the model for Freud, who most often treated women, and he found that many of them were sexually preoccupied, often with older men. They "transferred" these feelings to Freud, the therapist, leading him to investigate the matter further with his psychoanalytic technique.

In this version of childhood events, the sexual impulses emanate from the child toward the parent, not vice versa. Similarly, the sexual feelings originate entirely in the patient and not the doctor. The victim, a child or adult female, is blamed and the adult male is exonerated. The Oedipus complex theory is a monument to the extremes to which men will go to blame even small children for the passion that men themselves so often indulge irresponsibly.

Freud found that many of his female patients told stories of being sexually abused as children. How did Freud get from their reports of child abuse to a theory about children lusting after and even seducing their parents?

Like so many other things in the mental health field, Freud's Oedipus theory in its final form was motivated by political expediency. While others had suspected and even charged Freud with covering up child abuse in Victorian Europe, Masson found the smoking gun. As director of the Sigmund Freud Archives and as a respected young analyst, Masson gained access to many of Freud's unpublished papers that were stashed away in a cupboard in the house in London where Freud spent the last years of his life.

The letters confirm that Freud originally perceived the situation of the female correctly. Grown women were often suffering the aftereffects of childhood sexual abuse. Freud gathered this information and then presented it in a paper to a medical meeting in Vienna. Instead of applause and praise, he was met with stony, scornful silence. These gentlemen, some of them no doubt child abusers in their own right, wanted nothing to do with disclosures about the dark, sexual underside of family life.

Overwhelmed by their rejection, Freud wrote to a friend and colleague about his despair. Masson was able to show how Freud's disappointment led him, a short time later, to make a theoretical about-face. Little girls weren't being lusted after and abused by their fathers and other older men. Little girls generated their own sexual fantasies toward these men and then made up stories about their sexual contacts. Sometimes little girls even went so far as to seduce older men. Although common sense would locate responsibility for the problem within the sexually mature and powerful adult male, it was assigned instead to the sexually immature and powerless female child.

It is no exaggeration to say that psychoanalysis, much like psychiatry in general, was founded on the betrayal of women and children. Masson proves that Freud betrayed his patients and betrayed women and children in general, and like many other male betrayers, he became a fabulously honored man.

Invalidating the Patient's Viewpoint

Masson believes that he had threatened more than Freud's image,* and even more than the Oedipal theory. He had challenged the psychoan-alyst's habitual pattern of invalidating the personal or subjective viewpoint of the patient. If he was right in criticizing the Oedipus complex, Masson observed in 1988 and 1989 personal conversations with me, the patient's communications and reality could no longer be dismissed as fantasies and irrational wishes.

The fundamentals of both psychiatry and psychoanalysis—the use of diagnoses and biological or pseudoscientific "psychodynamic" explan-ations—tend to alienate the patient from his or her own words and real-life experiences. Instead of trying to understand what the patient is saying, the professional translates the patient's experience into a language that would be alien and unrecognizable to the patient. Where the client means one thing, the therapist can draw on concepts like "the unconscious" or "projection" to show that the client really means another thing.

One evening not long ago I was chatting informally with several na-tionally known psychotherapists. I casually suggested that patients ought to be shown clinical descriptions of themselves before publication in order to comment on their validity or accuracy. I was greeted with silence, punctuated by one dismayed "Really!"

Why not share our viewpoints openly with our patients? Beyond un-dermining the therapist's authority and empowering the client, it would provide too big a glimpse into the disparity between the clinical viewpoint and the client's own personal viewpoint.

---

*Masson was assaulted violently. He was fired from his directorship of the Sigmund Freud Archives. Then he was caricatured and misquoted in a magazine article and a book. (See David Gonzalez, "Plaintiff and Publishers Say They Are Satisfied," and other coverage, in the June 21, 1991, *New York Times*.) Finally, he found it impossible to get teaching jobs. A renowned Sanskrit scholar, he couldn't even get work in a field that remote from psychiatry and psychoanalysis. Masson tells the story in *Final Analysis: The Making and Unmaking of a Psychoanalyst* (New York: Addison-Wesley, 1990). In Masson's opinion, expressed to me personally, he was ridiculed and dismissed "like a woman" for taking the side of women and children.

A Patient Fights Back Successfully

Masson followed his unmasking of Freud with an attack on the very concept of psychotherapy in *Against Therapy* (1988). While not focused specifically on women's issues, his vignettes make clear that women are by far the gender more frequently injured by the psychotherapy process. An especially poignant and revealing story is that of Sally Zinman, now a leader in the ex-inmate movement, whose alternative approaches will be discussed in chapter 16. As she reconfirmed in an interview with me in 1989, Zinman was physically and sexually assaulted, virtually turned into a mental patient slave, by psychiatrist John Rosen. Rosen was one of the most famous psychotherapists in psychiatry during the 1950s and 1960s, often lecturing to impressed colleagues, and he is still cited and praised in the literature.

Many of Rosen's patients were being tormented by him in the isolated cottages in which he imprisoned them under guard. Most of them were women sent to him by parents and husbands. Even when Rosen's outrageous behavior became apparent to the profession, psychiatry did absolutely nothing about it. Finally Sally Zinman recovered sufficiently from her trauma to begin to look into Rosen's activities. When she discovered a whole pattern of abuse, she took action. Eventually her efforts led to other women coming forward and Rosen at last surrendering his medical license in 1983 in order to avoid facing charges. Few such stories of psychiatric oppression end as righteously. Even so, Rosen was never criminally charged with sexual assault, kidnapping, or false imprisonment. Nor was he ever diagnosed and psychiatrically treated for his "antisocial behavior."

Feminist Critiques of Freud and Psychoanalysis

For decades feminists have criticized Freud's hostile and degrading attitudes toward women. As early as 1963, Betty Friedan's *The Feminine Mystique* offered a lengthy critique of the Freudian approach to women. According to Friedan, Freud reinforced the age-old male prejudice against women as "animals, less than human, unable to think like men, born merely to breed and serve men. . . ." Friedan recounts how Freud showed no remorse in his biographical account of how the piano disappeared from his parents' home when his sister's playing interrupted his studies. The piano's disappearance admittedly removed all hope for her musical career.

Freud's prejudices, stated as scientific theories, reinforced the image of women as physically deficient (lacking a penis), passive, helpless, and irrational. The aspirations of women were condemned as "penis envy," a phrase that became a potent weapon in the hands of men eager to dominate women and to keep them from competing in the professional world. Friedan concludes, "The feminine mystique, elevated by Freudian theory into a scientific religion, sounded a single overprotective, life-restricting, future-denying note for women."

In *Sexual Politics* Kate Millett provides another of the earliest and most detailed critiques of Freud's views on women. She documents how Freud focused on negative traits produced by the male oppression of women, such as helplessness and self-destructiveness, and then attributed them to the inherent nature of women.

John Stuart Mill and the Medical Doctors

Freud cannot be excused on the grounds that he was inevitably culture-bound in his insensitivity toward women. In 1869 John Stuart Mill already had published one of the most important essays in Western literature, "On the Subjugation of Women." It can be found in *Essays on Sex Equality* (1970), by Mill and by Harriet Taylor, a woman who profoundly stimulated and molded his awareness. Mill straightforwardly confronted the question of the biological nature, and especially the supposed biological inferiority, of women:

. . . I deny that anyone knows, or can know, the nature of the two sexes, as long as they have only been seen in their present relation to one another. If men had ever been found in society without women, or women without men, or if there had been a society of men and women in which the women were not under the control of the men, something might have been known about the mental and moral differences which may be inherent in the nature of each. What is now called the nature of woman is an eminently artificial thing—the result of forced repression in some directions, unnatural stimulation in others. (P. 148)

Ruth Peachey: A Rare Psychiatrist

Ruth Peachey is a psychiatrist who, among other things, testifies on behalf of battered women in Tennessee. Well trained by the "hierarchical system" she rejects, she retains what she calls her "lower-class" identity as well as her profound empathy for abused women. She is a social psychiatrist, a subspecialty in which only a few were educated in America (but more in Europe) in the 1960s. She is concerned with the socio-economic and political context in which people get diagnosed and treated. From early in her career she was repulsed by the psychiatric oppression of women, the use of brain-damaging treatments, and the labeling of patients that frequently obscures underlying psychosocial and economic causes.

Peachey tells me that it remains commonplace in her experience for husbands and male partners to institutionalize women in order to control or get rid of them. The psychiatric establishment and the courts tend to side with the husband and to view with hostility any advocacy on behalf of the victimized wife. The problem is even more extreme in the South, where Peachey lives. According to Peachey, the oppression of women by psychiatry is rampant and often takes place in the context of men dominating women in their personal and family relationships.

Peachey tells the story of a woman who began to resist her husband's growing attempts to control her. As she rebelled, he carefully spread rumors in their social circle that she was going crazy, and then he had her committed. Using her alleged insanity as an excuse, he took off with their children. She became understandably distraught, which made it easier for him to keep her committed.[13]

"I knew this woman personally," Peachey says, "and there was nothing wrong with her. It started with her resisting her husband's attempts to control her."

Now labeled a mental patient, the woman lost custody of her children. After becoming more despondent, she was given electroshock.

"It fried her brain," psychiatrist Peachey observes. "She was never the same again. Now she alternates between the streets and psychiatric institutions."

When we talked, Peachey had returned recently from a conference on battered women. Stories of extreme abuse of women by men, with psychiatric participation, are common, Peachey finds. Yet each time a new story is told, people greet it as an outrage without precedent. "Unfortunately," she says, "it happens all the time."

Hope in Psychotherapy

While psychotherapy, particularly Freudian psychoanalysis, has abused women and men and will continue to do so, the talking therapies also have helped to liberate many women. Phyllis Chesler, as noted earlier, believes that many women have come to appreciate themselves and even to become feminists through psychotherapy. This is my experience as well.

Psychotherapy is one of the channels that has brought an ameliorating measure of women's values into our culture. It has encouraged a focus on feelings and a greater awareness of vulnerability in both men and women. Through psychotherapy, many women and men have gained a better appreciation of the value of subjective feelings, nurturance, co-operation, love, and receptivity. I wish that more therapists had a firm grounding in feminist principles, because without it there are grave limits, and many pitfalls, in the help that psychotherapy can offer.

There are a number of things that women or men can do to protect themselves from authoritarianism and chauvinism when they seek a psychotherapist. Personal recommendations from happy clients and a willingness to shop around are basic. Asking therapists about their views on feminist issues, perhaps in advance on the telephone, can weed out many of them.*

Choosing a female therapist doesn't necessarily protect the female client, since some women who become mental health professionals make an exaggerated attempt to compete on the same terms as men. Still, the odds of a client's being respected as a woman are probably better with a female therapist, especially if she has a feminist awareness. Men are also more likely to find these women more receptive to their tender qualities. On the other hand, many men, including some of my close friends, are caring therapists.

Choosing a nonmedical therapist—such as a psychologist, social worker, counselor, or family therapist—may increase the odds of a better therapy experience. Many of my referrals are to nonmedical female therapists, including lesbian feminists who sometimes show a special sensitivity to women's issues. However, it bears repeating that there are no guarantees in turning to any specific kind of therapist, since many have aligned themselves with the psychiatric establishment.

Many women find it lifesaving to join a female peer group that meets regularly, especially if it encourages an awareness of feminist principles and insights. Whether or not a woman is also in psychotherapy, these groups are valuable, and for women who are involved in psychotherapy, such a group can provide a needed sounding board for concerns about the experience.

Be hesitant to follow a therapist's warning or prohibition against talking about therapy with any other people. One of your best protections against abuse in therapy is to communicate freely about your experience with

---

*I also suggest asking ahead of time about a therapist's views on involuntary treatment, biological and genetic theories, drugs, and electroshock. Even if these alternatives seem unlikely for you, the potential therapist's views on them will be informative. I believe, for example, that if a therapist favors electroshock for any patients, his or her viewpoint on people in general should be suspect. See chapter 16 for further discussion of choosing a therapist.

people you trust, such as friends and family. If possible, share your concerns with someone who's had a good therapy experience of his or her own or someone who loves and respects you very much. Checking with another therapist can be self-defeating, since many therapists feel obliged to defend their colleagues and to blame the client sooner than the other therapist for any discord. Also, anyone who has a vested interest in your subservience, such as an abusive parent or spouse, may give you the wrong advice either by promoting an oppressive therapy or by discouraging a liberating one.

Remember that the buyer of mental health services must be very wary and highly selective. Like choosing a lifelong companion, it can be the most important choice, for better or worse, that you'll ever make.

Chapter 15

Psychiatry and the Psycho-Pharmaceutical Complex

The contacts of psychiatry with the pharmaceutical industry have been so overwhelmingly beneficial that it would be well-nigh criminal to jeopardize them.

>—*Psychiatrist and psychopharmacologist Nathan S. Kline*[1]

"In Bed Together at the Market: Psychiatry and the Pharmaceutical Industry."

>—*Title of an editorial by Matthew Dumont, M.D., in the* American Journal of Orthopsychiatry, October 1990

As we saw in chapter 11, Upjohn produces the most frequently prescribed minor tranquilizer, Xanax. Despite its drawbacks and dangers, Xanax recently became the first drug to win approval from the FDA for use in so-called panic disorder or recurrent anxiety. Since panic disorder is a faddish diagnosis among psychiatrists and patients, this FDA imprimatur is worth a fortune. How did this happen? The previously untold story of how Upjohn has curried favor with organized psychiatry provides a model for understanding what I call the psycho-pharmaceutical complex.

The American Psychiatric Association

The best way to influence psychiatry is to earn the goodwill of the American Psychiatric Association. APA represents more than thirty-five thousand of the approximately forty-thousand American psychiatrists. In recent years APA has developed legislative and promotional departments to increase the power and influence of psychiatry. It spends money to win over the public, the press, and state and federal governments. As we have seen, it periodically issues task force reports on such subjects as shock treatment and tardive dyskinesia, formulating the conclusions to support the profession against lawsuits, public criticism, and nonmedical competition. The task forces that deal with treatment never include skeptics or even mild critics. APA publishes journals and a newspaper which usually support a biopsychiatric orientation.

APA and the Pharmaceutical Industry

The drug companies provide the backbone of financial support for APA and for most of organized psychiatry. The psychiatric newspapers and journals, including those published by APA, are largely paid for by drug company advertising. In 1987, for example, the APA newspaper *Psychiatric News* had a surplus of $1,311,554, largely the result of drug ads. In recent years, according to its annual reports published each October in the *American Journal of Psychiatry*, 15 to 20 percent of APA's total revenue has come from drug company advertising.

That 15 to 20 percent is but the tip of the pharmaceutical iceberg. APA's national conferences are underwritten by drug company monies to the tune of several million dollars a year. They literally could not take place without the drug company booths and drug company–sponsored seminars and entertainment. The drug companies also support special political projects, such as APA's annual meetings on how to lobby for favorable legislation. They underwrite conferences in which biopsychiatric leaders get together and promote themselves as well as drug products. The "President's Fund," the APA Auxiliary, and even individual psychiatrists on fellowships at the national headquarters are supported by drug company funds.

Of course, as physician Stanley Wohl points out in *The Medical Industrial Complex* (1984), organized medicine in general is underwritten by the drug companies. This was recognized even earlier by Morton Mintz in *The Therapeutic Nightmare* (1965), when he excoriated the American Psychiatric Association for failing to speak out "on the abuses of psychiatric drugs, abuses affecting millions." And this was before the plague of tardive dyskinesia had been discovered.

While it's true that the American Medical Association collects its own unholy share of drug company funds, there is something even more insidious about APA's ties to the pharmaceutical houses. First, it is more intimate and more thorough. Second, the "illnesses" being treated with drugs are not, in reality, diseases. Third, the APA–drug company collusion sponsors a very narrow band of approaches, namely the psychoactive drugs and shock treatment, which also requires the use of medications. And finally, while many medical drugs have great worth, psychiatric ones have few redeeming features.

If any picture is worth a thousand words, it is the photograph of a smiling APA president Robert Pasnau on the front page of the January 2, 1987, *Psychiatric News*. The caption explains that Pasnau is taking a check for an unspecified amount from a representative of Smith Kline and French, who is smiling even more broadly than the APA president. More significant than the check itself, the transaction took place at the annual meeting of the APA board of trustees; not even the deepest recesses of the association are off limits to influence peddling.

APA and the Upjohn Company

The Upjohn Company manufactures and sells only two psychiatric drugs, the minor tranquilizers Halcion and Xanax. Both are noteworthy in being short-acting and therefore highly addictive, and both have drawn more than their share of adverse publicity in the media for their dangerous side effects, including mental dysfunction and death (see chapter 11). But Upjohn spends multimillions to guarantee that its two products are well received by psychiatry.

The April 3, 1987, *Psychiatric News* reports that APA held a Public Affairs Institute, a conference on how to get more influence, money, and patients for psychiatry. It was underwritten by several drug companies, including Upjohn. Upjohn produced an expensive 35-mm slide show used by psychiatrists to woo referrals from other doctors. As a part of the same outreach PR program, APA's Division of Public Affairs created a calendar with cartoons aimed at helping psychiatrists relate to the colleagues who might refer patients to them. The calendar was produced by Upjohn.

APA president Pasnau then sent out a letter on May 4, 1987, to all APA members telling them about the calendar and making it easy for them to meet with the Upjohn sales representatives in order to get it:

Soon, your local Upjohn Representative will call on you to deliver your free copy of the calendar, which supports my presidential theme, "Psychiatry in Medicine/Medicine in Psychiatry.". . . For your convenience in establishing a suitable meeting date with your Upjohn Representative, I have enclosed a self-addressed, stamped postcard.

It is astonishing that Pasnau, in his official capacity as APA president, could affront the principles of conflict of interest by serving a company's interests in this manner. It indicates the degree to which organized psychiatry has come to accept this kind of back scratching as routine business.

Following the 1988 APA national convention, now former APA president Pasnau sent out a twenty-page expensively packaged glossy booklet on *Consequences of Anxiety*. In the letter to all APA members, written by Pasnau as professor of psychiatry at UCLA, he boasted that three breakfast symposia on anxiety at the recent national convention had drawn more than twelve hundred psychiatrists. The free events were sponsored by UCLA with financial support from Pasnau's old friend, the Upjohn Company. The fancy booklet itself was "made possible by an educational grant from The Upjohn Company."

Upjohn also pays for something called the Anxiety Disorders Resource Center, "as a service to science writers." An August 1987 press release from the center is written by professor of psychiatry Arthur Rifkin, who states that panic attacks "have been solidly related to biological or genetic factors." As a treatment for panic attacks Rifkin, not surprisingly, singles out an Upjohn product, alprazolam (Xanax), from among the many available and mostly interchangeable minor tranquilizers. He makes the nearly miraculous claim that the drug "completely eliminated panic attacks in 85% of a group of 27 patients"; but we can't corroborate his statement, because he does not identify the study.

The editorial board of the center includes such biopsychiatric luminaries as former NIMH director Gerald Klerman and drug advocate Donald Klein, director of research at the New York State Psychiatric Institute. Presumably these individuals are compensated for their services.

Following their seminars on anxiety at the 1988 APA national meeting, Upjohn sent out still another promotional packet for its medication. The package, sent to all thirty-five thousand APA members, came with a "Dear Colleague" letter from two former directors of NIMH, Shervert Frazier and Gerald Klerman. Frazier and Klerman, two leading psychiatrists, cochaired the Upjohn-sponsored APA workshop. The large envelope contained four glossy reprints of articles favorable toward Xanax as well as an eighteen-page booklet with many charts.*

Upjohn continues to cement its financial relationship with APA. The January 20, 1989, issue of *Psychiatric News* reports:

A recent $1.5 million agreement between APA and the Upjohn Company will bear fruit in the form of three public audience mental illness videos, a new medical education workshop for nonpsychiatric physicians and

---

* My research assistant at the time, Wade Hudson, obtained estimates on the cost of printing the materials that came to roughly $70,000. This did not include producing the materials (editing, design, and so on) or collating, packaging, and mailing. Nor did it include any possible payments to the physicians involved.

health-care gatekeepers, an exhibit and symposia program that will reach out to other medical specialty societies, and faculty support for the 1989 APA Public Affairs Network Institute.

On top of all this, Upjohn advertises heavily in APA and other medical and psychiatric publications.

Upjohn Pays Top Dollar for a Psychiatrist

Upjohn's Xanax is probably the most addictive drug commonly used in the United States today, by one estimate causing 1.5 million addictions a year (see chapter 11). As suggested in chapter 11, the Xanax studies that led to FDA approval for panic disorder should have led instead to its rejection as a treatment. The investigations showed that the main effect of the drug is sedation and that it produces many alcohollike side effects, such as slurred speech and impaired coordination, as well as a withdrawal syndrome similar to that following chronic alcohol abuse. Moreover, the overall results of the eight-week drug trial were so negative (placebo did better) that Upjohn ended up citing only the first four weeks of the trial in its advertising. Despite the short trial period, *most* of the patients had withdrawal problems getting off the drug, including a worsening of anxiety.

In late 1990 Upjohn nonetheless got FDA approval. The key figure in promoting the Xanax studies does not appear among the long lists of official investigators. He is Gerald Klerman,* former director of NIMH (1971 to 1975) and former director of the superstructure that includes NIMH and NIDA, the Alcohol, Drug Abuse, and Mental Health Administration (ADAMHA) (1977 to 1980). Klerman is now professor of psychiatry at Cornell University. This is the same man who was associated with Upjohn projects as an editorial board member of the company's Anxiety Disorders Resource Center and as an expert at Upjohn-sponsored seminars at the annual meetings of the APA.

Years earlier Klerman was responsible for the badly flawed NIMH studies that led the profession and the public mistakenly to believe that

---

*I first met Klerman around 1957–58 when I was working with the Harvard-Radcliffe Mental Hospital College Volunteer Program and he was a young psychiatrist at the Massachusetts Mental Health Center. We talked amicably about my interests in going to medical school to become a psychiatrist, and I explained my desire to learn more and eventually to contribute to our knowledge about human nature, human psychology, and psychosocial therapy. He advised me that I was headed in the wrong direction and that psychiatry was moving toward drugs and computerized diagnosis and treatment. At least in regard to drugs, he helped make that prediction come true. Meanwhile, despite much experimenting, computerized psychiatry has as yet failed to materialize.

neuroleptics have a specifically helpful impact on the symptoms of so-called schizophrenia, such as delusions and hallucinations (see chapter 3). Now Klerman was hired by Upjohn to organize and promote the Xanax studies required by the FDA.

Klerman wrote a lengthy introductory statement to the FDA Xanax studies in the May 1988 *Archives of General Psychiatry* describing the apparent great lengths to which Upjohn had gone in order to guarantee objectivity and high scientific quality. Entitled "Overview of the Cross-National Collaborative Panic Study," Klerman's report is really an un-qualified, enthusiastic endorsement of both Upjohn and its studies. What the reader has no way of knowing is that it was a *paid endorsement* in the sense that Klerman is a highly paid consultant to Upjohn. The only credential listed by Klerman in the appropriate footnote at the beginning of the article is his affiliation with Cornell University Medical School. There is no mention of his financial arrangements or his longstanding relationship with Upjohn. Within the article itself, however, there is a passing mention of "G.L.K." (Klerman) as one of three members of a "steering committee" for the Xanax project.

It was rumored from several professional sources that Klerman was paid $1 million by Upjohn for his role in the Xanax panic disorder studies required by the FDA. Klerman himself, in a lengthy telephone interview with me on January 8, 1991, specifically denied that he had been paid "anywhere near a million dollars" but refused to divulge the actual figure. He explained that the rules at Cornell University, where he has been a professor for several years, specify that faculty members are allowed to work only one day per week as outside consultants. He said that he has had an "ongoing" relationship as a consultant to Upjohn for "no more than one day a week" since 1982 or 1983, and that he was hired specif-ically to help develop the overall package of Xanax studies for FDA approval.

Klerman at first said to me that he had identified himself as a paid consultant to Upjohn in the *Archives* report, but on reflection he decided he has begun to do so only more recently. Klerman said, however, that he had "never hidden" his relationship to Upjohn. Nonetheless, as late as July 1989 Klerman defended the Xanax studies in a lengthy letter published in the *Archives* without mentioning the existence of his ongoing financial agreement with Upjohn. Klerman sees no inherent conflict of interest in his role and defends it on the grounds that "our society" wants drugs and other medical therapies developed "in the private sector gov-erned by the profit motive."

Klerman's introductory assessment of the Xanax studies in the *Archives of General Psychiatry* is especially important because his stance is that of a disinterested scientist writing a report in a medical journal. Since he is not listed as one of the actual participants in the drug studies, the reader gets the impression that this well-known psychopharmacologist, professor, and former director of NIMH and ADAMHA, is lending his independent, objective support to the research and its conclusions. Indeed, I have spoken to well-informed researchers who to this day know nothing about Klerman being on the Upjohn payroll.

Klerman remains one of America's most esteemed psychiatrists. The American Psychiatric Association awarded him its 1990 Distinguished Service Award.[2]

The good-old-boy network that connects medicine in general to the pharmaceutical industry is illustrated again by Upjohn, whose chief executive officer, president, and board chairman is Theodore Cooper. Cooper is former assistant secretary for health in the Department of Health, Education and Welfare (DHEW) and former dean of Cornell Medical School. Klerman attributes to Cooper, a fellow physician, what Klerman calls the company's "progressive" attitude in utilizing consultants like himself.

The May 18, 1990, *American Medical News*, put out by the AMA, reports that Upjohn's first-quarter earnings increased 10 percent to $114 million on sales of $773 million.

Upjohn and the Archives

But what about the journal itself in which the studies were published? Could Upjohn money have reached into the *Archives of General Psychiatry* as well? In fact, Upjohn money greased the biggest wheel of all at the *Archives*, psychiatrist Daniel X. Freedman, its editor in chief for the past twenty years. Fifteen years earlier, when the first report on the seriousness of the tardive dyskinesia epidemic had come out in the 1973 *Archives*, Freedman had appended a most unusual editorial, warning people not to exaggerate the importance of the drug-induced disease or to allow the negative publicity to interfere with the federal funding of psychiatry. Now in 1988 Freedman took on a remarkable dual role: editor of the journal publishing the Upjohn-sponsored Xanax studies and *paid consultant to Upjohn* as chairman of the company's oversight committee supervising "ethical and safety issues" in regard to the studies.

In an "Editorial Note" at the conclusion of Klerman's report on Xanax, Freedman informs us that his self-described role as *consultant and assistant* to the "Division of Medical Affairs of the Upjohn Company" in no way influenced the journal's handling of the papers. But psychiatrist Isaac M. Marks of the Institute of Psychiatry in London believes otherwise. Marks is one of the world's most respected researchers in the field of anxiety and drugs, and indeed, a book and an article of his are cited in Klerman's report. He is the senior author of the letter written by the international group of eleven psychiatrists and psychologists to the *Archives* in July 1989 in criticism of the Xanax studies (see chapter 11). In a telephone interview with me in January 1991, Marks said that Freedman had tried to obstruct publication of the letter in his journal. According to Marks, at first Freedman refused to look at the letter and later turned it down, despite its distinguished group authorship. When Marks called to find out what the problem might be, Freedman's secretary informed him that the margin settings were not standard and that the names of all eleven authors did not appear on the same page. Freedman then wrote a letter to Marks that Marks characterized as "insulting" in tone. The letter attempted to discredit the criticism made by the experts. After that Freedman refused to publish the most important part of the letter, what Marks called a "damning table" showing that Xanax was "almost ineffective" at eight weeks. Publication of the letter was delayed until fourteen months after the original article, significantly reducing its impact.

Freedman himself has his own version of the story surrounding the publication of the letter and an entirely different viewpoint on the overall relationship between drug company money and drug company influence. In a February 27, 1991, interview with me, Freedman stated that the "damning table" had not been included in the original letter received from Marks; but Freedman could not explain why the table was not included for publication along with the letter when the alleged mistake was corrected by Marks months ahead of the publication date. He emphatically denied obstructing publication of the letter and dismissed Marks as a "complainer."*

Freedman rejected as unfounded any skepticism about his own dual role as a consultant to Upjohn and editor in chief of the journal publishing the Upjohn-sponsored research. At first he said he wrote the editorial note mentioning his business relationship to Upjohn in order to avoid any "appearance of conflict of interest"; but then he denied there was even an appearance. He is a "scientist," he said, and "the three P's in science are far more powerful and compelling than money." The three "P's," he explained, "are priority, prestige, and publicity."† While he admitted to being a paid consultant to Upjohn for three years during the Xanax studies, the amount of money involved, he said, was "trivial" compared to his overall income. He would not, however, venture to estimate the amount he was paid or the percentage of his income it represented.

---

*I found Marks sincerely concerned about the problem of drug company influence in psychiatry. I also agreed with him that the tone of Freedman's letter to him was insulting.
†When I described Freedman's "three P's" to one of my students at George Mason University, Louise Massoud, she declared with dismay, "He didn't include *patients* in his 'three P's.'" Indeed, patients do seem far removed from the motivation of psychiatric researchers.

I pointed out to Freedman that the 1988 *Archives* publication on the efficacy of Xanax—under his editorship—seemed misleading because the introductory abstract described only the more encouraging first four weeks of the study without even mentioning that it had gone on for an additional month with much less promising results. Freedman replied that he was sure there was no intention to mislead anyone; but he could not explain how or why the abstract had been written in that manner. He ridiculed the idea that readers of the journal might sometimes rely on the abstract without studying the complete text. Then, as if to exonerate his journal, he reminded me that the FDA had approved the drug.

During the interview, without personally criticizing me, Freedman applied the labels "Marxist" and "paranoid" to concerns about drug company influence over research. He felt that Upjohn should be praised for establishing the oversight committee that he chaired. Overall, Freedman believes that the funds pumped into the psychiatric profession by drug companies such as Upjohn do not encourage any bias on the part of investigators or psychiatry in general.

APA Joins the Xanax Celebration

Given Upjohn's bountiful financing of the American Psychiatric Association, it's no surprise that the January 4, 1991, issue of *Psychiatric News* describes the approval of Xanax for panic disorder in terms at least as laudatory as the drug company's own advertising.[3] The drug is reported effective at four weeks. *No mention is made of the fact that the study went eight weeks.* The thousands of psychiatrists who regularly read the APA newspaper would have no idea that the drug became ineffective within eight weeks and, compared to placebo, produced many severe side effects, including an increase in anxiety and panic. Gerald Klerman is cited as calling for gradual drug reduction in order to avoid withdrawal symptoms, but the study itself shows that this was of little or no help. Klerman is described as a "researcher" and not as a paid employee of Upjohn.

The Xanax Doctors Are Not Alone

I had the opportunity to discuss the funding of the Xanax doctors with a nationally known American psychopharmacologist,* who freely ad-

---

*He gave me permission to use his name, but I don't believe he is aware of the extent of the potential backlash, and so I have withheld his name.

mitted to receiving money from another pharmaceutical company with a competing product. Somewhat defensively, he told me, "I believe it's okay to take the money, but I speak the facts as I see them." He explained about psychopharmacology researchers in general: "We're all supported by somebody. The question is how much do you let it blur your judgment." He went to great lengths to explain to me that the payments he received did not affect his views on the drug; and yet throughout the conversation he minimized the dangerousness of his product while freely discussing the negative effects of its competitors. Indeed, one of his research reviews concludes with several paragraphs of near idolatrous praise for his patron drug company's product, and as usual, there's no footnote to indicate that he is a paid consultant to the company.

Nonetheless, this psychopharmacologist was critical of others in his field for their excessive devotion to the products of their sponsors. "Listen, I'll tell you that 'my drug' isn't *always* the best choice, but he [a Xanax study author] acts as if his drug is the only one. He gives lectures on how Xanax isn't anywhere near as addictive as it really is."

The psychopharmacologist went on to describe professional conferences as competitions at which the various doctors take sides on behalf of their patron drug companies. One expert would be defending Xanax while another was promoting Valium or BuSpar, and each was known to be a paid consultant to the respective drug company.

An extremely well known European psychiatrist and psychopharmacologist (who asked not to be named) told me that Upjohn "paid tens of millions of dollars" worldwide in consulting fees, honoraria, research grants, and gifts to influence psychiatrists around the world in order to affect the outcome of the Xanax studies and their reception by the profession. "Money talks," he said, adding that sometimes it seemed as if "the entire profession was working for Upjohn in one way or another." Nonetheless, he said that Upjohn's spending spree, while perhaps more extreme than many other pharmaceutical companies, is typical of drug company sponsorship of psychiatry and psychopharmacology.

Upjohn Is Not Alone

Most pharmaceutical firms that produce psychiatric medications are much larger than Upjohn and some very likely spend even more on making friends with the profession. Companies that help to support psychiatry include Smith Kline and French Laboratories, Mead Johnson (a Bristol-Meyers company), Dorsey (a division of Sandoz), Merrell Dow, Roerig (a division of Pfizer), Ives Laboratories, ER Squibb and Sons, Dista Products (a division of Eli Lilly), Boots Pharmaceuticals, Burroughs

Wellcome, and Lederle Laboratories. In defense of Upjohn, Klerman cites Mead Johnson as an example of other companies that also spend lavishly on the psychiatric community. Not surprisingly, Mead Johnson is a competitor to Klerman's patron company. It makes the minor tranquilizer BuSpar as well as an antidepressant.

APA Decides to Take From the Drug Companies

The American Psychiatric Association's governing body made a conscious decision to rely more heavily on drug company funding for its activities, and that decision most likely influenced individual doctors to line up as well for the handouts. In the early 1970s APA was in financial trouble. It was losing membership and its total income was $2 to $4 million per year, compared to its current income of over $21 million. The newspapers and journals were operating in the red instead of generating huge surpluses through drug company advertising. In general psychiatry was losing badly in the competition with psychologists, social workers, counselors, family therapists, and other nonmedical professionals who charge lower fees for psychotherapy patients. Psychiatric journals and newspapers were filled with gloom, lamenting that psychiatrists could no longer easily fill their workweeks. At the same time, psychiatry was coming under increasing criticism about psychosurgery, electroshock, and the newly publicized drug-induced disease, tardive dyskinesia.

A turning point was the conflict over whether or not to divest from drug company influence. In April 1974 the *American Journal of Psychiatry* reported that "the matter of APA's relationship with industry, especially the pharmaceutical companies," was becoming a concern for some members of the board of trustees, who felt that "APA's relationships with pharmaceutical companies were going beyond the bounds of professionalism, were compromising our principles, and in some instances were involving members in conflicts of interest." These doubts were being raised about a degree of involvement that looks petty by today's standards.

In response to the doubters, APA formed the Task Force to Study the Impact of the Potential Loss of Pharmaceutical Support. Its very title suggests the fear that independence from the drug companies struck in the hearts of the leadership. The task force concluded that many local APA member organizations as well as various training programs would fold without the "lifeblood" support of the drug companies. Continued support for seminars at the national conventions also was found acceptable, provided that it was not credited directly to individual drug companies.

The floodgates of drug company influence were opened and would grow wider each year. Nowadays dozens of seminars are supported by the drug companies, and the individual names of the companies are honored conspicuously with advertisements in psychiatric journals and newspapers prior to the meetings.

A lonely voice, Robert Seidenberg, clinical professor of psychiatry at the State University of New York, Upstate Medical Center in Syracuse, protested the APA's decision to cozy up to the drug companies in a November 2, 1979, letter to *Psychiatric News*. He calls the policy of drug company dependence "the nadir of ethical behavior."

Still struggling to make ends meet, in 1980 the APA board of directors threw ethical caution to the winds and "voted to encourage pharmaceutical companies to support scientific or cultural activities rather than strictly social activities as a part of the Annual Meeting program. . . ."[4] In other words, give us more than coffee and entertainment; give direct support to our major professional and scientific activities.

In the following years, APA went on to develop a Political Action Committee (PAC) and special departments aimed at influencing Congress, state legislators, the media, and the public to hold psychiatry in higher esteem and to support its economic interests. Many of these promotional efforts are now supported by drug companies.

Some of the motivation for psychiatry's new political thrust was expressed by the speaker-elect in his report published in the October 1984 issue of the *American Journal of Psychiatry*. The PAC, he tries to explain, was not "buying votes," but trying to better public policy. Meanwhile, he compares the rivalry between psychiatrists and psychologists to Star Wars, lamenting "an oversupply of competitive practitioners" that resulted in "a galaxy of turf wars."

Whatever function APA had ever fulfilled as a professional organization was now superseded by its function as political advocate for the advancement of psychiatric and pharmaceutical business interests. Continually reiterated is the conviction that only a medical or biological image can enable psychiatry to compete economically.

Protesting the Selling of Psychiatry

As organized psychiatry and individual leaders in psychiatry became increasingly intimate with the drug companies, a few voices of concern were expressed within the establishment. In the October 1984 *American Journal of Psychiatry* the APA speaker-elect, Fred Gottlieb, entitled his report ironically, "Better Living Through Chemistry: Industry Money for Education and Amenities." In it he notes that APA's Scientific Program Committee had written recently to the APA president about drug company influence on scientific programming. The committee questioned drug company funding of many aspects of the national conferences, including payment to members who participate in drug company–sponsored events.

Gottlieb cited research demonstrating "the powerful influence of commercial [drug company] sources on the nonrational prescribing behavior of physicians." In taking money from the pharmaceutical industry, he pointed out, "Our inherent conflict of interest is obvious" (p. 1333).

Gottlieb went on to subtitle one of his commentaries "Implications of APA's Expanded Funding Sources: He Who Pays the Piper . . . You Can't Have Your Cake and . . . or Can You, With Continuing Vigilance?" He declares, "The issue is to make sure such conflicts of interest are not hidden but are openly and carefully examined, as well as kept to a minimum" (p. 1333).

One year later, in October 1985 Gottlieb continued his warnings in his speaker's report. He says he previously "wrote about the *millions* of dollars of drug house money we receive annually from advertising and commercial exhibits and for awarded lectureships and social functions." Now he has been "startled to learn that our [APA] Federal Legislative Institute is similarly supported." He explains:

I do not suggest that either they [the drug companies] or we are evil folks. But I continue to believe that accepting such money is, in the long run, inimical to our independent functioning. We have evolved a somewhat casual and quite cordial relationship with the drug houses, taking their money readily. . . . We seem to discount available data that drug advertising promotes irrational prescribing practices. We seem to think that we as psychiatrists are immune from the kinds of unconscious emotional bias in favor of those who are overtly friendly toward us. . . . We persist in ignoring an inherent conflict of interest. (P. 1248)

Gottlieb voices regret over the APA's use of a Political Action Committee on the grounds that PACs serve a narrow self-interest rather than the long-range good of the profession or the public.

While Gottlieb was a significant voice of protest, the 1985 annual report makes clear that the APA board of directors has launched itself headlong into the era of dependency on the drug companies. It authorizes accepting money from a drug company to support subscriptions for one of its journals and most incredibly tightens up its policy on giving members information on financial and budget matters, including "pharmaceutical industry support" (p. 1247). Indeed, such information became and remains largely unavailable. The board also voted to hire a "marketing" consultant at $150,000 per year.

Gottlieb's concerns were steamrollered by APA leadership—no further criticisms were made by APA officals in following years, and drug company dependence has grown ever more rapidly. So has the APA policy of financial aggrandizement. The motivation was made clear in the report by treasurer George Pollock in the October 1986 *American Journal of Psychiatry*. He warns that "the national economy has placed pressure on APA through the field of psychiatry as a whole as well as through our individual members." The treasurer then unabashedly declares, "In fact, the field of psychiatry has become an economically driven profession" (p. 1340).

The "economically driven profession" now devoted increased expenditures for "various economic affairs," including "government relations, public affairs, and education," always with a biopsychiatric thrust aimed at regaining dominance in the mental health field. One direct result has been the swell of positive media coverage in response to pronouncements from APA and NIMH about alleged breakthroughs in biopsychiatry. Another has been increased federal support for psychiatry. While other federal budgets are being cut, NIMH's has again been growing.[5] Still another is the public's growing acceptance of catchword phrases like *biochemical imbalance* and *genetic predisposition*.

A Drug Company Circus

By 1987 the APA annual meeting had become a drug company circus.* Everywhere one turned there was drug company sponsorship. The *Daily Bulletin* for the conference was provided by one drug company and the "Message and Information Locator" by another. Even the shiny silver package of registration materials handed to each participant was marked "Provided by a grant from McNeil Pharmaceuticals, makers of Haldol (haloperidol) Decanoate." The CME seminars, where APA members can obtain their required continuing medical education credits, were credited as being supported by the drug companies. One irate psychiatrist, H. Steven Moffic, wrote to *Psychiatric News* on June 19, 1987, suggesting that APA was beginning to stand for the "American Psychopharmaceutical Association."

Psychiatrist Loren Mosher wrote an unpublished letter in August 1987 to APA treasurer Alan Levenson in reflection on his membership. Mosher observed about APA:

Its dependence on drug company support for its annual meeting, journals, newspaper and organization itself has reached, as far as I'm concerned, an

---

*Subsequent meetings have grown still worse.

unacceptable level. This organizational behavior is leading psychiatrists to be perceived by outsiders as principally prescription writers. The narrowing of our professional role that occurs in part as a result of dependence on drug company money will, I believe, be harmful to the profession in the long run. Hence, I believe APA's policies with regard to accepting drug company money should be changed. At the very least the membership should receive a complete accounting of drug company income and how it is expended.

That accounting of drug company influence has never been given. Nor will it ever be—without the intervention of Congress or the courts.

Debating the APA President on Oprah

Psychiatry's contempt for conflict of interest was brought home to me when I debated APA president-elect Paul Fink on television on the "Oprah Winfrey Show" on August 17, 1987. In my opening remarks I focused on the scandal of drug company funding of APA and pointed out that Fink himself had been head of APA's Public Affairs Division, which was drug company funded.* We then had the following exchange:

DR. BREGGIN: No, the Psychiatric Association is not beholden to the patients now, it's beholden to the drug companies. And we need a "Psychogate" investigation of this. Congress should investigate this, Oprah, and I ask Dr. Fink as the president to come clean next year and talk about the millions of dollars being channeled through the American Psychiatric Association.

WINFREY: Well, Dr. Fink is fuming now.

DR. FINK: Yes, he is.

WINFREY: He is fuming.

DR. FINK: I'm glad you said that.

WINFREY: Okay, okay, go ahead.

DR. FINK: Well, I think the—

DR. BREGGIN: Can you deny anything I just said?

DR. FINK: Can I deny that we get money—

DR. BREGGIN: Millions of dollars are being pumped through the Psychiatric Association by the drug companies.

DR. FINK: No. I can't deny that we get millions of dollars of support from the drug companies. I also can't deny that that seems to be tangential to the issue of whether the drugs that are used are of value, and they are—

---

*I didn't mention that he was chief medical editor of a glossy monthly magazine put out by Merrell Dow.

DR. BREGGIN: Your *scientific* meetings are funded by the drug companies.

DR. FINK: I don't—that's irrelevant. That's irrelevant.

DR. BREGGIN: How is that irrelevant?

DR. FINK: It's absolutely irrelevant, because the doctor on the street, the psychiatrist in the communities, is not affected by the fact we get some support—minimal, I might add, in terms of the entire budget—

DR. BREGGIN: Twenty percent is from drug company advertising.

DR. FINK: Ten percent.

DR. BREGGIN: Twenty percent in the last three budgets, and if you want, I'll go out and get the figures during the next segment.

I had the official APA reports ready in the waiting area. The actual figures for the previous two years had been 19.69 percent in 1985 and 19.92 percent in 1984.[6]

DR. FINK: Go ahead. I have the figures, as the president-elect.

DR. BREGGIN: Twenty percent of the revenues.

DR. FINK: The point is, whether it's 10 percent or 20 percent. . . .

WINFREY: Let him speak, Dr. Breggin, please.

DR. FINK: It's not really the relevant issue. The relevant issue is, are the drugs valuable? Yes, they are.

Judi Chamberlin had been invited by me to participate on the show as a psychiatric survivor representative. A short time after my exchange with Fink she brought us back to the topic, declaring, "But how can you have a scientific debate as to whether drugs are good or bad if the drug companies are underwriting the discussion? It skews everything."

DR. FINK: The assumption is that we're unconscionable and therefore we don't—we don't—

DR. BREGGIN: But you're a psychiatrist, you understand self-interest. If you go to a convention and everywhere it says "Supported by this drug company, supported by that drug company—"

DR. FINK: I don't understand. I don't understand.

Indeed, Fink seemed not to understand. He came back to the subject later in the show, displaying visible frustration:

DR. FINK: . . . you're worried about a couple million dollars from the drug companies, and that 33,000 psychiatrists are *just a bunch of rats* who are just thinking we got that money from the drug companies. It's kind of outrageous, it's very outrageous that the first thing you want to talk about is the fact that we are underwritten to a certain—

DR. BREGGIN: The *profession* is now underwritten—

DR. FINK: —to a certain extent, by a faction of the pharmaceutical industry.

Fink may have understood more about money and self-interest than he was letting on. Here is what he had declared in his candidacy statement for the APA presidency, published in the December 19, 1986, *Psychiatric News*: "It is the task of APA to protect the earning power of psychiatrists."

As the president of APA, Fink went on to sign the previously mentioned ground-breaking 1989 contract with Upjohn that delivers $1.5 million to APA's coffers for the promotion of psychiatry.

NIMH and the Psycho-Pharmaceutical Complex

In recent years the National Institute of Mental Health has become dominated by biopsychiatry. When I was a full-time consultant with NIMH in 1967 and 1968, biological psychiatry was a relatively small section within the institute; now it *is* the institute. The outgoing head, psychiatrist Lewis Judd, like his immediate predecessors, was wholly devoted to the brain rather than the mind as the legitimate subject of psychiatric research and treatment.[7] Politically he moved NIMH very close to becoming a lab science institute; and inside sources during his tenure were unanimous in telling me that he wanted to get rid of those services that defend patients' rights (protection and advocacy programs) or support innovative consumer approaches (community support programs).

NIMH exerts control over the mental health marketplace by setting trends, pushing biopsychiatric treatments, giving grants to individuals and institutions for research, supporting training, holding conferences, conducting its own research, and generally promoting biopsychiatry through the media. For example, when one flimsy study suggested that manic-depression might be linked to a gene, NIMH leaped forward to hold a press conference. As we saw in chapter 7, the study's status and value among researchers quickly dwindled, but its media impact did not. Similarly, the media have also promoted the DART program, which aims at getting more people to consider themselves depressed and to take drugs and shock treatment.*

---

*The National Institutes of Health (NIH), a separate bureaucracy from NIMH, uses drug companies to sponsor some of its continuing-education programs. For example, NIH periodically holds updates in psychopharmacology for the practicing psychiatrist. In October 1987 its program at the Hyatt Regency in Bethesda, Maryland, acknowledged the support of Abbot Laboratories, Bristol-Meyers, Hoechst-Roussel Pharmaceuticals, and Warner Lambert.

The FDA

As attorney James Turner wrote in *The Chemical Feast* (1970), it has long been known that the FDA is hardly the consumer watchdog it's supposed to be. It gets thrown too many bones from the pharmaceutical industry to bite the hand that feeds it. Earlier, in 1965, Morton Mintz of the *Washington Post* wrote *The Therapeutic Nightmare*, documenting the mutual, supportive relationships among the FDA, APA, and the drug companies. As an example, the FDA came close to permanently withdrawing Parnate, an MAOI antidepressant, from the market, because the drug was proving to be extremely dangerous with little evidence for effectiveness; but the FDA reversed itself under pressure from the APA and cancelled its planned hearings. Nonetheless, many psychiatrists rejected the drug and it fell into disfavor for a few years. However, in the current biopsychiatric climate Parnate and similar drugs are enjoying a brisk revival (see chapter 8).

In general the FDA has done little to monitor or control the use of psychiatric technologies or to highlight their damaging effects. It has backed off from requiring research on the safety of electroshock (see chapter 9) and it never did do anything about lobotomy and other forms of psychosurgery. While an unusual FDA regulation has required that drug companies show more honesty about the dangers of tardive dyskinesia, it was too little, too late. The 1985 intervention by the FDA came many years after the drug-induced disease had become a documented epidemic. And patients and doctors reading the FDA-mandated drug company advertising for neuroleptics would have no idea that rates of the disease approach and exceed 50 percent in long-term use.[8]

Mostly the FDA lends authority to the use of psychiatric drugs and electroshock by approving them, and in the case of psychosurgery it gives tacit legitimacy by not even investigating it. The public is lulled into believing that regulatory agencies are busy at work protecting them. In depositions when I am critical of the use of a specific psychiatric drug, opposing attorneys sometimes challenge me, "But wasn't it approved for that by the FDA?" When I am being deposed by the drug companies themselves, their attorneys always try to relieve their clients of responsibility by pointing to FDA regulation. The pharmaceutical companies and their attorneys hope that people sitting on juries will exonerate companies because they operate under the FDA umbrella.

Furthermore, as we've seen in regard to Prozac and Xanax, FDA approval of a drug misleads the public into thinking that thousands of patients have been tested in controlled studies for months or years, when in reality a few hundred are tested for a few weeks. In regard to the neuroleptic Clozaril (clozapine), the recent FDA approval is especially misleading. Parents, doctors, and patients anticipate that this drug is to be administered for years at a time, even for the lifetime of many patients, and frequently against the patient's wishes. Yet the FDA controlled trials for this extremely brain-disabling and sometimes life-threatening drug *lasted only six weeks!*[9]

Similarly the newly approved drug for obsessive-compulsive disorder, Anafranil (clomipramine), was studied for only ten weeks, when it, too, frequently will be administered for months or years. The FDA warns: "Because clomipramine has not been systematically evaluated for long-term use (more than ten weeks), physicians should periodically reevaluate the long-term usefulness of the drug for individual patients." Published in the obscure *FDA Drug Bulletin*, this warning will go unheeded.[10]

As we've also seen in regard to Xanax, FDA approval does not mean that the drug trials have really demonstrated either safety or efficacy. The FDA can bend over backward to accommodate the drug industry and its financially captive psychiatric experts.

Regulatory agencies are notorious for coming under the control of the industries they regulate because the giant corporations have the power and money with which to buy influence and to obtain favors from government bureaucrats and politicians. By comparison, the consumers have almost no voice at all. Recently Washington was rocked by disclosures of corruption in HUD, including housing industry influence over decision-making processes. Less known was a similarly outrageous scandal at the FDA, described by John Schwartz in "Corruption and Chaos Uncovered in the FDA Generics Approval Process," in the July 1989 issue of the *Psychiatric Times*, and by an ongoing series of disclosures in the general press.[11] It is tempting to retell the lurid details of drug companies buying favors from FDA bureaucrats, but "corruption" really isn't the main problem. The real problem, as we have seen, lies in the normal functioning of the FDA as it misleads the public into believing that psychiatric drugs are safe and efficacious when in fact they are neither.

"Toxic Parents" Join Toxic Psychiatry

Finally, there is the growing family movement, led by the National Alliance for the Mentally Ill (NAMI), with a rapidly expanding membership surpassing 100,000. It and its state affiliates consider all severe psychosocial disorders to be biochemical in origin and advocate lobotomy, electroshock, and drugs. It resists the growing movement of psychiatric survivors and supporters of patients' rights in general.*

APA and NIMH work hand-in-glove with NAMI. They lobby Congress together and meet the press together. NAMI leaders have direct access to the leadership of APA and NIMH, and they help plan national campaigns on behalf of biopsychiatry. NAMI recently published a letter it received from outgoing NIMH director Lewis Judd in which he spoke of the "dedication and shared purpose which has forged a unique and strong relationship and collaboration between NAMI and NIMH."[12] With no apparent awareness of the inappropriateness of handing a federal agency over to a self-serving parent lobbying group, Judd declared, "NIMH, in a very meaningful sense, is NAMI's Institute." He then went on to repeat their shared but wholly unproven credo: "During the last 15 years, we have unequivocally established that mental illnesses are brain related disorders, which often involve strong genetic influences." The public's false impression of breakthroughs in biological psychiatry is based on the repetition of these unfounded slogans.

NAMI is not content to support its own viewpoint. As already noted, it personally attacks critics of biopsychiatry and advocates of psychosocial approaches. It lobbies against the funding of psychosocial research, most vehemently opposing any project that implicates parents in the problems of their offspring. Thus it has tried to stop funding of relatively non-controversial studies indicating that the improvement of communication in families helps in the recovery of their mentally disabled members.[13]

NAMI has helped to develop and direct several high-profile media campaigns whose hidden agenda is convincing the public that the children of NAMI parents have diseases that cannot be blamed on the parents. It has cofounded the National Alliance for Research on Schizophrenia and Depression, which funds research in psychiatry. Research investigators thereby become dependent for their livelihood on funding from an organization that compulsively opposes psychosocial viewpoints and vehemently supports biopsychiatric ones.

Like the APA and its local branches, NAMI and some of its state organizations actively solicit and obtain support money from the drug companies. The fall 1990 issue of the *Journal*, the official publication of California Alliance for the Mentally Ill (CAMI), expresses gratitude for "generous financial contributions" from Sandoz Pharmaceuticals, Eli Lilly, and Upjohn. Earlier we noted that Sandoz has given NAMI parents "scholarships" to pay for the newly approved and dangerous neuroleptic Clozaril (clozapine) for their offspring. The March 1990 issue of NAMI's

---

* Recently I have heard of at least one local exception to this rule. Furthermore, not all NAMI parents have caused their childrens' problems, but the NAMI *leadership* has aggressively sought to suppress those with whom it disagrees.

national journal *Advocate* has an ad for Clozaril, plus an article describing the Sandoz scholarships, promoting the drug, and providing phone numbers to make it easier for physicians to get started using it. However, pressure on Sandoz more recently has caused the company to make it somewhat easier and cheaper to prescribe the drug.[14]

Medical Schools and Professorships

Medical school departments of psychiatry have gone largely biopsychiatric and often take money from the drug companies. Nowadays some heads of psychiatry departments are biochemists and nearly all are heavily biopsychiatric. Psychologically oriented department heads have gone the way of the California condor. Naturally, as a central part of the medical establishment, medical schools want to support biological approaches.

The schools also receive money from the drug companies in the form of research grants, sponsored professorships, and support for various projects. Indeed, the amounts probably far exceed those involved in supporting the APA. Professors at medical schools sit on the boards or act as consultants to research and development companies attempting to create and market new psychiatric drugs. Bright young researchers may go directly from working on a drug company grant at the university to joining the drug company's staff.

Health Insurers

Health insurers play a largely unexplored role in reinforcing the psychopharmaceutical complex. They tend to reimburse well for drugs, electroshock, and psychiatric hospitalization. On the other hand, they pay relatively little or nothing for psychotherapy and other forms of social rehabilitation, such as halfway houses, crisis centers, and residential homes, which ultimately can be more effective and less costly. Private practitioners, including psychologists and other nonmedical therapists, increasingly find themselves pressured by health insurers to give or to encourage drugs rather than to lose reimbursement for the treatment of specific patients. One colleague of mine, a psychologist, has been told by an insurance company to give one of his patients drugs for anxiety or the patient's coverage for the treatment will be terminated.

The practice of psychotherapy has been vastly curtailed by insurance company policies and successful psychosocial innovations for severely impaired people have withered from lack of support (see chapter 16). There is hope, however. I talked to the director of a corporation that manages several health insurance programs. He was against psychiatric hospitalization as too costly and often damaging and was considering plans to pay for intensive, even daily, psychotherapy as an alternative. In my experience, a month's worth of very frequent psychotherapy would be much more useful to most acutely disturbed patients than hospitalization, and far less expensive or dangerous.

The Psycho-Pharmaceutical Complex

What we have been examining is a giant combine similar to the military-industrial complex and involving the psychiatric profession (APA), government (NIMH and FDA), private industry (drug companies and health insurers), education (medical schools), and organizations representing the parents of patients (NAMI and other family groups). But the psycho-pharmaceutical complex is not a "conspiracy" in the usual sense of a wholly secret or covert collaboration. Much of it involves aboveboard, frank cooperation among like-minded, self-interested parties. Nonetheless, much of it also remains largely hidden from scrutiny, including the amounts of money paid by the drug companies to the APA and to leading psychiatrists. And whether it constitutes a *legal* conspiracy remains untested.

The only interest group not included in the psycho-pharmaceutical complex is the true consumers—the patients and victims of biopsychiatry—as represented by the National Association of Psychiatric Survivors (NAPS; see appendix A). Not surprisingly, the patients and ex-patient leaders have no significant voice in the psychiatric power structure.

Given the power of the psycho-pharmaceutical complex, it is no wonder that the public hears so little criticism of the biopsychiatric approach and almost nothing about psychosocial, human service alternatives.*

The Psycho-Pharmaceutical Complex Zeros In

As reporter Vince Bielski discloses in "The Assault on Patients' Rights" in the July 4, 1990, *San Francisco Bay Guardian*, the psycho-pharmaceutical complex is willing to bring its weight to bear on local issues. A 1989 California court decision, Riese v. St. Mary's, expanded

---

*In December 1990 Senator Ted Kennedy held hearings on the buying of doctors by drug companies through "lavish vacations, gifts and cash payments." As reported by Warren Leary in the December 12, 1990, *New York Times*, Kennedy observed that pharmaceutical firms are spending four times what they did in 1975 to promote drugs. However, it appears that the psycho-pharmaceutical complex and psychiatry have escaped scrutiny at these hearings.

the right of *legally competent* psychiatric patients to give informed consent or to refuse antipsychotic drugs. Perhaps because California tends to be a trend setter, this decision brought much of the psycho-pharmaceutical complex into the fray. The California branch of NAMI (CAMI) put pressure on state legislators to reverse the patients' rights decision. CAMI's attempt to make it easier to control its offspring was not surprising. As expected, the California Psychiatric Society also lent its considerable lobbying weight to reversing the court decision with new legislation. According to Bielski, state assemblyman Bruce Bronzan, the leading advocate of gutting the Reise decision, turned out to be the recipient of vast psycho-pharmaceutical complex largess, including:

contributions and honoraria from dozens of psychiatric and hospital asso-ciations, and pharmaceutical manufacturers, the Northern California and Central California Psychiatric Society, CA Hospitals, the Pharmaceutical Manufacturers Association, Sandoz Pharmaceuticals Corporation (maker of the neuroleptic Mellaril); Ciba Geigy Corporation (maker of Ludiomil and other psychiatric drugs) and Parke Davis (maker of Nardil and other psychiatric drugs).

Thus even national pharmaceutical firms were supporting the assault on patients' rights. The psycho-pharmacentical industry is one of the few American enterprises heavily supported by totally involuntary consumers.

Why is there so much interest in preventing legally competent patients from rejecting highly toxic drugs? After mentioning the unrealistic fear of chaos on the psychiatric wards,* Bielski observes, "Moreover, now that drugs have become the basic tools of psychiatry, hospitals, psychi-atrists and drug companies stand to lose money if patients refuse to swallow their prescriptions."

Psychiatry as Big Business

Implicit in all of this is the reality that organized psychiatry is big business more than it is a profession. As a big business, managed by APA and NIMH, it develops media relationships, hires PR firms, develops its medical image, holds press conferences to publicize its products, lobbies on behalf of its interests, and issues "scientific" reports that protect its members from malpractice suits by lending legitimacy to brain-damaging

---

*As I describe in *Psychiatric Drugs: Hazards to the Brain* (New York: Springer, 1983), the fear of psychiatric wards going wild has never materialized in states like Massachusetts that recognize the right to refuse treatment. Yet it is raised frequently by the psychiatric establishment as a means of thwarting public support for increased patients' rights.

366

technologies. It tries to increase not only its share of the market, but also the size of the whole market.

One way to increase the overall size of the market is to convince the government, society, and individual citizens that its services are needed. From this motivation grows "official estimates" of the "prevalence of mental illness" that the media latch onto in their stories about the need for psychiatric treatment.

The APA's Division of Public Affairs and Joint Commission on Public Affairs have the task of increasing business. They publish a "Fact Sheet" to help psychiatrists sell themselves to the public. The Group for the Advancement of Psychiatry (GAP) is a private group made up of leaders in the field. In 1987 GAP published *Speaking Out for Psychiatry: A Handbook for Involvement with the Mass Media*, in which they reprint the "Fact Sheet." Here are the estimates for how many Americans are in need of psychiatric services:

> Anxiety disorders: 11.1 million
> Depression: 9.4 million
> Schizophrenia: 1.5 million
> Substance and alcohol abuse: 25.5 million
> Emotional and developmental problems in children: 12 million

These five estimates add up to 59.5 million Americans, and that's not including some of the more popular diagnostic categories, such as eating disorders, sexual dysfunctions, and organic brain disorders. Even assuming some inevitable overlap among the groups, 59.5 million potential consumers is a lot of business, more than enough to keep busy a mere forty thousand psychiatrists! Indeed, GAP's estimate that 15 to 25 percent of the elderly have "significant" mental illness would be enough to keep the entire profession occupied.

Perhaps not having added up its own figures, GAP estimates that a mere one in five Americans need psychiatric treatment; but that's 20 percent of the population, or approximately fifty million Americans. Not content with 20 percent of Americans, NIMH has recently decided that one in five Americans suffers a mental problem in any *six-month period*. A *Washington Post* staff writer passes this on as the gospel truth in the June 27, 1989, *Health* magazine supplement.

Too Many or Too Few Psychiatrists?

There is an especially misleading aspect to these repeated attempts to inflate the numbers of allegedly mentally ill in need of psychiatric treatment. The PR line is that there aren't enough psychiatrists to help all of these people and that the profession must continue to grow in size and importance in the coming years. Thus the December 1990 *Clinical Psychiatry News* displays the front-page headline SHORTAGE OF PSYCHIATRISTS EXPECTED TO CONTINUE.

But is there really a shortage of psychiatrists? That is, are psychiatrists overburdened with too many patients? No, the article admits, the opposite is true. Despite intensive promotional efforts by NIMH and APA to get people to go to psychiatrists, *there are too many psychiatrists vying for too few patients.* According to the *Clinical Psychiatry News* report, "the low demand for the services of adult and child psychiatrists may make it seem as if there is an oversupply of these physicians, but more Americans need to use their services, and would if they could afford them. . . ." This "low demand" for psychiatrists indicates that psychiatrists are continuing to fall behind in their competition with nonmedical therapists—psychologists, social workers, counselors, and family therapists.[15]

Thus while psychiatrists continue to have too few patients to maintain their professional incomes at the desired level, their national organizations speak of a shortage of psychiatrists in order to convince the public, the federal government, and health insurance companies to give more support to the profession. The continued failure of psychiatry to attract voluntary patients is the main impetus behind the biopsychiatric propaganda we have been examining in this book.

Enforcing the Psychiatric Monopoly

In addition to the psycho-pharmaceutical complex, psychiatry also draws support from its complex relationship to the state and the judiciary. Psychiatrists, as physicians, are licensed to practice medicine by the individual states. Within the mental health marketplace this gives psychiatrists the unique power not only to prescribe physical treatments, such as drugs and shock, but also to dominate mental health practices in the hospital system, including state hospitals, general hospital psychiatric wards, and private hospitals. It gives them the all-important authority to use physical force to make consumers accept their services through involuntary treatment.

No other professional, indeed no other person, in Western society can exert such personal power over clients or consumers. Imagine if other physicians could force patients into treatment on the grounds that they were in need of it. No one would be allowed to die of cancer without the "services" of the local surgeon or radiologist. Or imagine if lawyers or priests could exercise this kind of power over anyone they designated as their consumers or clients. Because psychiatry can compel patients into treatment, it frequently abuses them and loses its incentive to develop more appealing treatment approaches.

Some psychologists, with their Ph.D.s rather than M.D.s, are becoming increasingly envious of psychiatric medical power. Instead of promoting the psychosocial model and resisting the medical and biopsychiatric model, they are going to court and to legislatures to demand nearly all the rights of psychiatrists, including the right to prescribe drugs. The drug companies are underwriting some of these efforts by sponsoring seminars at national meetings to discuss the possibilities and advantages of psychologists prescribing drugs.*

Psychiatrists also have a pronounced advantage over nonmedical therapists when it comes to health insurance reimbursements for their services. In the past, especially, health insurers were prone to pay for bills generated by psychiatrists but not by other mental health professionals. In order to qualify for reimbursements from health insurers, these other professions have tried increasingly to make themselves over in the image of psychiatry. In a field where innovation and variety should have top priority, limiting health insurance reimbursement to traditional look-alikes stultifies the field.

The requirement for CME credits at first glance looks to be in the public interest. Continuing medical education is supposed to keep psychiatrists on their toes by requiring them to go to seminars each year in order to qualify for state licensure or membership in professional organizations. Actually the CME programs enforce conformity to the prevailing biopsychiatric viewpoint. The easiest way to get CMEs is to go to conferences sponsored by APA, NIH, mental hospitals, and medical schools—programs typically underwritten by drug companies.

Because the drug companies are not likely to pay for CME seminars that train doctors in psychosocial theories and practices, or that criticize drugs, the requirement for CME credits has become a powerful force toward biopsychiatric conformity.

Psychiatrists also exert enormous monopoly powers through the courts, where they are recognized as the experts in a variety of spheres, including the critical input on court decisions that declare people incompetent to stand trial or not guilty by reason of insanity.

When psychiatrists are sued for malpractice, who appears in court to

---

*As of January 1991 I became one of the few psychiatrists accepted for full membership in the American Psychological Association. One of my aims in joining the American Psychological Association was to encourage it to remain free of the psycho-pharmaceutical complex. Another was to help support the independence of psychologists from psychiatrists in conducting psychosocial therapies. Psychiatry has always tried to limit the rights of psychologists to practice independently. Meanwhile, as a psychiatrist, I have been a member of the American Psychiatric Association for several decades.

testify as to whether or not the accused doctor actually performed in a negligent manner? Other psychiatrists. Since professional retaliation can be brutal, trying to get one psychiatrist to testify against another is like trying to get Mafia members to rat on one another. I have seen cases where dangerous combinations and gross overdoses of psychiatric drugs have nearly killed patients, leaving them comatose or crippled, but no psychiatrists within the state could be found to testify on the patients' behalf. Attorneys frequently complain, "Several psychiatrists have said that it was obvious negligence but that they didn't dare testify against their colleagues."

Biopsychiatrists have begun to turn on their psychosocial colleagues in a way not previously seen. In print they are recommending that doctors who fail to use drugs can be guilty of malpractice. Recently a famous private psychiatric hospital settled out of court for failing to give an antidepressant to a man who later claimed he was saved by the drug at another institution.

Threats of malpractice actions are intimidating social workers, counselors, psychologists, and other mental health professionals who are unable or unwilling to give drugs. More and more frequently nonmedical therapists are referring their clients to psychiatrists for medication, even though the use of drugs may be at odds with the psychosocial approach taken by these professionals.

The picture I have drawn looks overwhelming, yet it is not an exaggeration. Psychiatry is a giant industry, protected by a state monopoly and promoted by a psycho-pharmaceutical complex with multi-billion-dollar power.

Despite these enormous advantages, psychiatry is not doing well financially and must struggle continually to maintain its monopoly power. This clearly indicates that psychiatry would lose out entirely in a genuine competition with psychological and social alternatives. In almost every arena in which psychiatry operates, psychosocial interventions—to which we now turn—are much less harmful, often less expensive, and far more appealing and helpful to suffering human beings.

Part V

Psychosocial Alternatives

Chapter 16

Psychotherapy and Psychosocial Programs

In the treatment of nervous cases, he is the best physician who is the most ingenious inspirer of hope.
— *Samuel Taylor Coleridge (1833)*

In psychotherapy, enthusiasm is the secret of success.
— *Carl Jung, "On the Psychogenesis of Schizophrenia" (1939)*

The words, "secular pastoral worker," might well serve as a general formula for describing the function of the analyst.
— *Sigmund Freud, "Postscript to the Question of Lay Analysis" (1927)*[1]

The awareness of human separation, without reunion by love—is the source of shame. It is at the same time the source of guilt and anxiety. The deepest need of man, then, is the need to overcome his separateness, to leave the prison of his aloneness. The *absolute* failure to achieve this aim means insanity. . . .
— *Erich Fromm,* The Art of Loving *(1956)*

Thou shalt love thy neighbor as thyself.
— *Leviticus XIX*

In the rich experience of life, there are so many ways to heal and be healed, and they are inseparable from the overall process of learning to overcome fear and helplessness and to love life. Indeed, to *love* is to be healed: to take joy in life, to be reverent toward life, to be immersed in life, to cherish oneself and others, animals and plants, nature and existence itself. The paths along this way are infinite, and anyone who tells you differently is preoccupied with his or her own self-interest, and not with yours, and not with the good of all.

My friend Leonard Frank shared with me some of the ways he has grown in personal strength over the years and, in the process, how he has been healing himself from the brain damage inflicted on him by psychiatry. Leonard would not say that he is *healed*, but rather that healing is an ongoing process through the stages of our lives. * Leonard continues his process of self-realization through "contemplation—self-conversation" and through conversation with others. He is healing through meditation: "clearing the mind through the repetition of caring, calming words or phrases, allowing the deeper mind to set its own agenda." He is healing through Gandhi and Lao Tzu, Emerson and Thoreau, William James and Arnold Toynbee, Lincoln and Tolstoy, and Isaiah and Matthew. He is healing through the notebooks that he keeps to evoke his "inner teacher," through recording and reflecting on his ideas and dreams, through reading and studying, and walking, being in touch with nature, and transforming his diet and life-style. And, I would add, he has been growing through his friendships, his moral life, and his devotion to liberty and love as expressed in his psychiatric reform work.

"But What Are the Alternatives?"

When I criticize toxic psychiatry, people often ask urgently about my alternatives. They want to know what I have to offer that's better. Throughout this book I have described psychosocial therapies and given examples of how they work in helping people overcome fear and helplessness, including so-called schizophrenia, depression, and panic attacks. I have contrasted them with technologies that disable the brain and biopsychiatric theories that foster helplessness and dependence. But the request for specific alternatives expresses the narrowness of our vision. We think there are one or two potential methods for overcoming the worst of our spiritual ailments; if one doesn't work or if it's too dangerous, we quickly want to know the other. If someone dares criticize one of our previously accepted approaches, such as drugs or shock, then we demand that he or she immediately provide us with another.

Once we have begun to think in such a manner, we are already on the wrong track. We are turning for a solution to the critic, and that is bound to increase our feelings of helplessness, fear, and dependence. We are seeking *the answer*, which is likely to be too simple, too shallow, and in all likelihood too authoritarian and self-limiting. We overlook the truth that rejecting bad theories and practices is, in and of itself, a suf-

---

*In fact, Leonard would discard the term *healing* because of its medical connotations. He prefers the concept of self-realization.

ficient blessing—one that liberates us to imagine and to implement better ways of healing.

The search for healing processes in life should not be a competition between two opposing camps in the mental health arena. Indeed, I was tempted to write this book without discussing *any* alternatives to toxic psychiatry. *All of life* is an alternative to drugs, electroshock, lobotomy, involuntary treatment, and materialistic theories based on biochemistry and genetics. Almost anything and everything, including the whole spectrum of secular and religious philosophy, is better than biopsychiatry.

Psychosocial alternatives—including the ones we have discussed already and those we shall examine in this chapter—are but a few examples among many possible catalysts in the process of recovery. If and when I help people grow stronger and realize their potential, I have helped them tap their inner resources and the vast resources of life itself. No therapist should ever believe "My therapy is the way." Nor should we believe that therapy in general is the only way. There are many paths of psychospiritual growth, all of them exploring the delicate harmonies between helplessness and independence, skepticism and faith, reason and emotion, self and other, human beings and nature, and, in religious terms, between all life forms and God. Professional therapy of any kind can be but a slender reed, and one that cannot possibly claim to be the only staff to be used along the path.

What Is Therapy?

The word *therapy* comes from the Greek *therapeutikos*, meaning attendant or one who takes care of another, while *psycho* comes from the Greek *psyche*, meaning soul or being. Psychotherapy means ministering to the soul or being of another. It is psychiatry that has medicalized and corrupted the word to mean "the treatment of mental illness." Because therapy involves healing the spirit or the soul—the whole essence of the person—it must draw on all of the wisdom and human potential of the therapist. Individual practitioners may be very good at providing therapy—at least to some clients with whom they feel rapport and find shared values. But can this "therapy" be made into a profession? Can it be taught? Can it even be defined? Can any two or three professionals even agree on what it is? Should the state try to regulate it by granting licenses to psychiatrists, psychologists, or counselors? These are tough questions, and I will not shirk them. But I will put them off until I've further examined what I believe therapy can and should be.

A few years after going into private practice in 1968, I interviewed a number of former and current clients to ask them what they found most useful about our work together. I expected them to cite various psychological insights and discoveries about their childhood. One and all they told me, in effect, "Peter, you *cared* so much about me that I learned to care about myself." Therapy is, above all else, a form of caring, and caring is a form of love.

In his introductory textbook *Understanding Human Behavior* (1989), psychologist James V. McConnell summarizes the relevant research:

Psychological change almost always occurs in a supportive, warm, rewarding environment. People usually "open up" and talk about things—and try new approaches to life—when they trust, admire, or want to please the therapist. Criticism seldom changes thoughts or behaviors, and it often kills all chance of improvement. (P. 509)

Understanding is an aspect of caring and love. To understand is to hear the other person's viewpoint, to comprehend or grasp it as fully as possible, to acknowledge it, and to recognize its reality for that person. We may then wish to share our own reality, to contrast it with our client's, and to make helpful contributions to the other person's understanding; but first and foremost, we must care and understand.

For a relationship to be caring and understanding, it also must be *safe*. In order to open his or her heart, the client must feel free of any potential harm. The relationship must be limited to the office or other circumscribed boundaries, it must not involve the whole life of the individual, and it must be guarded by professional ethics. This, hopefully, will make the therapy safer than the client's conflicted personal relationships. *

A caring, understanding relationship—made safe by professional ethics and restraint—is the essence of psychotherapy.

A Mini-Utopia

A safe, caring, understanding relationship—easier said than done.

Good psychotherapy should be *safer*, more protected by specific principles, than is friendship. The limitations placed on the therapy relationship allow therapists to be more caring and understanding than they otherwise might be. The limitations permit the client to be more open, vulnerable, and real than he or she might be ordinarily. And they permit a special focus on the client's thoughts and feelings.

---

*When the therapist uses involuntary treatment, physical interventions, medical diagnoses, or authoritarian approaches, therapy becomes one of the *least safe* places in the world. Especially since the ascendancy of biopsychiatry, going to a psychiatrist has become one of the most dangerous actions a person can take.

In psychotherapy, many things go on other than caring and understanding, and there's considerable variation in emphasis from therapist to therapist. I try to help my clients discover their childhood, especially its influence on their self-defeating patterns in adulthood. I encourage them to look inward, to experience and to express their feelings, and to find better ways of communicating their viewpoint. Sometimes I share whatever wisdom I've accumulated and I encourage the development of values that promote an ethical and satisfying life. I invite them to define and discuss self-determination, liberty, and love. Sometimes I urge people to read books about overcoming childhood oppression and about feminism. Most of all I try to ask, again and again, "Tell me more. Tell me more about your thoughts and feelings and experiences."

When I work with couples I try to help them learn to focus on and to listen to each other. They learn to feel safe and cared about with each other, and they learn to communicate about whatever seems important to each other and to the relationship. The aim, however, is not to "fix the relationship," but to help each person enter into it as fully as he or she desires.

The principles I've been describing apply equally to helping relatively strong, mature individuals and to helping very disturbed people diagnosed as schizophrenic. When people are deeply injured, frightened, or helpless, deviations from the principles of a safe and caring space become especially destructive. Yet we've already seen that the most vulnerable patients, those labeled psychotic, are typically victimized by the most severe, disabling treatments.

Liberty and Love

In therapy, as in life, people must be helped to respect one another's rights and never to use force or the threat of force except in self-defense. Even in self-defense, the minimum amount of force must be used, with care not to harm the aggressor more than absolutely necessary. The therapist, while firmly resisting verbal or physical assault, must not overreact or retaliate, or try to hurt the client in order to get even, to prove a point, or to enforce his or her authority. Nor should the therapist use force "in the client's best interest." Force must be limited to protecting oneself against attack. When it is not, as we have seen throughout this book, it becomes a dangerously uncontrolled weapon in the hands of the therapist.

We also must learn to love—to feel connected and to care about one another in a joyful, reverent manner. Love is more than respect, more than appreciation of the other's accomplishments, achievements, or ethical conduct. Love reaches to the spiritual heart of the other and says, "I treasure you *as you are.*" My working definition of love is "joyful, caring, reverent awareness of another human being."

When we love another person, even force used in self-defense seems objectionable to us. We would at times rather endure pain than risk injuring the other in self-defense. Love creates an abhorrence of all force.

It is not always possible for the therapist to esteem or respect the conduct of the client. In life it can be hard at times to respect our loved ones, and conversely it may be hard for them to always respect us. But love is unconditional—it finds the *inherent worth* of the other human being. It says, "I'm happy knowing you are alive." It says, "I cherish your life and will do everything I can to protect and to promote it."

Love transcends the distinction between self and other. Love is the most ethically consistent experience, because selfishness and altruism no longer seem opposed or in conflict. When we take such joy in the existence of the other, his or her interests begin to approximate our own. When we promote the happiness of a loved one, we promote our own as well.

Treating People Against Their Will

Without going extensively into the legal and moral arguments against involuntary treatment—so admirably discussed in the writings of Thomas Szasz—experience shows that it's difficult if not impossible to help people against their will. It's like the old joke about how many psychotherapists it takes to change a light bulb: Only one, but first the bulb has to want to change.

When people are "treated" against their will, they mainly learn one thing—how to adjust to being bullied. Inmates in mental hospitals learn to be "good patients" in order to avoid punishment and to stay out of trouble. Battered or abused spouses who can't escape tend to do the same thing. Trapped people frequently become deceptive and manipulative, or slavish and dependent, or all of those things, in order to keep from getting even more hurt.

For people to become truly visible to one another, to trust one another, to grow to love one another, first they must feel safe, and only the assurance of liberty provides that kind of safety.

So while I'm against involuntary treatment on moral and constitutional grounds, I'm also against it as a practical matter. If we want to strengthen and to empower people, if we want to help them learn mutual respect and love—then forcing our help on them must interfere directly with the achievement of our goals.

Liberty and Suicide

Anyone who wants to commit suicide can find a way to hide the impulse long enough to carry it out. Furthermore, the threat of being locked up scares people away from getting help at the very moment they could benefit from it most. People in despair sometimes become afraid to discuss suicidal feelings with their friends or therapists for fear that a psychiatrist will be called in to commit them. We'd "save" a lot more people if we offered all of our help on an exclusively voluntary basis.

When we know we can use force to make people accept our "services," we have little motivation to offer better ones. If psychiatrists could not treat people against their will, they might try harder to develop something more appealing to potential consumers than drugs and electroshock.

Honest communication becomes impossible when the suicidal client is afraid of getting locked up or, conversely, wants the therapist to take over responsibility for his or her life. If the therapist shows a willingness to resort to involuntary hospitalization, then psychotherapy—as a safe, caring, understanding relationship—is virtually abolished.

But when the therapist refuses to enter that power struggle, both participants are liberated to focus on the most important question of all—how to help the client understand and overcome his or her self-destructive feelings.

In my career I have never had a patient commit suicide. This includes several years of volunteering in state mental hospitals, several more years of training in psychiatric hospitals, and more than twenty years of full-time private practice. Partly it's luck; suicides can occur in the practice of any psychiatrist or psychotherapist, because ultimately our clients are responsible for their own lives. Partly it's a blessing. And partly, I believe, it's because I don't threaten to lock up my clients when the going gets rough. The therapist who refuses to use involuntary treatment is forced to think and work harder, to be more creative, to care more, to try harder to understand, and to pay greater attention to the client's needs.

Psychiatry and Love

Nowhere in my formal psychiatric training was there a serious discussion of caring, compassion, or love. Psychiatrists, more than most nonmedical therapists, are taught to be aloof, objective, and authoritative. Yet what do clients learn if, after hours of being with their therapist, no bond of affection develops? They learn that no one, including the person who is supposed to understand them best, will spontaneously feel love for them.

Not to allow therapy relationships to mature into an affectionate or loving bond—within professional boundaries—is to stifle the human spirit. It is natural for people to feel friendly and caring toward each other when they spend time together, especially when they are talking so intimately with each other. Not to acknowledge this is to perpetuate the client's original feelings of unlovability, alienation, and worthlessness.

The inherent power imbalance between the professional therapist and the client makes it difficult for the client to become fully empowered. In a hospital setting, surrounded by medical trappings and under the shadow of involuntary treatment, empowerment of the patient becomes nearly impossible.

Having summarized the most basic principles of psychotherapy, we'll look first at the treatment of the most seriously disturbed people, so-called schizophrenics, in institutional settings. If a safe, caring, understanding human service works best for them—even better than the "miracle drugs"—then it will be easy enough to believe in the same liberating principles of psychotherapy for all people. Then we'll look at perhaps the most ideal psychosocial approach to empowering people—self-help programs, including those run by psychiatric survivors. And finally, we'll evaluate psychotherapy in general.

Giving Love and Support to the Patient

In chapter 1 we learned about the Harvard-Radcliffe Mental Hospital Volunteer Program in which college students became case aides and even psychotherapists for individual mental patients on the back wards of a state mental hospital. We saw how these students, working one afternoon a week with group supervision from a social worker, were able to help nearly all of their patients leave the hospital. In our jointly authored book about the program, *College Students in a Mental Hospital*,[2] we make clear that casual friendship was not the goal of our work, but neither was alienated professionalism: "You must, at all times, aim at giving support and love to the patient. Make him feel that he is important to you, the worker; this may be the most important goal of all relationships" (p. 74).

That we reached such conclusions was partly due to our sensitivity as young people, as well as to social worker David Kantor's supervision. We saw the patients with eyes unclouded by professional bias, and so we saw them as human beings with the same feelings and needs as any other human beings, including ourselves. We were beginning to learn something that continues to impress me on ever-deeper levels as the years go on: all human beings have the same basic needs for love, recognition, personal empowerment, self-determination, and self-esteem.[3]

A Growing Disillusionment

Seven years after it began, the volunteer program received its most important affirmation from the major mental health planning and strategy report of the 1960s, the federal government's *Action for Mental Health: The Final Report of the Joint Commission on Mental Illness and Health* (1961). After describing the volunteer program in detail, the report officially recommends: "The volunteer work with mental hospital patients done by college students and many others should be encouraged and extended." Similar projects, the commission suggests, would relieve understaffing, provide young people with incentive to become mental health professionals, and encourage the public to be more tolerant and sympathetic toward the mentally disabled.

The joint commission report was one of the last gasps of psychosocially oriented psychiatry within the establishment. Despite the volunteer program's enormous success and this ringing endorsement, organized psychiatry, under increasing biopsychiatric domination, rejected the widespread use of volunteers. Untrained college students conducting psychotherapy and getting patients out of hospitals! Clearly too threatening to biopsychiatric authority. Nonetheless, the Harvard-Radcliffe Mental Hospital Volunteer Program demonstrated over many years that untrained college students can outperform trained professionals and drugs in helping the most difficult patients in state mental hospitals.

Moral Psychiatry

There is a historical precedent for helping severely disturbed patients in institutions through love, kindness, understanding, and moral support. It was called "moral treatment."

As long as we consider psychiatry a "science," it will seem odd to go back in time to an era when the basic principles, if not the practices, often surpassed our own. Most of us like to believe in straightforward progress, especially in fields we identify as scientific or medical. That's why we tend to accept each pronouncement from organized psychiatry about its latest biological discovery or newest miracle drug. It rings of the technological advancement we expect. But as we've seen, psychiatry is neither pure science nor medicine. It's a mishmash of philosophy, psychology, religion, law enforcement, and politics as well as social engineering and big business, and occasionally science and medicine. So in the case of psychiatry we cannot hope so naively for progress, and in fact we are now undergoing a regressive period. Modern psychiatry is suffering a moral decline under the psycho-pharmaceutical complex (chapter 15). Psychiatry has had a better past than present.

From the late-eighteenth through the mid-nineteenth century, a few small private psychiatric hospitals, and even some larger ones, consciously tried to implement the values of the Enlightenment. The Enlightenment drew on rich sources, from the writings of John Locke to those of Thomas Jefferson. In principle, at least, it promoted individual rights, self-development, tolerance, and optimism about the human being's rational and moral capacities. In moral treatment this was combined with Judeo-Christian love, charity, and kindness. Unlike today, these principles were espoused openly as the basis for psychiatry.

Moral treatment sought to correct the abuses heaped upon institutionalized patients—the squalid living conditions, physical tortures, and restraints—and to replace them with a caring and humane attitude. These doctors weren't perfect; they reflected the authoritarianism of the times. And in most hospitals, violent abuses remained. But what they promoted as an ideal was far better than anything since, and in limited ways they sometimes succeeded in practicing their principles.

Statistics gleaned from relatively small hospitals of the moral era indicate that they performed as well as modern ones in the percentages of patients they rehabilitated, often with a gentler hand. Their accomplishments are chronicled in *Moral Treatment in Psychiatry* (1963) by Sandor Bockoven, himself a state mental hospital superintendent.

Almost everyone has heard of psychiatrist Philippe Pinel and his grand gesture of removing the chains from dozens of inmates in state hospitals of Paris beginning in 1793. Pinel tried to bring the liberating spirit of the times into the lives of the patients, and he understood them to be suffering from moral despair. In his *Treatise on Insanity* (1806)[4] he dramatically describes how desperately deluded inmates could at times be calmed through persistent gentleness and rational persuasion.

Pinel's successor, Jean Etienne Dominique Esquirol, wrote *Mental Maladies* (1845), a classic document of moral psychiatry. Esquirol declares, "The insane are, as Locke remarks, like those who lay down false principles, from which they reason very justly, although their consequences are erroneous." In his view, the "insane" also suffer from social isolation; they are too resistent to the soothing influences of other people. "This moral alienation is so constant, that it would appear to me to be an essential characteristic of mental alienation." The patient is not biologically defective but developmentally disturbed: "So many points of resemblance do they bear to children and young persons, that it will not be surprising, if both one and the other should be governed by similar principles."*

As managers of giant lockups, both Pinel and Esquirol continued to inflict cruelties on many of the inmates under the guise of treatment. A more gentle nature is exemplified in the less well known psychiatrist W. H. O. Sankey, the author of *Lectures on Mental Diseases* (1866). A fellow of the Royal College of Physicians and proprietor of Sandywell Park Private Asylum, Sankey's writings embody the best principles of moral treatment as it hopefully was implemented in some smaller mental hospitals like his own.†

Sankey lamented the routinely wretched treatment of mental patients throughout the world and sought to foster the principles of "non-restraint"—supplanting physical and chemical controls with kindness, patience, and love. One of his dictums coincides exactly with the theme of this book: "Speaking generally, it is almost universally admitted by all experienced practitioners, that depressing or debilitating agents are contraindicated in the treatment of insanity."

Instead of drugs and chains, Sankey offered loving moral support:

The moral treatment consists in the action or influence of the sane mind on the insane mind. The principle of the non-restraint is therefore mental, not mechanical. . . . The principle of non-restraint was founded on Christian charity, and its doctrines find their best exposition in the significance of that word. It is the feeling carried out towards the patients which suffereth long and is kind. . . .

The "old system," he observes, worked "by bringing the unsound mind into subjugation, by depressing it, or by acting through the depressing passions." This "old system" is of course the same system that we have today—biological psychiatry. That's why I call it the new-old psychiatry. According to Sankey,

The aim of the newer system is to cheer, to conciliate the patient, to produce good feelings toward his custodian; to raise, not to depress him, to fill his mind with the pleasurable emotions of hope, love, thankfulness. . . .

*Those wishing to dominate and control other people often compare them to children. Esquirol was certainly paternalistic and authoritarian and at times promoted the medical model; but he also attempted to take a more humanitarian attitude than had been prevalent within institutional psychiatry, and his views remain in many ways more sensitive and aware than those of today's biopsychiatrist. Overall, however, historians generally agree that the practices of the moral era were far more oppressive than its stated principles.

†I know of no source of information other than Sankey's own descriptions of his principles and practices.

Sankey acknowledges that restraint remained a part of the system, since the patient was forced to remain in the institution. But despite this inherent coerciveness, he explains, treatment must be geared toward making patients feel welcome, comfortable, and cared for.

How did a hospital like Sankey's control its inmates without heavy reliance on chemical or physical restraint? Sankey says that it was accomplished through moral persuasion, through love. Although he seems to have treated patients as disturbed as those seen today in hospitals, he rarely found the need to resort to anything but firm, kindly personal influence. With that most difficult patient, the manic who is totally out of control, he warns us to avoid force whenever possible and to unite the staff to exert a caring moral influence on the patient. He greeted all new patients personally to assure them of a proper welcome to his institution.

Eventually moral treatment was swept away by gargantuan state mental hospital systems. With growing urbanization, the mass incarceration of the homeless poor became psychiatry's chief mandate. The function of sweeping the streets clean rapidly supplanted any therapeutic policy. As the inmates deteriorated and died during lifelong exposure to these inhumane institutions, the optimism of the moral era was replaced by medical cynicism. The conviction grew that psychiatric inmates suffer from incurable brain diseases.

Seventy years after Sankey implored the profession to be gentle stewards of the mentally disturbed, electroshock, lobotomy, and other brain-damaging therapeutics would become the standard.[5]

Soteria House: A Safe Therapeutic Haven

Psychiatrist Loren Mosher is a keeper of the flame of moral psychiatry. He developed Soteria House, a haven for individuals undergoing their first "schizophrenic" crisis. It is described in *Community Mental Health* (1989) by Mosher and his coauthor from Italy, Lorenzo Burti, and is thoroughly documented in many journal articles and book chapters by Mosher and various collaborators.[6]

To house Soteria, Mosher chose a home on a busy residential street. For the staff he sought people who had sincere interest in listening to the seemingly irrational communications of the patients. They were egalitarian and nonauthoritarian, individuals who didn't seek a hierarchy in which to feel superior and who didn't insist on artificial distinctions between themselves and their clients.

Mosher found that professional training was of no particular help in relating in a caring or understanding fashion, and the staff was chosen and trained on the job without regard for credentials. Most of those selected turned out to have no professional training, confirming that psychotherapy can be provided at a relatively low cost by not relying on highly paid professionals.

In the September 1978 *Hospital and Community Psychiatry*, Mosher and Alma Menn, a social worker and colleague at Soteria House, write, "Because they lack the preconceived notions of professionals, our non-professional staff members have the freedom to be themselves, to follow their visceral responses, and to be a 'person' with the psychotic individual." Mosher and Menn advocate recognition of the psychospiritual nature of the acute crisis:

At Soteria House the disruptive psychotic experience is also believed to have potential for reintegration and reconstruction, resulting in a more stable sense of self, if it is not prematurely aborted or forced into some psychologically strait-jacketing compromise. . . . Basically psychotic persons are to be related to in ways that do not result in the invalidation of the experience of madness. . . . Because "irrational" behavior and mystical beliefs are regarded as valid and as capable of being understood, Soteria staff try to provide an atmosphere that will facilitate integration of the psychosis into the continuity of the individual's life.

A series of carefully controlled studies demonstrate the superiority of Soteria for people undergoing their first schizophrenic break compared to a control group sent to a regular mental hospital. As reported by Mosher and Menn, Soteria clients did stay longer initially than the hospitalized patients, but the homelike setting was far preferable and less expensive to run.

In one series only 8 percent of patients received drugs during their initial stay at Soteria, while *all* of the hospital patients were medicated with the dangerous neuroleptics. In a two-year follow-up, according to Mosher and Menn, "experimental subjects significantly less often received medications, used less outpatient care, showed significantly better occupational levels, and were more able to live independently."

In another group of Soteria patients, *none* were given any neuroleptics during the first six weeks and only 10 percent eventually received them. Again they did better than the matched controls, all of whom were drugged in the regular psychiatric system.

Perhaps in an effort to conform to expectations about "scientific articles," the published reports do not emphasize some of the human values that Mosher and Menn focus on in private communications. Soteria clients gained a much greater sense of self-understanding, self-esteem, and personal empowerment. Instead of learning to accept brain-disabling drugs and humiliating hospital regimens, they often came through Soteria feeling *more independent* and *stronger* for the experience, and better in touch with their feelings and aspirations.

And They Didn't Get Tardive Dyskinesia

While Soteria House produced better results than hospital and drug psychiatry, it did not produce miracles. Frightened, confused, and disturbed people are not easy to work with. But in addition to helping patients, Soteria avoided hurting them. Patients put through the regular psychiatric system often remain on neuroleptics for several months or more, exposing them to a high risk of tardive dyskinesia, tardive dementia, and other permanent disabilities (see chapter 4).

The Fate of a Psychiatric Success Story

By almost any standard, Soteria is a success story. It would be relatively easy to set up hundreds of similar havens around the country, since they utilize residential housing and nonprofessional staff. How, then, do you locate a Soteria House to send your friend or relative to for help? You can't, except in Berne, Switzerland. Despite many published papers demonstrating the success of Soteria in California, and despite Mosher's superb credentials for many years as the head of schizophrenia research at NIMH, Soteria has had no significant impact on the treatment of patients. No money could be found to continue the project or to mount others like it around the country. NIMH decided not to continue funding it and the Department of Mental Health of California would not pick up the tab. Health insurance companies—oriented to hospital treatment and the medical model—would not reimburse Soteria patients for the cost of treatment. Needless to say, the drug companies—who support almost everything else in psychiatry—did not offer any help.

Again we find that the psychiatric monopoly and the psycho-pharmaceutical complex must be broken before significant progress can be made in developing humane, caring, nonmedical alternatives. We have a blueprint for easy-to-develop, effective programs, if only they could get funded.

Other Residential Innovations

Burch House, in Littleton, New Hampshire, is run by psychotherapist David Goldblatt, who apprenticed with R. D. Laing in England. In its newsletter Burch House describes itself as "a sanctuary for eight to ten individuals experiencing emotional crisis. Housed in an old farmhouse, with four to six live-in staff and five senior staff, the House offers an approach based on harmlessness, relationship and community." As at Soteria House, the feelings and communications of the clients, however seemingly irrational, are respected and taken seriously. Even more than Soteria, it provides clients the opportunity to take their time and to reach out to the staff and others at their own pace. A small portion of the residents are on psychiatric drugs, usually from earlier facilities, and Burch House supports the client's own choice about taking medications.

But how can anyone afford such a highly intensive psychosocial intervention? Get ready for a shock. The fee is $85 per day—a tiny fraction of the cost of a psychiatric hospital stay and less than the cost of some one-hour consultations with a psychiatrist. ("And the food is great!" adds one staffer.) And 35 percent of the services are delivered free to needy clients!

How can it be done? Many noncredentialed staffers are grateful to work in such an inspiring, if sometimes stressful, environment for meager pay. In an unpublished paper delivered in 1986 Goldblatt wrote eloquently:

As therapists, we must be completely present, yet at the same time our own problems must not intrude. We cannot afford to be too affected by what the person goes through or too invested in a particular outcome. Such attachment becomes interference. Clients show tremendous courage if allowed to suffer in the presence of an accepting, compassionate other. We need to have complete faith in the healer which is within our clients and within each of us. If we ourselves know that basic experience of faith and hope, then we can sit with someone who is in despair and know that hope is possible for them.

Spring Lake Ranch is another psychosocial alternative in the form of a cooperative community of more than thirty residents in the countryside of Cuttingsville, Vermont. There's no "professional staff," and distinctions between therapists and clients are blurred. According to Spring Lake Ranch, "Inherent in the life we live here is the expectation that everyone will contribute to the common good, even if that contribution is, because of disability or illness, of a relatively modest nature. It is through each person's contribution that all members of this community begin to experience a feeling of being needed and of belonging." A work program, including its lucrative maple syrup production, is central to the rehabilitation of its chronically disabled clients. Its 1989 annual report proudly asserts, "P.S. This year our syrup took third prize at the Vermont State Fair."

While some residents are on drugs, the doses are often relatively small, and a recent visitor was surprised that individuals with chronic psychiatric histories were seemingly so normal in their social relations as well as relatively free of zombielike drug effects. Spring Lake Ranch considers itself a model low-cost, communal-oriented approach.

Few innovative programs get state licensure as mental health facilities. Spring Lake Ranch was grandfathered into the state mental health system. As a more radical alternative, Burch House has no establishment connections or support. Soteria House, as already noted, collapsed because insurance companies would not reimburse clients for their costs. As long as the psychiatric and medical monopoly controls the delivery of mental health services, creative alternatives will be rare. Yet they are by far the least expensive and the most effective.

Into the Home with Noncredentialed Advocates

Probably nothing is as useful as direct psychosocial interventions into the home. When involuntary they pose a serious civil liberties and privacy threat; when sought voluntarily they can be the single most effective way of delivering help to disturbed or failing individuals and families.

Jerome Miller, president and founder of the National Center for Institutions and Alternatives (NCIA), whose headquarters are in Alexandria, Virginia, has inspired many psychosocial rehabilitation innovations. Miller, who holds a doctorate in social work, used volunteer advocates working with families as part of an overall strategy that eventually emptied and closed Massachusetts's juvenile detention centers.

Miller's assistant at the time was Thomas L. Jeffers, who in 1975 went on to found Youth Advocate Programs (YAP), a private not-for-profit agency with programs in five states and a central office in Harrisburg, Pennsylvania. Working with probation, child welfare, and mental health departments, YAP delivers intensive family-oriented services directly into the homes of children and young adults who might otherwise be institutionalized. Many of the youngsters, as well as their parents, carry the most severe psychiatric diagnoses, such as schizophrenia, as well as histories of severe delinquency. Many of the families are from a "hard-core inner-city" culture. Some of the children are so difficult that they have been rejected by residential facilities.

Echoing themes throughout this book, YAP bypasses traditional mental health approaches and often uses noncredentialed part-time advocates to work with the families. On occasion a responsible and loving neighbor may be hired and trained as the family's advocate. In an interview Jeffers told me that the first criterion for selecting an advocate is, "Would we want this person to work with our own children?"

When offering help to families, the first question the advocate asks is, "What does the family feel it needs?" It may want help with landlord-tenant relations, time out for Mom (day respite care), a job for one of the potential wage earners of the extended family, or "life skill training" in how to handle oneself more effectively in the world. Often the advocates work as liaisons with schools and various public agencies. If the youngster is having "behavioral problems" in class, the advocate may accompany him right into the classroom, an intervention that can calm student and teacher alike.

YAP advocates are not traditional psychotherapists, but they do meet regularly with the children and their families to provide emotional support and counseling. Often the children are involved in therapy groups outside the home as well. Typically children reduce any drugs they are on while in the program, and according to a YAP representative, "Kids on medication can't function well enough to benefit fully from the program."

The advocate spends an average of fifteen hours a week working face-to-face with the child and the family, usually for six to nine months. By psychiatric standards this is an enormous amount of personalized direct involvement, but it's exactly what's needed for these last-ditch efforts with down-and-out children and their families.

The cost of so much human service? Because the advocates are not traditional professionals, the cost is a relatively low $6,000 per year, compared to $40,000 to $100,000 or more per year for the traditional psychiatric inpatient services the program attempts to supplant. Effectiveness? According to Jeffers and his staff, 75 percent of the young clients remain in the care of their own families following YAP's intervention. The enormous help offered to the entire family cannot even be calculated.

In chapter 13 we found that psychiatric incarceration not only humiliates children and abrogates family responsibility, it costs more than putting a full-time professional into the home. Family intervention programs like YAP bolster the esteem of children, empower the family, and cost relatively little. They could largely eliminate any need for psychiatric hospitalization for children and for adults alike, while doing a lot more good and a lot less harm.

The alternatives we have been looking at—the Harvard-Radcliffe Mental Hospital College Volunteers, Soteria House, Spring Lake Ranch, Burch House, and YAP—function without relying heavily on mental health professionals. Even though they serve patients and clients who are considered very difficult to help, they have proven to be effective. Relatively unencumbered by psychiatric ideology and training, the therapists or advocates in these programs are able to work with people in more direct, personal, and practical ways, and at a lower cost.

Professional Psychotherapy with Hospitalized Patients Labeled Schizophrenic

Another approach that has been rejected by the "new psychiatry" is professional talking therapy in the treatment of hospitalized schizophrenic patients. In *The Psychotherapy of Schizophrenia: The Treatment of Choice* (1981), Bertram Karon and Gary VandenBos review the most well-controlled research studies and present the results of their own Michigan project as well. Even under the disadvantageous conditions of psychiatric hospitalization, often in state hospitals, about half a dozen relatively sound scientific studies confirm the efficacy of psychotherapy for individuals diagnosed as schizophrenic.

Patients who received psychotherapy as compared to those receiving medication showed less thought disorder (that is, they were more able to think logically when they wanted to), spent much less time in the hospital, and were able to live their lives more like human beings in a wide variety of ways. Furthermore, these effects became more marked the longer the patients were followed, and psychotherapy proved to be less costly in the long run. (P. 371)

Karon recently published a thorough, updated review in Seymour Fisher and Roger Greenberg's *The Limits of Biological Treatments for Psychological Distress* (1989). In his final remarks Karon states that psychosocial interventions reduce dosage levels and "improve the overall level of functioning of medication-treated patients." Furthermore, "the conclusion that schizophrenic patients must be treated with medication, whatever else is done, is based on poorly designed studies. . . ." He makes clear that "the optimal treatment for a schizophrenic is psychotherapy, from a competent therapist, without medication, if the patient, the therapist, and the setting can tolerate it."

Typically the patient is forced to take toxic drugs because of low levels of tolerance for the patient's conduct rather than because of his or her own wishes and needs. In my own experience this intolerance frequently greets any expression of resentment or anger toward the family or doctor, however justified it may be.

Karon believes that biopsychiatric politics, rather than facts, govern current treatment standards for schizophrenia:

Unfortunately, political and economic factors and a concentration on short-term cost-effectiveness, rather than the scientific findings, currently seem to dictate the type of treatment. The data seem to clearly indicate the value of psychosocial treatments, including individual psychotherapy, as opposed to medication. (P. 146)

In personal conversations Karon has confirmed his belief that neuro-leptic drugs should be used as little as possible in therapy: "I think patients are better off without them. Diminished affect [emotion] is what you get from the medications, and affect is what you work with in therapy." He informs patients that the drugs "don't cure anything. They only make the pain more tolerable. What really helps is understanding."

Karon told me that he advises therapists, "When in doubt, act like a human being." The patient must feel that "the therapist is really on my side and really wants to help." More important than any specific method is the therapist's personal *way of being* with the patient.

According to Karon, "People gain more from each hour of therapy if they don't have medication." If the medication makes both the patient and the therapist feel more comfortable talking with each other, Karon believes it may be used as a stopgap measure; but it should be given for the shortest possible time.

Karon is the leading American researcher in the field of professional psychotherapy for patients labeled schizophrenic.

Treating the Families of People Diagnosed as Schizophrenic

Many professionals who work with very disturbed people have felt that family therapy is the most effective. Often these therapists approach the whole family as the true "patient"; they locate the problem in the family including its relationship with the person identified as mentally ill. While I've found this to be the most effective way of helping people through their first episode of "schizophrenic" overwhelm, until recently there were no objective evaluations to support my impressions.

Recent family therapy research has focused on Expressed Emotion (EE) in the family of people labeled schizophrenic.[7] The aim is to diminish emotionally painful communications made within the family and to encourage more warmth among its members. Not surprisingly, a number of studies have found that negative communications directed at the identified patient worsen his or her upset and symptoms. Family therapy can reduce painful reactions generated by emotionally charged discussions, and this, in turn, can cut down significantly on the relapse rate. Because it is relatively straightforward, the type of help offered in the EE studies could be delivered especially easily by noncredentialed therapists.

The disturbed offspring of the family can often be understood as a victim of abusive or destructive communications. These new studies of EE tend to confirm this; but in the era of collaboration between organized psychiatry and the family movement, the investigators of Expressed Emotion usually have been careful not to implicate parents as contributing to their children's distress. The parents are asked to help make the family life more harmonious and hence conducive to the patient's recovery, but they are specifically exonerated of any fault in causing the patient's original problems.

What Do Patients Want for Themselves?

While most psychiatric patients in hospitals get drugs and almost no conversation from their doctors, my impression is that the great majority wish it were the other way around. A study by Keith McIntyre and his colleagues, published in the January 21, 1989, British Medical Journal, confirms this. Among ninety-nine psychiatric inpatients, more than half of them labeled schizophrenic or manic, "being able to confide in a member of the staff" or "simply talking to a care giver" was "widely regarded as the most helpful aspect of care." It was much superior, in the patients' opinion, to hospitalization or drug treatment. The authors felt it necessary to remind doctors that talking with their patients was valued by them, even though in most cases it amounted to less than an hour per week.

McIntyre's team also reports, "Ironically this study shows that the thing psychiatric inpatients value the most about being in hospital is their ability to leave." When I used to work in hospitals during my training, I found that many, and probably most of the inmate-patients wanted above all else to get out speedily with the minimum amount of interference with their bodies and lives. I concluded that my most important service to them lay in making that possible.

The Personal Skepticism of Biopsychiatrists

We have found strong evidence for the efficacy of psychotherapy and social therapy with acutely and chronically disturbed people labeled schizophrenic. So why don't biopsychiatrists recognize that psychotherapy often helps? Indeed, why are they so insistent that it cannot possibly help?

There is a personal reason why most biopsychiatrists cannot accept psychotherapy as something useful: they are not good at doing it. Naturally enough, if they failed time and again to help their patients by talking with them, they would conclude that it doesn't work. Few young psychiatrists would have the courage or honesty to conclude instead, "I wasn't good at being a therapist," "I wasn't personally suited to the work," or "As my wife complains about me, I never did care much for talking."

Why would so many young psychiatrists turn out to be poor therapists? In general, medical training is the worst possible way to select and prepare psychotherapists. To become a medical student you undergo your undergraduate years as a lab mole and a bookworm, subterranean creatures most unsuited to working with people. The whole premedical and medical training is so competitive and authoritarian that much of the student's humanity is washed out. Indeed, the problem of producing too many stilted, socially inept physicians with narrow interests is now generally recognized in medicine and frequently discussed in professional publications. Plans are being set in motion for bringing more humanistic, caring students into medical programs. Sadly, psychiatry has not been a leader in recognizing the need for people-oriented physicians. Instead it is going in the opposite direction.

Even warm, loving, insightful people find themselves losing their humanity during their psychiatric training. As college volunteers in the state mental hospital we had the advantage of working in a system that lacked the capacity to monitor what we were doing. We could be as friendly and caring as we wished, because there was no one around to notice. Besides, as "college kids," we could be forgiven our tendency to "get involved." But the young psychiatric resident in a training center is sure to be noticed if he or she starts acting "unprofessionally" by caring a great deal about his or her patients.

Psychiatric residents, who are already biased in favor of biopsychiatry, are especially unlikely to do well at psychotherapy. They believe that their patients' problems are genetic and biological and that their words are products of disease. This alienates these young doctors from their patients and makes meaningful communication impossible. They favor giving drugs or even shock when the emotions of the patient become intense, thereby suppressing the person, discouraging further passionate communication, and obliterating what could have been the most productive moments in psychotherapy. Furthermore, biopsychiatrists tend to be more authoritarian and more protective of their role as medical doctor—exactly the opposite profile of the one sought after in innovative psychosocial programs. Indeed, if we were trying to select the worst possible psychotherapist, we might choose a physician fresh out of medical school who was laboring under a biopsychiatric viewpoint. It is no wonder that they become discouraged and decide that psychotherapy doesn't work.

"On Our Own"—The Making of a Psychiatric Survivor Network

The most exciting and potentially important alternative of all is self-help. Judi Chamberlin, the author of *On Our Own* (1978), is one of the leaders in developing patient-run approaches. Chamberlin's personal exposure to psychiatry began in 1965 when she had a miscarriage. Twenty-one years old, unhappily married, and a secretary without much of a future—the loss of the baby was one blow too many for her. She became depressed. Her first psychiatrist, she told me recently, turned out to be "ineffectual and bland. I hardly remember what we talked about." What does an ineffectual, bland male psychiatrist do with a passionate, depressed, but brilliant and attractive young woman who might somehow threaten him? He drugs her.

A naive youngster in those days, Chamberlin didn't know any better than to take the medication. She told me, "He was the expert. He was supposed to know. He said that the drugs were going to make me feel better, so he ought to know. I was very trusting."

When she only got worse, Chamberlin tried to admit herself to a private hospital. Its beds were full, but instead of sending her home, as she wished, the doctors whisked her off to the psychiatric ward of New York City's Bellevue Hospital. She arrived there, was held incommunicado, and realized to her terror that no one in the world knew where she was. Among other things, they took away her glasses, leaving this frightened young woman nearly blind in her new environment.

Petrified, and brain-disabled by neuroleptics, Chamberlin became progressively more irrational. She explained, "They took somebody who was going through a depression in reaction to losing her baby and made a 'schizophrenic' out of her." She began to believe and even to see her face "collapsing." The bones were caving in on themselves, painfully, right in front of her eyes. But the "delusions" and "hallucinations" were filled with meaning. "I was being dehumanized. Losing my face was a representation of what was happening to me. I was being turned into something else, something other than myself."

Between March and October 1966, Chamberlin was in six different hospitals. "I'd become totally demoralized—like my life was over. I was told I was a chronic schizophrenic and would never be able to survive outside an institution." She went home to live with her parents.

At home Chamberlin happened to visit her internist, who referred her to a psychologist. "He turned out to be a great guy—someone who built me up and made me feel there was no reason why I couldn't do anything

I wanted to do." When she told him that she'd been diagnosed "chronic schizophrenic, with no future," he didn't buy it.

Of the good qualities that this therapist displayed, it was his respect for her that mattered most. Chamberlin worked with him for about a year, at first in individual therapy and then in group as well. She's had no therapy since then.

Chamberlin observes, "It really is the luck of the draw who you end up with. You can get someone who believes in shock or drugs, or in talking; you just don't know. You're in a very vulnerable state when you seek help."

Finding Other Survivors

Despite her successful therapy, Chamberlin still harbored profound doubts about herself. Why had she become "mentally ill"? Why had she "failed" to benefit from all of those treatments that were supposed to help?

Then in 1971 she learned about the MPLP, the Mental Patients' Liberation Project, in New York City. One of the first people she met was Ted Chabasinski, who later moved to California and organized the Berkeley ban against shock. (Chabasinski's story was recounted in chapter 9; he is the lawyer who had been electroshocked at the age of six and locked away for most of his childhood.)

"It was like a door opening," Chamberlin says of her first meeting with MPLP former inmates. "It was a confirmation of all my most heretical ideas." By 1974 she was actively involved and had met Leonard Frank at the Second Annual Conference on Human Rights and Psychiatric Oppression. It was inspiring to meet someone "so knowledgeable and determined to do something—strength, knowledge, power." People would soon be describing Judi Chamberlin in the same terms.

Like so many other survivors, Chamberlin found the understanding and empathy she needed with people who had suffered through the same psychiatric abuse. She learned that what seemed inexplicably psychotic to the psychiatrists often had profound meaning when understood in the context of the individual's life. Her emotional crisis, her new allies confirmed for her, was psychospiritual and not medical in nature. The survivor network gave new meaning to her life, and in return, contributing to the network has become one of Chamberlin's greatest satisfactions—"serving as a catalyst" to help other survivors feel understood and supported in their recovery from psychiatry and their reentry into the world.

In the mid-1980s, the ex-inmate leadership formed an official national organization, the National Alliance of Mental Patients (NAMP). Recently it was renamed the National Association of Psychiatric Survivors (NAPS). NAPS, which has its headquarters in Sioux Falls, South Dakota (see appendix A), aims at developing self-help programs and at stopping all involuntary psychiatric treatment.

Developing Self-Help Alternatives to Psychiatry

A large portion of Judi Chamberlin's time is now devoted to the Ruby Rogers Advocacy and Drop-In Center in Cambridge, Massachusetts, which she founded several years ago. With a state Department of Mental Health grant of $80,000 per year, this survivor-run drop-in center provides a refuge for an average of twenty people a day, both current and former psychiatric inmates.

With no professionals on board, clients don't risk being committed or pushed into taking drugs. Says Chamberlin, "If the drop-in center is just one more place from which they can cart you away, you're negating its whole purpose." Most of the visitors are barely functioning from day to day, and in Chamberlin's words, "life is difficult for them most of the time."

The Ruby Rogers Center provides a safe space where survivors can talk with other people, many who have suffered at the hands of psychiatry. It's a "little community" where people can be themselves. The only rules are no violence, no alcohol, and no drugs. Sometimes parties or cookouts are set up. There are self-help discussion groups and a women's group.

Serious incidents at the center are rare. There's no need for locked doors to keep people in and the police have never been called to handle a disturbance. Patients who seem to be "losing it" usually are calmed by care and attention from other former inmates. While some choose to get help by going to a hospital, no one is pressured to do so.

The survivor-run drop-in center is an important innovation. Successful variations are in existence around the country, including one in Berkeley headed by psychiatric survivor Sally Zinman and another in Oakland run by Howie the Harp, who is both a survivor and a former street person. They are staffed by former homeless people and ex-psychiatric inmates.

When I met with staff and clients at these two California centers, their themes were remarkably consistent: "We can do it on our own. We never want psychiatric treatment forced on us, and we don't want to be drugged or electroshocked under any circumstances. We are voting with our feet to stay out of the mental health system, even if we have to sleep outdoors on the ground." During one meeting that I attended a woman said she might go to a mental hospital for shelter if she were cold and hungry enough, but no one agreed with her, and several members of the group shouted anxious warnings to her not to risk it.

While most of the street people I talked with in California had little contact with psychotherapy or counseling, some did say they'd been helped by it at one time or another and very few felt animosity toward "talking doctors." Their fear and outrage was directed at psychiatrists who use drugs, shock machines, mental hospitals, and involuntary treatment.

Sally Zinman, Howie the Harp, and Sue Budd have edited an excellent book about the survivor self-help movement, *Reaching Across: Mental Health Clients Helping Each Other* (see appendix B). Their approach has a similar ring to that of the Harvard-Radcliffe College Volunteer Program and Soteria House.

Most importantly, we believe that clients should act in a way that empowers and validates each other. We should all be equals, treating each other with respect and tolerance as responsible, capable adults. Everyone has something to offer the group.

We believe we should view our peers not as diagnostic symptoms but as people—people with real problems and with real needs—needs common to everyone. We should provide assistance and support to each other—not treatment or therapy. (P. 5)

Like most psychiatric survivors, the authors of *Reaching Across* are wholly against involuntary treatment.

We are against anything which is in any way involuntary, forced, or coerced. Therefore, we believe participation in client-run alternatives should be *completely voluntary and that client-run alternatives should never involuntarily commit people to treatment situations.* (P. 5)

The Future of Survivor Self-Help

As Judi Chamberlin and other ex-inmate leaders point out, drop-in centers are only a partial measure. The mental health profession allows these alternatives an uneasy coexistence because they don't wholly undermine establishment psychiatry.* What's really needed will be far more threatening to organized psychiatry—overnight crisis centers where psychiatric survivors can help people get through psychospiritual crises without doctors, drugs, or shock machines. So far none have gotten off the ground, both because of lack of funding and because of the liability involved in

---

*Prodded by Congress, a reluctant NIMH has recently given grants to some of these drop-in centers, but the political trend probably will be against future NIMH support.

"practicing medicine without a license." The psychiatric monopoly again prevents innovation in psychosocial services.

Another big need, from Chamberlin's viewpoint, is for various levels of affordable housing, from closely supervised to barely supervised, where former inmates can live together and lend one another moral and practical support. Nearly all of those offered within the present system are so bad that only destitute, helpless people will turn to them, typically under threat of commitment to a state facility. As we saw in chapter 3, the clients of these board-and-care facilities usually are kept heavily drugged. The few supervised homes that provide any semblance of human service have waiting lists.

The psychiatric survivor movement has a long way to go before transforming public opinion and making a dent as a service provider. As Judi Chamberlin puts it, "If you hope that psychiatrists are human beings with a special knowledge about what makes people tick, then you may want to hand over to them all the difficult people in our society. That's what has happened. Psychiatry is enshrined in our society."

A Rae of Hope

We have found that psychosocial programs staffed by caring, understanding nonprofessional people are less expensive to run and more effective than traditional ones. Similarly, if we change our standards for who can deliver psychotherapy to the general public, the fees would drop precipitously for the average person seeking "talking therapy," and the services may improve as well. Rae Unzicker exemplifies the value of therapists who lack formal accreditation.

Unzicker, the coordinator of NAPS, is a woman of boundless energy and great heart. As a youngster she was shuffled around to a number of therapists, but none of them could or would help her with her problem: she needed to escape her parents. In her first year of college she had a spiritual crisis and a breakdown. Throughout a very oppressive childhood, she had not been allowed to make her own decisions. Now she couldn't handle college.

"I had no idea how to be on my own; I was terrified." She entered an "altered state of consciousness" and, trained to submit to authority, she sat in her room expecting a message on the college intercom system that would give direction to her life. And if not direction, then some much-needed support—maybe the voice that would say, "I'm here for you. I love you."

In the fall of the year, Unzicker agreed to admit herself to a state mental hospital, where she got "drugs, volleyball, and a doctor who couldn't speak English." She had entered voluntarily, but when she asked to leave, she was committed.

Eventually she learned to be compliant, and five months later, barely twenty years old, she returned home. Shortly afterward, on Mother's Day, her mother took her to Kansas City, gave her fifty dollars, and dropped her off on the street. There she was raped, became pregnant, and ended up going through the psychiatric system one more time, this time to justify an abortion when they were otherwise illegal. Despairing, Unzicker attempted suicide many times during this period.

The turning point for Unzicker came when a woman in a hotel heard her crying through the walls. Heidi knew a minister in Sioux Falls who was willing to be of assistance, and she helped Unzicker with the transportation costs. The minister arranged for Unzicker to live with a family for a year, and it became her first exposure to "real family life." She lived and worked free of psychiatric drugs for a year.

Then Unzicker took one of the biggest steps of her life: "I divorced my biological family." She severed all connections with her family and began to build a new network of family for herself, one that was chosen freely.

Of course, it's ideal to have a good and loving relationship with one's parents and to work out any misunderstandings or abuses from the past. But despite the best efforts of the now-grown child, it sometimes turns out to be impossible. And too often mental health professionals are reluctant to encourage a firm stand toward abusive parents.

Unzicker met and married Jim, a cinematographer, and after being together for six years, they began having some problems. Unzicker, with her robust optimism, again sought professional help. But this time she made specific demands on the psychologist, setting conditions under which almost all psychiatrists and many other mental health professionals would have refused to work—no drugs, no "mental illness" diagnosis, and no involuntary treatment. Her therapist agreed. At last she had met someone who would respect her freedom and dignity, and her need for safety. Her therapist also agreed to include anyone Unzicker wanted involved in the therapy and no one she didn't want. For the first time in her experience, Unzicker's therapist helped her to focus attention on the harm done to her in childhood.

"Rae's Madness Marathon"

As a part of her new therapy, in December 1981 Unzicker put together what she calls "Rae's madness marathon." She hoped she could go through one of her acute states of emotional overwhelm "without drugs, seclusion, restraint, labeling, or invalidation," and to come out a more alive and self-aware person. For thirty-six hours she was accompanied by her husband, several female friends, her psychologist, a friend of her psychologist, and the woman who was becoming her new personally selected mother. A lot of folks to help one person? Yes, but many were unpaid friends; and it was the last time she would turn to professional psychotherapy.

During "Rae's madness marathon," she relived the worst of what she had experienced at the hands of her parents. At dawn the next day she went through a "rebirthing" experience in which she was brought into the world in a gentle and loving manner. She now knew in her heart that "Some Higher Being or Someone has places for me to go in my lifetime, and that to take my own life would be to desecrate my spirituality." Her "parent" in this rebirthing process was a spiritual healer, wholly untrained in traditional mental health.

Unzicker finally had received the help she needed and wanted. It wasn't the kind officially approved by the American Psychiatric Association. Many professionals would view it as bizarre. For Rae Unzicker, it was a spiritual triumph.

Becoming a Therapist

Unzicker's own career as a helping person began in 1978, before her madness marathon. She had stayed in casual touch with her last traditional therapist, a psychologist who had terminated her therapy after she attempted suicide. Unzicker had returned home one evening to find him sitting in her living room, sobbing. She invited him to stay with her and her husband for awhile.

Over the years Unzicker has developed a wide variety of helping relationships, often with escapees from the state hospital system, people identified by psychiatry as hopelessly schizophrenic. She has conducted a new kind of underground railroad. According to Unzicker, many of these survivors are not only "functioning in the world," they are thriving. In ten years, more than five hundred people have lived with her and her husband, Jim, for periods spanning a few days to several years. No wonder *Woman's Day* gave her a Woman of the Year Award in 1987.

Like many other helpers, Unzicker draws on an eclectic repertoire, especially reparenting, body work, and various methods for reducing rage. About once a year she takes seminars at Esalen Institute in Big Sur, California, where she studies bioenergetics, gestalt therapy, spiritual healing, and other alternative therapeutic approaches.

Uncredentialed people can take seminars at institutes like Esalen or Omega in Rhinebeck, New York, or at meetings of the Association for Humanistic Psychology.[8] People who participate in these activities easily can become better informed and more experienced with the latest psychosocial and spiritual healing techniques than are most psychiatrists.

While some schools of therapy require a professional degree before giving advanced training leading to a certificate, many techniques are taught to anyone who is interested through private institutes, group seminars, New Age retreats, and psychology conferences. These opportunities make nonsense of the notion that the public needs to be protected by a monopolistic mental health profession dominated by psychiatry.

In recent years Unzicker has asked fewer and fewer people to live with her. She's become somewhat more formal in her work and has a growing practice with individuals and groups. A psychologist and a psychiatrist have become supportive of her work. After sitting in on her groups, they have encouraged the participation of their own patients.

The experience of Rae Unzicker demonstrates the value of noncredentialed therapists. They charge lower fees and encourage diversity. Often they provide better services.

Unfortunately, the mental health establishment continually attempts to tighten state licensing requirements. These laws supposedly are aimed at protecting the public from unqualified practitioners, but their main aim is to encourage health insurance companies to pay for costly services. Overall, licensure laws enable groups of professionals to monopolize the psychotherapy market by locking out unlicensed competitors while guaranteeing a steady flow of clients and high fees for themselves. Since psychiatry has tried to corner the entire market for itself, I cannot blame other professional groups, such as counselors or family therapists, for trying to get licensed. But nonmedical therapists would better serve themselves and the public by coming out against state licensing for "talking therapy." Fees in general would hopefully decline, but the lower fees charged by less-establishment therapists might rise once the licensure monopoly was ended. Then each group—such as psychiatrists, psychoanalysts, psychologists, or counselors—could concentrate on training its own members and on enforcing high ethical standards within that particular profession.

Psychotherapists as Secular Ministers

Psychotherapy is an educational, spiritual, and moral endeavor that should lie outside the realm of state licensure and control. Even Freud called psychotherapists secular moralists and was against requiring them to have medical licenses.*

Psychotherapy should exist much as religion does, unfettered by state control. If you want to go to a Methodist minister for counseling, you can find one through a Methodist church. If you want a Jewish rabbi, you can find one through a synagogue. Similarly, if you prefer a charismatic preacher who's founded his own church, you're equally free to choose him. The U.S. Constitution prohibits state control of religion, and so the establishment religions qualify and monitor their own ministers, priests, or rabbis; and the nonestablishment ones are freely available to anyone who leans in their direction.

Much as people now do with religion, clients seeking Freudian psychoanalysts can check with the local psychoanalytic association. Similarly, clients can contact institutes representing Adlerians, Jungians, transactional analysts, gestalt therapists, behaviorists, and so on. People desiring a psychiatrist can call the American Psychiatric Association, the AMA, the local medical school, or their family doctor. And people seeking a psychotherapist in their local community who is experienced and who has undergone psychotherapy can call the headquarters of the American Academy of Psychotherapists in Decatur, Georgia.

In a limited way, a free market already exists in the field of psychotherapy, with many people seeking talking therapy from outside the medical, academic, or professional establishment. But fees for services generally are inflated and a false sense of security is created, encouraging the public to trust therapists because they are licensed. Meanwhile, the licensing monopoly is increasing from day to day as new groups become certified.

What About the Risk of Unlicensed Therapists?

People are permitted to give over the care of their *souls* to religious counselors without the state monitoring the process. Should it be any different in regard to the care of their *minds* by psychotherapists? Besides, the line between the spiritual and psychological—the soul and the mind—is becoming increasingly blurred in the professional practice of psychotherapy. With little or no additional training, many ministers provide psychological counseling, and with little religious or ministerial background, many psychotherapists provide essentially spiritual services. The journal *Common Boundary: Between Spirituality and Psychotherapy*, published in Chevy Chase, Maryland, exemplifies this joining of roles.

* See the Freud quote at the beginning of this chapter.

The annual meeting of the Association for Humanistic Psychology, for example, typically provides a potpourri of healing practices that span the secular and the religious, often combining the two. You might begin at sunrise with Moslem Sufi dancing, Yoga, or American Indian ceremonies and go on to a full day of seminars on a variety of often-conflicting psychotherapy philosophies and techniques (such as Freud, Jung, Maslow, Perls, or Satir), concluding at sunset with an encounter group of several hundred people or perhaps a more silent retreat to learn more about Christian or Hindu meditation. Meanwhile, there will be opportunities to get acquainted with various forms of massage, martial arts, painting and drawing, or creative writing—all with a therapy orientation. After the several days of meetings, many therapists will return home to incorporate one or another of these experiences into their own work. The balance between psychological and spiritual practices will depend on each therapist's philosophy of life.

The prospect of trying to license all of these "specialties" boggles the mind! It becomes a matter of who obtains the political clout to claim the status of a bona fide psychotherapy specialty.

Meanwhile, some nonprofessional self-help groups, such as Alcoholics Anonymous (AA), Narcotics Anonymous (NA), and Adult Children of Alcoholics (ACoA), offer psychospiritual services to millions of clients without state control. There is no way to distinguish between an AA group and a psychotherapy group except by the absence of a paid, professional leader. Similarly, Re-evaluation Co-counseling (RC), headquartered in Seattle, provides a form of nonprofessional self-help counseling advocated by some psychiatric survivors. It offers a carefully defined approach to psychotherapy, as described, for example, in its book *Fundamentals of Co-Counseling Manual*.[9] Another self-help group, Recovery, draws on psychiatrist Abraham Low's ethical and therapeutic principles, described in his book *Mental Health Through Will-Training* (1950). The Chicago-based self-help organization does not promote itself as offering psychotherapy, but its groups, intended for "schizophrenics," operate on Low's psychotherapeutic principles without a professional leader.

The dangers involved in ending state control over psychotherapy would be outweighed by the advantages. Many more people would be able to afford help and to go as often as they actually need or wish. And in a more free market, the services offered would be much more imaginative, varied, and tailored to meet the demands of the consumer.

An "Inner-City Psychotherapy Institute"

Without state licensing and its inflated academic requirements, even poor people could stake a claim to becoming psychotherapists. Schools for teaching psychotherapy could open within the inner city, much as churches do, to cater to the needs of the poor.

If Harvard and Radcliffe college student volunteers could do therapy with state hospital patients, if Soteria House was staffed by untrained but caring people, and if psychiatric survivors can run drop-in centers—then surely many other people could be *trained* in two years to be psychotherapists. After graduation from the therapy school, an additional year or two of supervision could be required for certification by the psychotherapy institute, while the therapist earns a living by providing relatively low-cost services.

Think of how many housewives, retired people, and just plain folks would love to become psychotherapists with a two-year program that required no special educational background. Think of how many good people would enter the profession and how the cost of psychotherapy would fall. The trouble is, the professionals are thinking the same thing, and doing their best to make sure it doesn't happen. Again, the pressure for reform will have to come from the public.

Demonstrating the Value of Psychotherapy in General

In this and earlier chapters we have looked at studies confirming the efficacy of psychotherapy in schizophrenic overwhelm and in depression. But what about psychotherapy for the average person looking for help with emotional problems? What's the evidence that it works?

The issue became a hot one in the late 1970s, when insurance companies began to cut back on psychotherapy coverage and Congress held hearings to determine if psychotherapy works. In 1980 the Office of Technological Assessment evaluated research on the efficacy of psychotherapy. REPORT FAVORABLE ON THERAPY OUTCOME, summarizes the headline in the December 5, 1980, issue of *Psychiatric News*. After reviewing the scientific literature, the government agency concludes rather tentatively, "Although the evidence is not entirely convincing, the current literature contains a number of good-quality research studies which find positive outcomes for psychotherapy."

In the same year, Elliot Marshall reported on the controversy in the February 1 issue of *Science*, under the title "Psychotherapy Works, But for Whom?" Marshall observes that only 20 percent of mental health expenditures are for psychotherapy, confirming the dwindling role of the talking therapies as well as the dominance of hospitals, drugs, and electroshock. He cites various studies indicating efficacy, but a quote from psychiatrist Jerome Frank is more to the point:

To try to determine by scientific analysis how much better or worse, let us say, gestalt therapy is than transactional analysis is in many ways equivalent to attempting to determine by the same means the relative merits of Cole Porter and Richard Rogers. To ask the question is to reveal its absurdity.

Frank opined that a good therapist, like an artist, is unique.

Nonetheless, the search for proof has continued, and so has the debate. In *The Clinical Psychology Handbook* (1983), edited by Michel Hersen, Alan Kazdin and Alan Bellack, Kazdin reviews the myriad problems surrounding any attempt to evaluate the therapeutic value of conversation. His conclusions confirm the impressions of many experienced therapists: various schools of therapy have more in common than meets the theoretical eye. When therapists are observed at work, their techniques are much more similar than their differing theories suggest. While there's evidence for good outcomes from a number of studies, in general there's not much difference in success rate among the various schools.

In his 1989 textbook *Understanding Human Behavior*, psychologist James V. McConnell does a good job covering many of the issues surrounding the efficacy of psychotherapy. Spontaneous recovery rates hover around 30 to 50 percent, while recovery rates from all forms of therapy approximate 70 percent in most studies. *This leaves plenty of room for skepticism about the superior effectiveness of any type of intervention, including psychotherapy.*

Overall, the problem of evaluating therapy runs into seemingly insurmountable problems of individual differences among therapists and among clients. It also is difficult to reach agreement on the criteria for "improvement." A psychology that promotes "adjustment" sets different goals for its clients than one that encourages self-actualization. Biological psychiatrists tend to focus on the reduction of symptoms, such as "insomnia" or "weight loss," while psychosocial therapists are likely to look for changes in the client's personal relationships or more positive attitudes toward life. A Catholic counselor may believe that "saving a marriage" represents the ultimate success, while a secular therapist may put a higher priority on each individual's personal growth, regardless of the outcome for the marriage.

Even the concept of treatment is itself highly controversial. A shock doctor believes that a patient who is euphoric from brain damage has been "treated" and is "improved," but many critics of shock believe that the same person has been violently assaulted and badly injured.

Since psychotherapy is inherently more like education and religion than medical treatment, evaluating psychotherapy becomes as difficult as deciding what kind of schools or churches are most effective. There will be as many differing opinions about psychotherapy as there are about the meaning of life and how best to live it.

Abolishing Psychotherapy as a Profession?

In *Against Therapy: Emotional Tyranny and the Myth of Psychological Healing* (1988), Jeffrey Masson challenges the basic concept of a *profession* of psychotherapy. After documenting many cases of severe abuse by psychotherapists, some of them highly renowned, Masson concludes that there is something inherently wrong with the idea of a profession made up of healers of the human spirit. He points out there's no way to determine in advance who will become a good psychotherapist, because we cannot measure or evaluate such qualities as compassion and understanding. In his view, there's no way to *select* good candidates for therapy training. Furthermore, there's no way to *train* adults to become more loving or more able to listen. Since very few people have the necessary qualities, and since good therapists cannot be preselected or trained, there is no way to justify a profession of psychotherapy. Worse still, by making believe we can select or produce good psychotherapists, we mislead the public into seeking professional help from people who may not be personally qualified or able to provide it.

Masson's arguments are cogent, and the situation is in some ways even worse than he describes. Training programs for psychotherapists—such as psychiatric residencies or graduate schools of clinical psychology—are not even *trying* to screen their applicants to find good, kind people who will become loving and understanding therapists. They are competing with other programs for the students with the highest test scores, the best college grades, and the most impressive academic recommendations. Furthermore, as we have already seen, few, if any, psychotherapy programs are trying to teach people to be more loving and understanding. Often they teach "objective," manipulative, and sometimes dehumanizing techniques, especially in the psychiatric training programs. Besides, there is such divergence among "schools" of psychotherapy that being "trained" by itself says very little about the therapist's viewpoint or approach. The individual could be a behaviorist or a psychoanalyst, a biopsychiatrist or a spiritually oriented minister, an authoritarian or a feminist.

Many good psychotherapists would agree that they acquired little that was helpful in their training and that, if anything, they had to *recover* from the process of being schooled. The most valuable learning experiences typically come after the formal training is complete and involve privately purchased supervision, specialized seminars, personal discussions with colleagues, and experience. Psychotherapy exemplifies the axiom that experience is the best teacher, and in psychotherapy that experience is too often gained at the expense of unwitting clients.

I am not yet ready to reject the concept of a profession of psychotherapy. Many good psychotherapists do share somewhat common values and approaches, approximating or overlapping with the ones espoused in this book, and many clients are helped by them. But I do believe we must demystify the whole area. Psychotherapists are people, and they suffer from all of the shortcomings of human beings in general; and they are trained in a variety of often-conflicting approaches, some of which are outright damaging. The buyer of psychotherapy services must be extremely cautious.

Whether or not therapy can and will help you is ultimately a matter for you to evaluate for yourself. If you decide to look into the possibility, be sure not to be entrapped by an authoritarian or manipulative therapist. If one therapist doesn't seem to be helpful, try another. Remember that you should have rapport with your therapist: the two of you should grow to genuinely like and appreciate each other.

Shop around among the many psychotherapists who probably work within traveling distance of you. You should be able to get a good idea about the personal chemistry between the two of you and about the usefulness of the sessions within a few hours or less, without an excessive expenditure of time and money. Especially beware of doctors who offer drugs before they've gotten to know you and, in my opinion, stay away from anyone who believes in electroshock.

Approach psychotherapy with skepticism and yet with a measure of hope and enthusiasm. Many people have found their lives changed for the better by a safe, caring, and understanding relationship with a psychotherapist. But always remember that you, and you alone, can determine if your therapist is helping you.*

The Future of Psychiatry

We want to know more about how stress affects the body and how the body recovers from emotional overwhelm and chronic tension. We need to know whether, and in what ways, the immune system can really be affected by our mental or spiritual state. It is important to continue

*Chapter 14 contains additional thoughts about how to choose a therapist.

learning about how brain damage or disease affects mental function and how the person can try to overcome or transcend an impaired central nervous system. Indeed, there are things to learn about the brain and the mind that we have not yet begun to imagine. For example, I suspect that the kind of neuronal relationships that produce the mind remain, as yet, beyond our most creative guesses. So there is a worthwhile role, now and in the future, for the medically trained psychologist or the psychologically trained physician.

For some people, at least, there also will be a desire to investigate and to use drugs that seemingly soothe the mind and calm the spirit. Thus there will be a public demand for physicians specializing in psycho-pharmacology, even though some of us may question the value of their services.

But in reality psychiatry is much more than an academic discipline or a therapeutic approach. Psychiatry is the political center of a multi-billion-dollar psycho-pharmaceutical complex that pushes biological and genetic theories, as well as drugs, on the society. It is a political institution licensed by the state, financed by government, and empowered by the courts. Its "diagnoses" carry enormous legal weight and have vast political implications. Psychiatric labels allow parents to lock up their children in psychiatric hospitals and allow the state to do the same to homeless people.

Psychiatry's political power has permitted it to perpetrate the harm documented throughout this book, from drugging millions of children to shocking tens of thousands of the elderly. Its power has allowed the profession to go largely uncriticized and unimpeded while producing an epidemic of brain damage.

There is no place for the *political* institution of psychiatry in a free society, and it should be abolished. The first step requires stripping the profession of its legal but illegitimate powers, including its right to lock up and treat people against their will and its authority in court to determine who is "not guilty by reason of insanity" after they have committed crimes.*

The second step involves disempowering the psycho-pharmaceutical complex. Psychiatric organizations, such as the APA, and individual psychiatrists must be stopped from collaborating financially with the drug companies while claiming to act as objective scientific bodies or scientists.

The third step will be even more difficult to attain, because it strikes at the heart of the psychiatric viewpoint. Psychiatry and psychiatrists must not be allowed to make false claims about the genetic and biological

---

*As Thomas Szasz and others have pointed out, psychiatry's legal capacity to determine if an individual's criminal conduct was influenced by "mental illness" has very negative consequences for society. It legitimizes psychiatric authority over what are essentially moral, social, and political problems.

origins of so-called mental illness. Such claims are unethical, if not fraudulent, and serve only to perpetuate the influence of the profession and individual practioners. But if it rejected its biopsychiatric claims, the profession would admit to being something very difficult to justify or defend—a medical speciality that does not treat medical illnesses.

Once psychiatry is separated from its illegitimate powers, its corrupt relationship with the drug companies, and its unfounded claims, then we shall see if people really want what it has to offer. Can psychiatry compete in a more free market with psychotherapy and psychosocial alternatives, as well as with all of the other ways people seek to heal their minds and their hearts and to grow? Would people rather talk through their problems and go to self-help groups, or take drugs? Would they rather think of themselves as struggling persons, or as defective biochemical devices? Would people prefer to seek the source of their personal problems within themselves and their lives, or within their genes? Would they rather go to nonmedical havens for moral and spiritual support, or to mental hospitals for medication and electroshock? Would they rather provide the homeless poor with better, more affordable housing, or shut them up and drug them in custodial state hospitals? Would people prefer to provide the elderly with more love and better social services, or with electroshock? Would they rather offer the nation's schoolchildren smaller and more stimulating classrooms, or Ritalin? Would people prefer to face the problems plaguing the American family, or drug and lock up its troubled or troubling members?

How you respond to some of those questions may depend on how closely you identify with other, less fortunate people. You may be tempted to protest, "But I'm different; there are people who really need drugs or shock or hospitalization." Then recall one of the most important lessons of life. We are, as human beings, all made of the same psychospiritual stuff. The needs for security and self-esteem are universal, as are the aspirations toward liberty and love. What's good for one of us is likely to be good for all of us.

Most important in regard to psychiatry, what seems harmful to you or me is likely to be harmful to any one of us, and what fails to help us is likely to fail to help other people. When we have personal problems or conflicts, we don't want authorities to force themselves and their solutions on us, and we would not expect their interventions to help us. So-called mental patients, being no different from us, also resent being coerced, and they, too, are not likely to be helped against their will.

I am not in favor of abolishing psychiatry as a medical specialty. Let there be doctors who are concerned with the relationship between the mind and the body, and let them offer their drugs to people on a strictly voluntary basis, provided that they thoroughly explain what the drugs really do. But I am in favor of holding psychiatry responsible for the damage it inflicts on its patients. Psychiatrists, their organizations, and the pharmaceutical industry should be held legally responsible when they fail to warn people about the addictive and damaging effects of their treatments. The psycho-pharmaceutical complex should be scrutinized in the courts and investigated by Congress as an unethical and possibly illegal combine.

Psychiatry will fight to the bitter end against any kind of reform. To this day, it resists even the slightest control over its most obviously abusive practices, such as state mental hospitals, involuntary drugging, electroshock, and lobotomy, and it fights against every attempt to increase patients' rights. If anything it tends, when criticized, to reaffirm its devotion to coercion and brain-disabling treatments. There is no reason to believe that psychiatry will change these attitudes in the future. But psychiatry's rejection of reform may, in the end, guarantee its own disempowerment and the flowering of freely chosen, more effective, caring alternatives.

Appendix A

Groups to Join, Periodicals to Subscribe to, Sources of Legal and Psychotherapeutic Help

To Learn About the Psychiatric Reform Movement
Center for the Study of Psychiatry

The Center for the Study of Psychiatry (CSP), based in Bethesda, Maryland, is a nonprofit research and educational network devoted to reform in psychiatry and to offering independent analyses of current psychiatric theories and practices. Founded in 1971 by Peter Breggin, the network includes more than seventy-five leading mental health professionals, attorneys, patient advocates, psychiatric survivors, and members of the U.S. Congress.* Anyone can keep abreast of CSP activities by joining the National Association for Rights Protection and Advocacy (NARPA), which issues a quarterly newsletter called *The Rights Tenet*. A CSP report, "News and Views on Psychiatry," appears in each issue of the NARPA newsletter. Write directly to NARPA (see the next entry) to join the organization and to get the newsletter with the CSP reports. Individuals can also network with and hear talks by many Center members at the annual NARPA conference each fall. The annual meetings are announced in *The Rights Tenet*.

National Association for Rights Protection and Advocacy
Mental Health Association of Minnesota, 328 East Hennepin Avenue, 2d Floor, Minneapolis, Minn. 55414

NARPA is open to all people interested in supporting the advocacy of patient and inmate rights. You do not have to be a mental health professional or an activist in order to join. NARPA publishes a newsletter, *The Rights Tenet*, and holds an annual convention on patients' rights and psychiatric reform, with workshops by lawyers, advocates, survivors, and reform-minded mental health

---

*See the acknowledgments for specific names.

professionals. It's worth joining to get the newsletter and to be reminded of the yearly conference, which is the best in the field. As mentioned above, the Center for the Study of Psychiatry makes a report in each NARPA newsletter. The annual NARPA membership fee is $20.

National Association of Psychiatric Survivors
P.O. Box 618, Sioux Falls, S.D. 57101

If you have been damaged by psychiatry and want to join other survivors for moral support, political action, and the development of client-run alternatives, this is your organization. Even if you are not a former patient, your membership and support are welcome. NAPS publishes a newsletter and can provide the addresses of local survivor groups around the United States and in many other countries. The NAPS annual membership fee is $25.

The Canadian survivor network can be contacted through the Ontario Psychiatric Survivors Alliance (OPSA), 3107 Bloor Street West, Suite 201, Toronto, Ontario M8X 1E3, Canada.

The British survivor network can be contacted through MIND, 22 Harley Street, London WIN 2E, England.

Dendron
P.O. Box 11284, Eugene, Oreg. 97440

Founded, edited, and published by David Oaks, this psychiatric survivor journal and newsletter offers articles on psychiatric oppression, human rights, and self-help alternatives. It is highly recommended for staying in touch with what's happening in psychiatric reform and the survivor movement. Individual annual subscriptions to Dendron are $10; institutional subscriptions are $20.

Joining NARPA and NAPS and subscribing to Dendron will keep you up with the latest activities in the psychiatric survivor and psychiatric reform movements.

To Obtain Legal Aid Against Psychiatric Abuse
National Association of Protection and Advocacy Systems
220 Eye Street N.E., Suite 150, Washington, D.C. 20001
Phone: (202) 546-8202.

If you are or have recently been an inmate subjected to abusive psychiatric treatment in any institution, public or private, and need help in protecting your rights, you can contact NAPAS. It can provide you with the addresses and phone numbers of federally funded protection and advocacy agencies in your state. Many of these state agencies are doing good work supporting patients' rights and investigating violations. The services are free. They may be able to provide referrals to sympathetic private attorneys as well.

To Find a Psychotherapist
American Academy of Psychotherapists
P.O. Box 607, Decatur, Ga. 30031
Phone: (404) 299-6336

The AAP central office can provide names from among its more than seven hundred members, some of whom may live in your area, including psychologists, psychiatrists, social workers, counselors, and other professionals. AAP members are trained and experienced in psychotherapy and have undergone psychotherapy themselves. Get several names and shop carefully for a person with whom you feel comfortable and confident. Membership in any organization does not guarantee that an individual is ethical or competent. AAP is not affiliated with the Center for the Study of Psychiatry, NAPS, NARPA, or any other psychiatric reform organization, and membership in AAP indicates nothing about a psychotherapist's views on psychiatry. It is up to the individual seeking help to question any potential therapist about his or her orientation and values. Chapters 14 and 16 contain some suggestions on choosing and evaluating therapists.

Appendix B

Additional Reading

I. General Critiques of Psychiatry

Breggin, Peter. *The Crazy from the Sane*. New York: Lyle Stuart, 1970. [A novel—the fictional story of a young psychiatrist's disillusionment with his profession.]

Cohen, David, ed. *Challenging the Therapeutic State: Critical Perspectives on Psychiatry and the Mental Health System*. Vol. 11, nos. 3 and 4 (1990) of the *Journal of Mind and Behavior*. [Highest recommendation. Contains many important articles on psychiatric reform by Center for the Study of Psychiatry members Judi Chamberlin, Leonard Frank, Peter Breggin, Lee Coleman, Ron Leifer, and Phyllis Chesler as well as Theodore Sarbin, George Albee, Thomas Szasz, Andrew Scull, David Cohen, Phil Brown, and others. Available in some libraries, it also can be purchased for $18 plus postage by writing the *Journal*, P.O. Box 522, Village Station, N.Y., N.Y. 10014.]

Coleman, Lee. *The Reign of Error: Psychiatry, Authority, and Law*. Boston: Beacon Press, 1984. [Excellent summary and analysis of the myths of modern psychiatry, with special focus on psychiatry and the law. Highly recommended.]

Kesey, Ken. *One Flew Over the Cuckoo's Nest*. New York: Viking, 1962. [A well-known classic.]

Leifer, Ronald. *In the Name of Psychiatry: The Social Functions of Psychiatry*. New York: Science House, 1969. [Excellent theoretical criticism of psychiatry in general.]

Masson, Jeffrey Moussaieff. *Against Therapy: Emotional Tyranny and the Myth of Psychological Healing*. New York: Atheneum, 1988. [Highly recommended for raising important, challenging issues and for examples of abuse within psychotherapy and psychiatry.]

————. *Final Analysis: The Making and Unmaking of a Psychoanalyst*. New York: Addison-Wesley, 1990. [Fascinating autobiographical account of his years in the cult of psychoanalysis. Challenges the assumptions that became the basis of much of modern psychotherapy.]

Morgan, Robert, ed. *The Iatrogenics Handbook: A Critical Look at Research and Practice in the Helping Professions*. Toronto: IPI Publishing, 1983. [Valuable studies in how treatment can hurt patients.]

Robitscher, Jonas. *The Powers of Psychiatry*. Boston: Houghton Mifflin, 1980. [Although wedded to the psychiatric establishment, Robitscher makes important criticisms. Weak on issues concerning drugs.]

Rosenhan, D. L. "On Being Sane in Insane Places." *Science*, January 19, 1973, pp. 250–78. [Using volunteers to masquerade as patients, this article documents the absurdity of diagnosis and treatment and the oppressiveness of typical mental hospitals. A classic.]

Scheflin, Alan, and Edward Opton, Jr. *The Mind Manipulators*. New York: Paddington, 1978. [A sweeping criticism of psychiatric theory and practice.]

Schrag, Peter. *Mind Control*. New York: Pantheon, 1978. [A popular, insightful critique of psychiatry.]

Szasz, Thomas. *Law, Liberty, and Psychiatry*. New York: Macmillan, 1963. [One of the better of many books Szasz has written contrasting the values of responsibility, freedom, and rationality to the philosophy and practice of psychiatry.]

————. *The Myth of Mental Illness*. Rev. ed. New York: Harper and Row, 1974. [The seminal book analyzing psychiatry as an offense against the western values of autonomy and liberty. A classic.]

II. Critiques of Public Hospitals, Contemporary and Historical

Brown, Phil. *Transfer of Care*. London: Routledge, Chapman, and Hall, 1988. [Historical analysis of deinstitutionalization as a political phenomenon rather than a triumph of treatment.]

Deutsch, Albert. *The Mentally Ill in America: A History of Their Care and Treatment from Colonial Times*. New York: Columbia University Press, 1949. [Documents the long history of psychiatric abuse in state mental hospitals.]

Dix, Dorothea. *On Behalf of the Insane Poor: Selected Reports*. New York: Arno Press and the New York Times, 1971. [Although deeply caring toward people labeled mentally ill, Dix inadvertently promotes the creation of giant psychiatric institutions and psychiatric authority over the poor.]

Foucault, Michel. *Madness and Civilization: A History of Insanity in the Age of Reason*. New York: Vintage, 1965. [How modern psychiatry evolved out of the industrial revolution and the need to control and incarcerate society's marginal citizens, including street people.]

Goffman, Erving. *Asylums: Essays on the Social Situation of Mental Patients and Other Inmates*. Garden City, N.Y.: Doubleday, 1961. [A classic, scholarly analysis of the demoralizing impact of mental hospitals and other "total institutions."]

Grob, Gerald. *Mental Institutions in America: Social Policy to 1875*. New York: Free Press, 1973. [A scholarly history that documents psychiatry's roots in incarcerating and controlling the urban poor.]

Kraepelin, Emil. *One Hundred Years of Psychiatry*. New York: Philosophical Library, 1962. [A psychiatrist's history of his profession inadvertently tells a story of unending torture and abuse in the guise of treatment.]

U.S. Senate, Joint Hearings Before the Subcommittee on the Handicapped of the Committee on Labor and Human Resources. *Care of Institutionalized Mentally Disabled Persons*. Washington, D.C.: Government Printing Office, April 1–3, 1985. [Documents the oppressiveness of contemporary public mental hospitals.]

III. Critiques of Psychiatric Drugs

Bargmann, Eve, Sidney Wolfe, and Joan Levin. *Stopping Valium: And Ativan, Centrax, Dalmane, Librium, Paxipam, Restoril, Serax, Tranxene, Xanax*. New York: Warner, 1982. [An indictment of the minor tranquilizers by a Ralph Nader organization.]

Breggin, Peter. "Brain Damage, Dementia and Persistent Cognitive Dysfunction Associated with Neuroleptic Drugs: Evidence, Etiology, and Implications." *Journal of Mind and Behavior* 11, nos. 3 and 4 (summer and autumn 1990): 425–63. [A detailed analysis with dozens of citations concerning permanent damage to the brain and mind by neuroleptics. See David Cohen in section 1 for information on obtaining.]

———. *Psychiatric Drugs: Hazards to the Brain*. New York: Springer, 1983. [In-depth analysis of neuroleptics, antidepressants, and lithium, providing citations and back-up information to this book.]

Brown, Phil, and Steven Funk. "Tardive Dyskinesia: Barriers to the Professional Recognition of an Iatrogenic Disease." *Journal of Health and Social Behavior* 27 (1986): 116–32 [Documents psychiatry's refusal to take responsibility for the damage it causes.]

Crane, George. "Clinical Psychopharmacology in its 20th Year." *Science* 181 (1973): 124–28. [A psychiatrist blows the whistle on tardive dyskinesia.]

Fisher, Seymour, and Roger Greenberg, eds. *The Limits of Biological Treatments for Psychological Distress: Comparisons with Psychotherapy and Placebo*. Hillsdale, N.J.: Lawrence Erlbaum Associates, 1989. [Very informative, scientific critiques of the alleged efficacy of antidepressants, minor tranquilizers, neuroleptics, and Ritalin as well as attention deficit disorder. Good discussion of psychotherapy of schizophrenia. Except for its pro-ECT chapter, recommended as a supplement to this book.]

Lehmann, Peter. *Der chemische knebel: Warum psychiater neuroleptika verabreichen* (The chemical cudgel: Why psychiatrists administer neuroleptics).

Berlin: Peter Lehmann Antipsychiatrieverlag, 1986. [By a leading European psychiatric survivor; highly recommended to anyone who can read German.]

Martensson, Lars. *Should Neuroleptic Drugs Be Banned?* RSMH-Malmo, Bergsgatan 12 B, S-211 54 Malmo, Sweden: circa 1984–85. [A booklet by a Swedish physician who discusses the damaging impact of the neuroleptics. Distributed in the United States by Alice M. Earl, Editor, *Peer Advocate*, P.O. Box 60845, Longmeadow, Mass. 01116–0845.]

Richman, David, with Leonard Frank and Art Mandler. *Dr. Caligari's Psychiatric Drugs.* 3d ed. Berkeley, Calif.: Network Against Psychiatric Assault, 1987. [Highest recommendation. This booklet offers a brief but detailed review of the side effects of psychiatric drugs by psychiatrist David Richman, written in down-to-earth language. Suitable for distribution to potential and actual psychiatric patients as well as to mental health professionals. Available from Leonard Frank, 2300 Webster Street, San Francisco, Calif. 94115. $6 postpaid.]

U.S. Congress, Hearings Before a Subcommittee of the Committee of Government Operations. *Federal Involvement in the Use of Behavior Modification Drugs [Ritalin] on Grammar School Children.* Washington, D.C.: Government Printing Office, September 29, 1970. [Documents that the controversy and outrage over drugging children has been going on for decades, while psychiatry has remained impervious to it.]

U.S. Senate, Hearings Before the Subcommittee on Health and Scientific Research of the Committee on Labor and Human Resources. *Use and Misuse of Benzodiazepines (Valium, Librium, and Other Minor Tranquilizers).* Washington, D.C.: Government Printing Office, September 10, 1979. [An important historical document with testimony on the hazards of these drugs.]

IV. Critiques of Electroshock

Breggin, Peter. "Disabling the Brain with Electroshock." In *Divergent Views in Psychiatry,* edited by Maurice Dongier and Eric Wittkower. Hagerstown, Md.: Harper and Row, 1981. [Detailed, documented discussion of ECT.]

———. *Electroshock: Its Brain-Disabling Effects.* New York: Springer, 1979. [The only medical book devoted to a critical examination of electroshock. Translated into German, French, and Italian.]

———. "Neuropathology and Cognitive Dysfunction from ECT." *Psychopharmacology Bulletin* 22 (1986): 476–79. [Paper presented at the 1985 NIMH-sponsored Consensus Conference on ECT, highly condensed, with many citations.]

Frank, Leonard. "Electroshock: Death, Brain Damage, Memory Loss, and Brainwashing." *Journal of Mind and Behavior* 11, nos. 3 and 4 (summer and autumn 1990): 489–512. [The most recent antishock review. Highest recommendation. See David Cohen in section 1 for information on obtaining.]

———, ed. *The History of Shock Treatment.* 1978. [By a shock survivor, a frightening record of fraud and violence with more than 250 chronologically arranged excerpts and articles by opponents and proponents. Highest recommendation. Available from Leonard Frank, 2300 Webster Street, San Francisco, Calif. 94115. $12 postpaid.]

Friedberg, John. "Shock Treatment, Brain Damage, and Memory Loss: A Neurological Perspective." *American Journal of Psychiatry* 134 (1977): 1010–13. [By the first physician to take an effective public stand against shock treatment.]

———. *Shock Treatment Is Not Good for Your Brain*. San Francisco: Glide, 1976. [Based on interviews with shock-damaged patients; an important, courageous book.]

Morgan, Robert, ed. *Electroshock: The Case Against*. Toronto: IPI Publishing, 1991. [A short book, useful as an introduction to the damaging effects of electroshock, with contributions from Bertram Karon, Peter Breggin, John Friedberg, Leonard Frank, and Berton Rouché. Highest recommendation.]

V. Critiques of Psychosurgery

Breggin, Peter. "Psychosurgery as Brain-Disabling Therapy." In *Divergent Views in Psychiatry*, edited by Maurice Dongier and Eric Wittkower. Hagerstown, Md.: Harper and Row, 1981. [A basic review with many citations.]

———. "Psychosurgery for Political Purposes." *Duquesne Law Review* 13 (1975): 841–62. [Documents the racist political motives behind the resurgence of psychosurgery in the late 1960s and early 1970s.]

———. "The Return of Lobotomy and Psychosurgery." In *Psychiatry and Ethics*, edited by Rem Edwards. Buffalo, N.Y.: Prometheus Books, 1982. [With a new introduction. The original 1972 paper from the *Congressional Record*, reviewed and criticized psychosurgery around the world and sparked the largely successful international campaign to prevent the resurgence of psychiatric brain surgery. There are many other interesting papers in this anthology.]

Chavkin, Samuel. *The Mind Stealers: Psychosurgery and Mind Control*. Boston: Houghton Mifflin, 1978. [Good on the politics of psychosurgery.]

Hansen, Heidi, et al. *Stereotactic Psychosurgery*. Suppl. 301 of *Acta Psychiatrica Scandinavica* 66 (1982): 7–123. [Lengthy in-depth study of how modern psychosurgery damages the brain and mind, producing a lobotomy syndrome.]

Valenstein, Elliot, ed. *The Psychosurgery Debate: Scientific, Legal, and Ethical Perspectives*. San Francisco: W. H. Freeman, 1980. [While Valenstein himself was hostile to the antipsychosurgery campaign and tried to co-opt it, his books have nonetheless brought public attention to the controversy. Many interesting pro-and-con articles.]

VI. Critiques of Biopsychiatric and Genetic Theories, Including Their Role in Nazi Germany and the Holocaust

Kevles, Daniel. *In the Name of Eugenics: Genetics and the Use of Human Heredity.* Berkeley: University of California Press, 1985. [A political and scientific critique of genetics and eugenics.]

Lapon, Lenny. *Mass Murderers in White Coats: Psychiatric Genocide in Nazi Germany and the United States.* Springfield, Mass.: Psychiatric Genocide Research Institute, 1986. [A psychiatric survivor documents the eugenic and psychiatric background of the holocaust in a lively, nonacademic style. Available from Psychiatric Genocide Research Institute, 55 Bryant Street, Springfield, Mass. 01108. $11 postpaid.]

Lewontin, R. C., Steven Rose, and Leon Kamin. *Not in Our Genes.* New York: Pantheon, 1984. [Debunks the genetic basis of psychiatric disorders. A classic. Highly recommended as a supplement to this book.]

Meyer, Joachim-Ernst. "The Fate of the Mentally Ill in Germany During the Third Reich." *Psychological Medicine* 18 (1988): 575–81. [A compact summary of the role of psychiatry and eugenics in helping to bring about the holocaust.]

Muller-Hill, Benno. *Murderous Science: Elimination by Scientific Selection of Jews, Gypsies, and Others in Germany, 1933–1945.* New York: Oxford University Press, 1988. [A German genetic researcher explains how psychiatric and eugenic principles and practices were indispensible in bringing about the holocaust. Very important and highly recommended.]

Proctor, Robert. *Racial Hygiene: Medicine Under the Nazis.* Cambridge, Mass.: Harvard University Press, 1988. [Excellent supplement on psychiatry's key role in the holocaust.]

VII. Women and Psychiatry

Chesler, Phyllis. *Women and Madness.* New York: Harcourt Brace Jovanovich, 1989. [Seminal book on the psychiatric abuse of women. Highly recommended.]

Martin, Del. *Battered Wives.* San Francisco: Volcano Press, 1981. [A groundbreaking book when first published in 1976, demonstrates how psychiatry blames and abuses battered wives. Highly recommended.]

Masson, Jeffrey Moussaieff. *The Assault on Truth: Freud's Suppression of the Seduction Theory.* New York: Atheneum, 1988. [Discloses how Freud betrayed women and children by abandoning his original observations on child abuse, instead concocting the Oedipal complex theory, which blamed and discredited the victim. Highly recommended.]

Millett, Kate. *Sexual Politics.* New York: Doubleday, 1970. [An early classic on the emancipation of women, with an incisive critique of Freud.]

Seidenberg, Robert, and Karen DeCrow. *Women Who Marry Houses: Panic and Protest in Agoraphobia.* New York: McGraw-Hill, 1983. [An excellent book on the psychological and political bases of so-called agoraphobia.]

Showalter, Elaine. *The Female Malady: Women, Madness, and English Culture, 1830–1980.* New York: Pantheon, 1985. [A scholarly, historical study.]

[Also see sections 8 and 9]

VIII. Children and Psychiatry

Coles, Gerald. *The Learning Mystique: A Critical Look at "Learning Disabilities."* New York: Pantheon, 1987. [Scientific analysis of the myths of hyperactivity, ADD, dyslexia, and other school-related diagnoses. Highly recommended as a supplement to this book.]

McGuinness, Diane. "Attention Deficit Disorder: The Emperor's New Clothes, Animal 'Pharm,' and Other Fiction." In Fisher and Greenberg (see section 3). [An excellent, recent scientific review of the myths of attention deficit disorder (ADD) and Ritalin; a useful supplement to this book.]

Plotkin, Robert, and K. Rigling. "Invisible Manacles: Drugging the Mentally Retarded." *Stanford Law Review* 31 (1979): 637–78. [A detailed analysis, with many citations to the medical and legal literature.]

Schrag, Peter, and Diane Divoky. *The Myth of the Hyperactive Child and Other Means of Child Control.* New York: Pantheon, 1975. [A classic, still relevant today.]

IX. Understanding the Abuse of Children and Its Impact on Them as Adults

Blume, E. Sue. *Secret Survivors: Uncovering Incest and Its Aftereffects in Women.* New York: John Wiley, 1990. [Many people diagnosed by psychiatry as mentally ill are in fact victims of outright sexual abuse. A self-help book. Very highly recommended.]

Bradshaw, John. *Healing the Shame that Binds You.* Deerfield Beach, Fla.: Health Communications, 1988. [Self-help.]

Breggin, Peter. *The Psychology of Freedom: Liberty and Love as a Way of Life.* Buffalo, N.Y.: Prometheus, 1980. [Chapters on the relationship between adult problems and childhood oppression.]

Forward, Susan. *Toxic Parents: Overcoming Their Hurtful Legacy and Reclaiming Your Life.* New York: Bantam, 1989. [Self-help.]

Gelles, Richard, and Murray Straus. *Intimate Violence: The Causes and Consequences of Abuse in the American Family.* New York: Simon and Schuster, 1988. [Documents the frequency of abuse and neglect and the consequences.]

Green, Arthur. "Physical and Sexual Abuse of Children." In Kaplan and Sadock (see section 13). [Demonstrates that problems attributed by biopsychiatry to biology and genetics are frequently the result of abuse and neglect.]

Jaffe, Peter, David Wolfe, and Susan Wilson. *Children of Battered Women.*

Newbury Park, Calif.: Sage Publications, 1990. [Summarizes scientific literature on the impact of child abuse.]

Middleton-Moz, Jane. *Children of Trauma: Rediscovering Your Discarded Self.* Deerfield Beach, Fla.: Health Communications, 1989. [Self-help.]

Miller, Alice. *For Your Own Good: Hidden Cruelty in Child Rearing and the Roots of Violence.* New York: Farrar Straus Giroux, 1983. [A classic. More academic than a typical self-help book, it has nonetheless helped many people understand their childhood trauma.]

Wolfe, David. *Child Abuse: Implications for Child Development and Psychopathology.* Newbury Park, Calif.: Sage Publications, 1987. [A scientific summary and analysis.]

X. Psychiatric Survivors and Client-Run Alternatives

[See appendix A for relevant organizations and newsletters.]

Burstow, Bonnie, and Don Weitz, eds. *Shrink Resistant: The Struggle Against Psychiatry in Canada.* Vancouver: New Star Publications, 1988. [Firsthand reports of psychiatric abuse, including hospitalization, drugs, and shock treatment. Survivors will feel inspired and validated by the poetry and prose of others with like experiences. Highly recommended.]

Chamberlin, Judi. *On Our Own: Patient-Controlled Alternatives to the Mental Health System.* New York: Hawthorn, 1978. [By a leader in the psychiatric survivor movement. A highly-recommended classic.]

Freeman, Huey. *Judge, Jury and Executioner.* Urbana, Ill.: Talking Leaves, 1986. [An autobiographic novel about being psychiatrically abused.]

Gotkin, Janet, and Paul Gotkin. *Too Much Anger, Too Many Tears: A Personal Triumph Over Psychiatry.* New York: Quadrangle, 1975. [A highly recommended classic by a psychiatric survivor and her husband.]

Hirsch, Sherry, Joe Adams, Leonard Frank, Wade Hudson, David Richman, et al. *Madness Network News Reader.* San Francisco: Glide, 1974. [Many interesting articles by survivors and professionals from the movement's first journal. Very lively and informative.]

Millett, Kate. *The Loony-Bin Trip.* New York: Simon and Schuster, 1990. [One of the first to write about the oppression of women, Millett now bravely recounts her oppression at the hands of psychiatry. Highly recommended.]

Plath, Sylvia. *The Bell Jar.* New York: Harper and Row, 1971. [A classic that describes a poetic soul's encounters with psychiatry.]

Zinman, Sally, Howie the Harp, and Sue Budd, eds. *Reaching Across: Mental Health Clients Helping Each Other.* California Network of Mental Health Clients, 1987. [The theory and practice behind psychiatric survivor self-help. This network is located at 1722 J Street, Suite 324, Sacramento, Calif. 95814.]

421

XI. Understanding the Psychology and Politics of Schizophrenia

Beers, Clifford. *A Mind that Found Itself: An Autobiography*. Garden City, N.Y.: Doubleday, 1908. [Psychiatric survivor Beers attempted to reform the psychiatric establishment from within and failed; but his autobiography confirms the psychospiritual nature of so-called madness.]

Boisen, Anton. *The Exploration of the Inner World*. Philadelphia: University of Pennsylvania Press, 1971. [A survivor who later became a minister explores the meaning of madness.]

Hill, David. *The Politics of Schizophrenia: Psychiatric Oppression in the United States*. Lanham, Md.: University Press of America, 1983. [A scholarly, philosophical, and thorough analysis.]

Kaplan, Bert, ed. *The Inner World of Mental Illness*. New York: Harper and Row, 1964. [Although the editor adheres to the medical model, his observations and most of the autobiographies confirm the psychospiritual essence of madness.]

Laing, R. D. *The Politics of Experience*. New York: Pantheon, 1967. [A well-known classic. Highly recommended.]

Lidz, Theodore, Stephen Fleck, and Alice Cornelison. *Schizophrenia and the Family*. New York: International Universities Press, 1965. [Describes the role of the family in causing and maintaining schizophrenia in its members.]

Peterson, Dale. *A Mad People's History of Madness*. Pittsburgh: University of Pittsburgh Press, 1982. [From the years 1436 to 1976, the writings of "mad people" give their viewpoints on themselves and their treatment.]

Sarbin, Theodore, and James Mancuso. *Schizophrenia: Medical Diagnosis or Moral Verdict?* New York: Pergamon, 1980. [A thorough, scholarly presentation.]

Szasz, Thomas. *Schizophrenia: Sacred Symbol of Psychiatry*. New York: Basic Books, 1976. [Discusses the role of the diagnosis of schizophrenia in justifying psychiatric authority.]

[Also see sections 10 and 12.]

XII. Psychotherapy and Psychosocial Approaches to People Labeled Schizophrenic or Mad

Breggin, Peter. *The Psychology of Freedom: Liberty and Love as a Way of Life*. Buffalo, N.Y.: Prometheus, 1980. [Provides some of the theory behind the author's practice of psychotherapy.]

Breggin, Peter, and E. Mark Stern, eds. *Psychotherapy and the Psychotic Patient*. A two-volume edition of the journal *The Psychotherapy Patient*, also to be issued as a hardcover book. To be published by Haworth Press, probably in 1992–93. [Contributions from across the spectrum of psychosocial approaches to helping people diagnosed as psychotic or schizophrenic, including traditional psychotherapy, new approaches to family therapy, and survivor-run and professionally run alternative havens.]

Christie, Nils. *Beyond Loneliness and Institutions: Communes for Extraordinary People*. Oslo: Norwegian University Press, 1989. [A wonderful little book about how mentally handicapped people live full lives in spiritually oriented communal villages throughout Europe. Distributed by Oxford University Press.]

Fisher and Greenberg (see section 3). [Good chapters on psychotherapy versus drugs in depression and in schizophrenia.]

Karon, Bertram, and Gary VandenBos. *Psychotherapy of Schizophrenia: The Treatment of Choice*. New York: Jason Aronson, 1981. [A scientific review of the effectiveness and superiority of psychotherapy over drugs with so-called schizophrenic patients in psychiatric institutions.]

Mosher, Loren, and Lorenzo Burti. *Community Mental Health: Principles and Practices*. New York: W. W. Norton, 1989. [An innovative book about psychosocial and community approaches to madness. Should be read by all professionals in the field.]

Walkenstein, Eileen. *Beyond the Couch*. New York: Crown, 1972. [Both a critique of psychiatry and a lively description of the author's own alternative psychotherapy approach.]

[Also see sections 9, 10, and 11.]

XIII. Commonly Used Sources of Drug Information in Psychiatry

[Most of the following books are used frequently in psychiatry, and they often reflect the interests of the psycho-pharmaceutical complex. Although they can provide useful information, they also can provide inaccurate or misleading information. When looking up the dangers and side effects of psychiatric drugs, it is important to check several sources, including those written from viewpoints not dominated by biopsychiatry. See section 3, as well as this book.]

American Psychiatric Association task force report. *Benzodiazepine Dependency, Toxicity and Abuse*. Washington, D.C.: American Psychiatric Association, 1990. [Contains useful information not routinely included in textbooks or drug company advertising.]

American Psychiatric Association task force report. *Tardive Dyskinesia*. Washington, D.C.: American Psychiatric Association, 1980. [The original APA report on tardive dyskinesia. Provides clinical descriptions and statistics.].

American Psychiatric Association task force report. *Treatments of Psychiatric Disorders*. 4 vols. Washington, D.C.: American Psychiatric Association, 1989. [The APA's controversial attempt to standardize various treatments.]

Goodman, Alfred, et al. *Goodman and Gilman's The Pharmacological Basis of Therapeutics*. 7th ed. New York: Macmillan, 1985. [A commonly used textbook.]

Gorman, Jack. *The Essential Guide to Psychiatric Drugs*. New York: St. Martin's Press, 1990. [A popularly written book, but sometimes more complete than textbooks regarding drug hazards. However, the author is strongly prodrug.]

Kaplan, Harold, and Benjamin Sadock, eds. *Comprehensive Textbook of Psychiatry*. Baltimore: Williams and Wilkins, 1989. [A commonly used textbook.]

Nicholi, Jr., Armand, ed. *The New Harvard Guide to Psychiatry*. Cambridge, Mass.: Harvard University Press, 1988. [A commonly used textbook.]

Physicians' Desk Reference (PDR). Oradell, N.J.: Medical Economics, published annually. [A product of the pharmaceutical companies, with FDA supervision. Lists many drug effects, while omitting or minimizing others.]

Talbott, John, Robert Hales, and Stuart Yudofsky, eds. *Textbook of Psychiatry*. Washington, D.C.: American Psychiatric Press, 1988. [A commonly used textbook.]

USP DI. *Advice for the Patient: Drug Information in Lay Language*. Rockville, Md.: U.S. Pharmacopeial Convention, published annually. [Not always complete, but still better than many sources of consumer information.]

———. *Drug Information for the Health Care Provider*. Rockville, Md.: U.S. Pharmacopeial Convention, published annually. [Often more helpful than the *PDR*.]

Wolf, Marion, and Aron Mosnaim. *Tardive Dyskinesia: Biological Mechanisms and Clinical Aspects*. Washington, D.C.: American Psychiatric Press, 1988. [Chapters vary enormously in quality, but 9 and 10 confirm the high tardive dyskinesia rates among children and older patients, respectively. Also see chapters 18 and 19.]

XIV. Audiocassettes by Peter Breggin

Audiocassettes of talks, testimony, and seminars by Peter Breggin on a variety of subjects can be obtained through: Breggin Audiocassettes, c/o James Turney, 2214 Hey Road, Richmond, Va. 23224. Phone: (804) 276-9255. The purchase price is $9.95 per cassette, including postage and handling. Titles include:

"Therapy and Psychosocial Rehabilitation as Better Alternatives"

"Psychiatric Drug Update"

"Electroshock Update"

"Psychiatry and the Abuse of Children"

"The Abuse of Women in Psychiatry and Society"

"Psychiatry as a Contributing Factor to the Holocaust in Nazi Germany"

"Psychiatry and the Homeless: A Long, Tragic Story"

"An Overview of Psychiatry: Past, Present, and Future"

"The Psychology of Liberty and Love"

"Communication as the Window to the Soul"

"How to Raise Independent, Happy Children"

"How to Improve Communication and Resolve Conflict Within Couples, Families and Friendships"

Notes

Acknowledgments

1. In 1987 the National Alliance for the Mentally Ill brought a complaint against my medical license in the State of Maryland, because I had criticized psychiatric drugs on Oprah Winfrey's national TV talk show. Although I was not aware of NAMI at the time, I soon learned that it is a large, powerful organization representing the parents of mentally disturbed or incapacited individuals. NAMI is closely connected to establishment psychiatry, and its leadership supports everything I have been criticizing for years: biological and genetic theories, involuntary treatment, heavy reliance on drugs, electroshock, and even lobotomy. (NAMI's positions will be elaborated throughout the book.) The NAMI attack became a major confrontation over my reform work.

After a hearing, the Maryland Commission on Medical Discipline completely exonerated me in a letter dated October 1, 1987, declaring that there was "no legal violation or ethical impropriety" on my part. The commission even expunged the record and said, "This entire matter is essentially a free speech issue." Its letter concluded by informing me, "We wish to thank you for having been concerned with [the] assurance of quality health care services in Maryland." In "Medical Probe: Penalty Is Ruled Out for Bethesda Psychiatrist," the October 1, 1987, *Baltimore Sun* quoted the chair of the Maryland Commission on Medical Discipline: ". . . we dismissed the whole affair and expunged it from the commission's records."

The publicity surrounding the attack proved to be a great boost to my reform efforts. At the time, I had been losing my enthusiasm after two decades or more of reform efforts; but the overwhelmingly positive response from individuals and groups throughout the country revitalized my efforts, made me many new friends and colleagues, and led to the writing of this book.

For further information on the attack, see three articles by Daniel Goleman in the *New York Times*: "Free Expression or Irresponsibility? Psychiatrist Faces

Test Today" (September 22, 1987), "Psychiatrist Says Panel Cleared Him" (September 24, 1987), and "Psychiatrist Is Cleared in Case" (October 13, 1987); and two articles by Susan Schmidt in the *Washington Post*: "Psychiatrist's TV Comments Prompt Md. Probe" (September 19, 1987), and "Doctor Says Md. Medical Panel Cleared Him" (September 23, 1990). Also see "Complaint Against Psychiatrist Critic of Biologic Therapy Dismissed," *Clinical Psychiatry News*, November 1987.

Chapter 1

1 Carter Umbarger, Andrew Morrison, James Dalsimer, and Peter Breggin, *College Students in a Mental Hospital: An Account of Organized Social Contacts Between College Volunteers and Mental Patients in a Hospital Community* (New York: Grune and Stratton, 1962). Also see P. Breggin, "The College Student and the Mental Patient," in proceedings of the *College Student Companion Conference*, November 7–9, 1962 (Connecticut State Department of Mental Health and NIMH).

2. Throughout the 1970s I devoted much of my time to creating the campaign to abort the return of lobotomy and newer forms of psychiatric brain surgery, such as cingulotomy and amygdalotomy. My efforts included founding the Center for the Study of Psychiatry; educating the public through the media; writing articles for the profession; publishing independent follow-up studies and holding press conferences about individual patients whom the neurosurgeons and psychiatrists had falsely claimed to cure; testifying in malpractice suits and in the landmark Kaimowitz decision (the suit was brought by attorney Gabe Kaimowitz) that ended psychosurgical experimentation in the state mental hospitals; disclosing the racist motivations behind some of the best-known surgical projects; and writing the legislation that created the federal Psychosurgery Commission, which declared the treatment experimental and unsuitable for routine clinical use. The campaign was largely successful, and probably fewer than two hundred operations a year are done in the United States at present. Descriptions of my efforts can be found in newspaper and magazine reports from that period, such as: B. J. Mason, "New Threat to Blacks: Brain Surgery to Control Behavior," *Ebony*, February 1973, pp. 63–72; J. Dietz, "Boston's Psychosurgery: Success and Controversy," *Boston Sunday Globe*, January 21, 1973, p. A1; J. Dietz, "Opponent Sees 'Grave Danger' in New Psychosurgery Effort by Hub Team," *Boston Globe*, May 24, 1973, p. 43; and R. Trotter, "Peter Breggin's Private War," *Human Behavior*, November 1973, pp. 50–77. A more complete list can be found in P. Breggin, "Brain-Disabling Therapies," in *The Psychosurgery Debate*, ed. E. Valenstein (San Francisco: W. H. Freeman, 1980). Also see chapter 3 for further citations on psychosurgery and the antipsychosurgery campaign.

Chapter 2

1. See H. Fireside, *Soviet Psychoprisons* (New York: Norton, 1979); and S. Block and P. Reddaway, *Psychiatric Terror* (New York: Basic Books, 1977).
2. For example, see A. Boisen, "Onset in Acute Schizophrenia," *Psychiatry* 10 (1947): 159–206; and A. Boisen, "The Genesis and Significance of Mystical Identification in Cases of Mental Disorder," *Psychiatry* 15 (1952): 287–96. For Boisen, not only does mysticism illuminate madness, but the study of madness clarifies the experience of Jesus and other prophets.
3. See D. Shutts, *Lobotomy: Resort to the Knife* (New York: Van Nostrand Reinhold, 1982); and E. Valenstein, *Great and Desperate Cures* (New York: Basic Books, 1986).

Chapter 3

1. An exception is T. van Putten and P. May, "Akinetic Depression in Schizophrenia," *Archives of General Psychiatry* 35 (1978): 1101–7. The quotes at the beginning of the chapter are typical of patient responses to the drugs. Additional graphic descriptions can be found in many books by survivors (see appendix B).
2. Heidi Hensen et al., *Stereotactic Psychosurgery* (Munksgaard Copenhagen, 1982), *Acta Psychiatrica Scandinavica* 66, suppl. 301.
3. As summarized in chapter 1, in the text and in an endnote, much of my time in the early 1970s was devoted to stopping the return of lobotomy and psychosurgery. My reviews and analyses, which describe the effects of this brain mutilation, include: "The Return of Lobotomy and Psychosurgery" (1973), reprinted with a new introduction in *Psychiatry and Ethics*, ed. R. B. Edwards (Buffalo N.Y.: Prometheus Books, 1982); "Psychosurgery for Political Purposes," *Duquesne Law Review* 13 (1975): 841–62; "Brain-Disabling Therapies," in *The Psychosurgery Debate*, ed. E. Valenstein (San Francisco: W. H. Freeman, 1980); and "Psychosurgery as Brain-Disabling Therapy," in *Divergent Views in Psychiatry*, ed. M. Dongier and D. Wittkower (Hagerstown, Md.: Harper and Row, 1981).
4. Thomas Szasz, "Some Observations on the Use of Tranquilizing Drugs," *Archives of Neurology and Psychiatry* 77 (1957): 86–92.
5. For further discussion of neuroleptic-caused lobotomy effects, see P. Breggin, *Psychiatric Drugs: Hazards to the Brain* (New York: Springer, 1983); and P. Breggin, "Brain Damage, Dementia and Persistent Cognitive Dysfunction Associated with Neuroleptic Drugs: Evidence, Etiology, Implications," *Journal of Mind and Behavior* 11, nos. 3 and 4 (summer and autumn 1990): 425–64.
6. I discuss the brain-disabling hypothesis in *Psychiatric Drugs: Hazards to the Brain*; and "Iatrogenic Helplessness in Authoritarian Psychiatry," in *The Iatrogenics Handbook*, ed. R. Morgan (Toronto: IPI Publishing, 1983).
7. For further analysis of deinstitutionalization, see L. Mosher and L. Burti, *Community Mental Health* (New York: W. W. Norton, 1989); P. Brown,

The Transfer of Care (Boston: Routledge and Kegan Paul, 1985); C. Warren, "New Forms of Social Control: The Myth of Deinstitutionalization," *American Behavioral Scientist* 24 (1981): 724–40; and Andrew Scull, *Decarceration: Community Treatment and the Deviant; A Radical View* (Englewood Cliffs, N.J.: Prentice Hall, 1977). For the APA's approach to the homeless, including involuntary drugging, see H. R. Lamb, ed., *The Homeless Mentally Ill* (Washington, D.C.: American Psychiatric Association, 1984).

Chapter 4

1. In addition to my 1983 book, a good source on the frequency and severity of neuroleptic-induced neurological effects are the research papers of Theodore van Putten in the *Archives of General Psychiatry*, pp. 67–72 and 102–5 (vol. 31, 1974), 1101–7 (vol. 35, 1978), and 187–90 (vol. 38, 1981); in *Comprehensive Psychiatry* (vol. 16, 1975): 43–47; and in *Psychopharmacological Bulletin* (vol. 16, 1980): 36–38. For one of the few comparisons between lethargic encephalitis and neuroleptic effects, see Henry Brill in the *American Handbook of Psychiatry* (vol. 2, 1959): 1163–74.
2. F. Ayd, Jr. and B. Blackwell, eds., *Discoveries in Biological Psychiatry* (Philadelphia: Lippincott, 1970).
3. The Mental Commitment of M. P., in the Supreme Court of Indiana, Court of Appeals no. 2–1185 A 355, Supreme Court no. 49S02–8707–CV–704, 1981.
4. C. Thomas Gualtieri and Robert Sovner, "Akathisia and Tardive Akathisia," *Psychiatric Aspects of Mental Retardation* 8, no. 12 (December 1989). This is a good source on tardive akathisia. My book *Psychiatric Drugs: Hazards to the Brain* (New York: Springer, 1983) contains a discussion of akathisia in general, with references. Current information also can be obtained from the survivor-founded Tardive Dyskinesia/Tardive Dystonia Foundation, 4244 University Way NE, P.O. Box 45732, Seattle, Wash. 98145.
5. The true rates are almost surely higher than those reported in the vast majority of studies. It generally is agreed that tardive dyskinesia rates have been going up since the original APA estimates. The increased rate may be due to the wider use of long-acting injections, which make it impossible for patients to avoid taking the medications, as they can when it is given out as pills. Except for those involving long-acting injections, all studies are likely to underestimate the rates for tardive dyskinesia, because a larger percentage of patients always manage to get away without taking their medications. Therefore, they are not being exposed to the risk of tardive dyskinesia, even though they are in the studies. Dilip Jeste and Richard Jed Wyatt note medication rejection rates of 25 to 50 percent in outpatient clinics. Joseph Comaty and Philip Janicak, in the July 1987 *Psychiatric Annals*, cite noncompliance rates of 11 to 19 percent in hospitalized patients. The rates are also artificially low, because most patients—up to 90 percent—deny their symptoms. If the patients won't report their symptoms, and if the researchers typically examine them for only five or ten minutes, many

cases are going to be missed. Frequently symptoms will appear or worsen when the patient is tired or stressed. Furthermore, as already noted, the drugs tend to mask the symptoms, and since most studies are conducted on drugged patients, the rates again will be too low. Also, the patients are followed for only a fraction of their lives, and even for only a fraction of the time during which they are exposed to the drugs. Many won't develop the tardive dyskinesia until after the study is over. Lifetime studies are not yet available.

6. *Journal of Mind and Behavior* 11, nos. 3 and 4 (summer and autumn 1990). See appendix B, section 1, David Cohen, for availability.
7. Igor Grant and Kenneth Adams, eds., *Neuropsychological Assessment of Neuropsychiatric Disorders* (New York: Oxford University Press, 1986).
8. Psychiatrist Larry Lehmann, quoted by Ron Winslow, "Sandoz Corp.'s Clozaril Treats Schizophrenia but Can Kill Patients," *Wall Street Journal,* May 14, 1990.
9. Daniel Goleman, "Schizophrenic Drug Hailed, Except for Cost," *New York Times,* May 15, 1990. The article provides further confirmation of psychiatry's unwillingness to take seriously the dangers of its drugs. According to Sandoz, the special monitoring program was necessary because "During our clinical trials we found that about 80% of psychiatrists, all at very good hospitals, became complacent about the blood tests and failed to keep them up, and the blood disease can occur at any point, even after months or years."
10. See, for example, "New Approaches to Treatment-Resistant Schizophrenia," a series of articles in the *Journal of Clinical Psychiatry*, monograph series, vol. 8, no. 1 (May 1990).
11. See, for example, John Waddington and Timothy Crow, "Abnormal Involuntary Movements and Psychosis in the Preneuroleptic Era and in Unmedicated Patients; implications for the Concept of Tardive Dyskinesia," in *Tardive Dyskinesia: Biological Mechanisms and Clinical Aspects,* ed. Marion Wolf and Aron Mosnaim (Washington, D.C.: American Psychiatric Press, 1988). While not denying the reality of tardive dyskinesia, the authors try to suggest that the picture is complicated by spontaneous dyskinesias in psychotic patients. The remainder of the volume contains studies demonstrating that tardive dyskinesia exists, that the rates are high, and that spontaneous dyskinesias are rare indeed, even among the elderly, where the highest frequency is to be expected.
12. See, for example, P. M. Schyve et al., "Neuroleptic-Induced Prolactin Level Elevation and Breast Cancer: An Emerging Issue," *Archives of General Psychiatry* 35 (1978): 1291–1301; and J. E. Overall, "Prior Psychiatric Treatment and the Development of Breast Cancer," *Archives of General Psychiatry* 35 (1978): 898–99. The 1990 *PDR* (see Thorazine, p. 2109) gives a surprisingly long discussion of the danger and mentions that chronic neuroleptic exposure increases mammary cancer in rodents. It also notes a menacing relationship between prolactin output, which is increased by the neuroleptics, and breast cancer. However, it finds that "the available evidence is considered too limited to be conclusive at this time." Similar data

in regard to a drug given to any group other than "female mental patients" surely would raise grave concern at the FDA and among physicians. Instead the danger goes largely unnoticed in psychiatry and is not mentioned in major textbooks.

13. David Hill, "Opinion: The Problem with Major Tranquillisers," *Openmind*, no. 13 (February/March 1985).

Chapter 5

1. Benno Muller-Hill, *Murderous Science: Elimination by Scientific Selection of Jews, Gypsies, and Others. Germany 1933–1945* (Oxford: Oxford University Press, 1988), 88. See appendix B, section 6, for other books and articles describing the role of psychiatry in the mass murder of mental patients and then in helping to bring about the wider holocaust.
2. I am grateful to Jeffrey Masson for pointing out the importance of this book to me.
3. J. H. Powell, *Bring Out Your Dead: The Great Plague of Yellow Fever in Philadelphia in 1793* (New York: Time Reading Program, Special Edition, 1965). I am grateful to Ginger Ross-Breggin for bringing this important book to my attention.
4. For a discussion of Heath, see Peter Breggin, "The Return of Lobotomy and Psychosurgery," in *Psychiatry and Ethics*, ed. Rem B. Edwards (Buffalo, N.Y.: Prometheus, 1982).
5. For a review of tardive dyskinesia and brain damage, see Peter Breggin, "Brain Damage, Dementia and Persistent Cognitive Dysfunction Associated with Neuroleptic Drugs: Evidence, Etiology, Implications," *Journal of Mind and Behavior* 11, nos. 3 and 4 (summer and autumn 1990): 425–64.

Chapter 6

1. In Heinz and Rowena Ansbacher, eds., *The Individual Psychology of Alfred Adler* (New York: Basic Books, 1956), 322–23. For a variety of contemporary views of elation and mania, see E. Mark Stern, ed., *Psychotherapy of the Grandiose Patient* (New York: Haworth Press, 1989).

Chapter 7

1. The interested reader may want to refer to any current textbook; S. Ankier and B. Leonard, "Biological Aspects of Depression," *International Review of Neurobiology* 28 (1986): 183–239; or L. Siever and K. Davis, "Overview: Toward a Dysregulation Hypothesis of Depression," *American Journal of Psychiatry* 142 (1985): 1017–31. As in every other aspect of psychiatry, there are many highly speculative hypotheses, but no firm ones, and no proof that mood disorders have a biological basis.

Chapter 8

1. Most textbooks do not give withdrawal problems as much attention as this book does. In addition to those already mentioned in the text, two sources of information on withdrawal are Barbara Geller et al., "Prospective Study of Scheduled Withdrawal from Nortriptyline in Children and Adolescents," *Journal of Clinical Psychopharmacology* 7 (1987): 252–54; and Steven Dilsaver, "Managing Withdrawal from Antidepressants Requires Keen Eye," *Psychiatric Times*, March 1989.

2. For example, see Steven Dilsaver et al., "Antidepressant Withdrawal Syndromes: Phenomenology and Pathophysiology," *International Clinical Psychopharmacology* 2 (1987): 1–19; and Steven Dilsaver et al., "Amitriptyline Supersensitizes a Central Cholinergic Mechanism," *Biological Psychiatry* 22 (1987): 495–507.

3. Ramzy Yassa et al., "Tardive Dyskinesia in the Course of Antidepressant Therapy: A Prevalence Study and Review of the Literature," *Journal of Clinical Psychopharmacology* 7 (1987): 243–46.

4. For a brief listing of studies of brain atrophy in affective disorders, see George Jaskiw, Nancy Andreasen, and Daniel Weinberger, "X-Ray Computed Tomography and Magnetic Resonance Imaging in Psychiatry," *American Psychiatric Association Annual Review* 6 (1987): 260–99. This team of investigators is radically biological, and their entire thrust is to blame the patient's supposed mental illness rather than the obviously damaging treatments. As if by fiat, individual studies sometimes declare, without further explanation, that electroshock and drugs are not the cause of the brain shrinkage. See Ronald Rieder et al., "Computed Tomography Scans in Patients with Schizophrenic, Schizoaffective, and Bipolar Affective Disorder," *Archives of General Psychiatry* 40 (1983): 735–39.

5. For further information on depression and suicide, see I. Oswald et al., "On the Slowness of Action of Tricyclic Antidepressant Drugs," *British Journal of Psychiatry* 120 (1972): 673–77.

6. The June 1990 *Health Letter*, published by the Public Citizen Health Research Group, lists many categories of drugs that can cause depression, including barbiturates, minor tranquilizers, numerous heart and blood pressure medications, ulcer drugs, corticosteroids, some antibiotics, anticonvulsants, antiparkinsonian drugs, diet pills, painkillers, and Antabuse. The Public Citizen Health Research Group tends to favor the more potent psychiatric medications and does not list three of the worst offenders: neuroleptics, antidepressants, and lithium.

7. See J. M. Strayhorn, Jr., *Foundations of Clinical Psychiatry* (Chicago: Yearbook Medical Publishers, 1982), 306; and Armand Nicholi, Jr., *The New Harvard Guide to Psychiatry* (Cambridge, Mass.: Harvard University Press, 1988), 509–10.

8. Seymour Fisher and Roger Greenberg, in their 1989 book *The Limits of Biological Treatments for Psychological Distress*, appendix B, section 3, underscore the necessity of control groups using active placebos that cause side effects. Their in-depth review suggests that antidepressants may have no

greater impact than an active placebo. They conclude that despite decades of clinical use, the therapeutic effect of the antidepressants remains unconfirmed and a matter of grave concern. In the July 1979 *Annals of Internal Medicine* (pp. 106–10), J. S. Goodwin and his associates write about the "Knowledge and Use of Placebos by House Officers and Nurses." They confirm that "the Placebo Effect has been responsible for the efficacy of the great majority of therapies throughout the history of medicine." But the power of placebo is even more evident in psychiatry than it is in medicine in general.

9. Also see, for example, Jerrold Rosenbaum, "The Media and the 'Miracle Drug': Risks, Benefits of Treating Depression," *Psychiatric Times*, October 1990; Anastasia Toufexis, "Warnings About a Miracle Drug," *Time*, July 30, 1990; John Kifner, "Police Say Kahane [Murder] Suspect Took Anti-Depressant Drugs," *New York Times*, November 9, 1990; and "More Cases Have Been Filed Against Manufacturer of Antidepressant," *Psychiatric Times*, October 1990.

10. In the February 1990 *American Journal of Psychiatry* (147:207–10), Martin Teicher, Carol Glod, and Jonathan O. Cole report on six depressed patients, previously free of recent suicidal ideation, who developed "intense, violent suicidal preoccupations after 2–7 weeks of fluoxetine treatment." The suicidal preoccupations lasted from three days to three months after termination of the treatment. The report estimates that 3.5 percent of Prozac users were at risk. While denying the validity of the study, Dista Products, a division of Eli Lilly, put out a brochure for doctors dated August 31, 1990, stating that it was adding "suicidal ideation" to the adverse events section of its Prozac product information.

11. See chapter 7 and studies and commentaries in the vol. 51, April 1990 issue of the *Journal of Clinical Psychiatry* entitled "Serotonin and Its Effects on Human Behavior" and in S. Brown and J. M. van Praag, eds., *The Role of Serotonin in Psychiatric Disorders* (New York: Brunner/Mazel, 1991).

12. See S. A. Welner et al., "Autographic Quantification of Serotonin$_{1A}$ Receptors in Rat Brain Following Antidepressant Drug Treatment," *Synapse* 4 (1989): 347–52; F. Sulser, "Serotonin-Norepinephrine Receptor Interactions in the Brain: Implications for the Pharmacology and Pathophysiology of Affective Disorders," *Journal of Clinical Psychiatry* 48 (1987): 12–18; and J. Wamsley et al., "Receptor Alterations Associated with Serotonergic Agents: An Autoradiographic Analysis," *Journal of Clinical Psychiatry* 48 (1987): 19–25.

13. Alfred Goodman et al., eds., *Goodman and Gilman's The Pharmacological Basis of Therapeutics*, 7th ed. (New York: Macmillan, 1985), 550.

14. Many people do not develop a "high" from Prozac, but their feeling of increased well-being may be a subtle high. Relatively small doses of any stimulant, including amphetamine or cocaine, may increase the sense of well-being without producing a gross high or euphoria.

15. Many sources report frequent signs of an organic brain syndrome in routine antidepressant treatment—for example, A. B. Wells and M. Mendelson, "Antidepressants," in *Mind-Influencing Drugs*, ed. M. Goldberg and G.

Egelston (Littleton, Mass.: PSG, 1978). They write, "Patients say that they forget what they are saying in mid-sentence, or forget where they placed things. Reassurance is necessary, especially for older patients, who may fear they are becoming senile." We shall find that ECT also causes memory dysfunction, but that shock doctors almost uniformly tell patients that it is due to their "mental illness" rather than to the shock.

16. M. Schou, A. Amidsen, and K. Thomsen, "The Effect of Lithium on the Normal Mind," in *De Psychiatria Progrediente*, vol. 2, ed. P. Baudiš, E. Peterová, and V. Sedivec (Plzen, 1968), 712–21.

17. For pediatric references, see Lawrence Kerns, "Treatment of Mental Disorders in Pregnancy," *Journal of Nervous and Mental Disease* 174 (1986): 652–59; Gordon Johnson, "Lithium," *Medical Journal of Australia*, October 27, 1984, pp. 595–601; and Peter Breggin, *Psychiatric Drugs: Hazards to the Brain* (New York: Springer, 1983), 194.

18. See Rose Salata and Irwin Klein, "Effects of Lithium on the Endocrine System: A Review," *Journal of Laboratory and Clinical Medicine* 110 (1987): 130–36.

19. An exception is Rudra Prakash, "A Review of Hematologic Side Effects of Lithium," *Hospital and Community Psychiatry* 36 (1985): 127–28.

Chapter 9

1. See C. Miller Fisher, "Neurologic Fragments. II. Remarks on Anosognosia, Confabulation, Memory, and Other Topics; and an Appendix on Self-Observation," *Neurology* 39 (1989): 127–32. Fisher describes how brain-injured patients tend to deny their mental losses and to "confabulate" or make up stories to cover their deficits. The general tendency, called anosognosia or unawareness of neurologic deficit, is so common that Fisher declares, "Indeed, it may qualify as one of the general rules of cerebral dysfunction." Yet shock advocates persistently claim that ECT-damaged patients exaggerate their memory loss.

2. APA task force report: *The Practice of Electroconvulsive Therapy: Recommendations for Treatment, Training, and Privileging* (Washington, D.C.: American Psychiatric Association, 1990). The task force, chaired by Richard Weiner and including Max Fink and Harold Sacheim, two other defenders of shock treatment, set out to exonerate the "treatment."

3. See James L. Bernat and Frederick Vincent, eds., *Neurology: Problems in Primary Care* (Oradell, N.J.: Medical Economics, 1987). In discussing "Minor Closed Head Injury" they state, "The patient who is not fully oriented at the time of evaluation and who demonstrates defective immediate recall and recent memory should be hospitalized for 24 to 48 hours." Shock patients are typically much more impaired and are suffering from what would be called severe head injury by neurological standards.

4. Edward Babayan, *The Structure of Psychiatry in the Soviet Union* (New York: International Press, 1985). For criticism of shock, see pages 36–37, 53, 134–35, and 294.

5. In the June 1960 *American Journal of Psychiatry* psychiatrist and shock advocate David Impastato describes the drama surrounding the first shock treatment in Italy. An involuntary patient had been subjected to one shock, which failed to make him convulse. "The Professor [Ugo Cerletti] suggested that another treatment with a higher voltage be given. The staff objected. They stated that if another treatment were given the patient would probably die and wanted further treatment postponed until the morrow. The Professor knew what that meant. [Presumably, that they would refuse to participate again.] He decided to go ahead right then and there, but before he could say so the patient suddenly sat up and pontifically proclaimed no longer in jargon, but in clear Italian, "Non una seconda! Mortifere!" (Not again, it will kill me.) This made the Professor think and swallow, but his courage was not lost. He gave the order to proceed at a higher voltage and a longer time; and the first electroconvulsion in man ensued. Thus was born EST out of one man and over the objection of his assistants."

6. Gary Aden, "The International Psychiatric Association for the Advancement of Electrotherapy: A Brief History," *American Journal of Social Psychiatry* 4, no. 4 (1984): 9–10.

7. Alison Bass, "McLean Hires Back Doctor Ordered to Quit," *Boston Globe*, February 10, 1989.

8. The $200 to $300 figure was given by psychiatrists at the Alioto hearings.

9. The availability of dangerous but remunerative technology encourages exploitation in other fields of medicine as well. See the Associated Press, "Doctors Owning Machines X-Ray Patients More Often: Study Shows Some Evidence of Exploitation," *Washington Post*, December 6, 1990, p. A7.

10. Deposition of Glen N. Peterson in John Doe vs. D. Michael O'Connor et al., Defendants, vol. 2, in the Superior Court of the State of California in and for the County of Los Angeles, no. C 646 194, CSR no. 3081, March 18, 1988.

11. Peterson said in his deposition that the woman had received four series of shock treatments prior to his administering 130–140 more. A series usually consists of at least six or eight treatments, and sometimes more. He also said that he was using the "upper end of the scale" of electrical energy, 150–170 volts. Depending on other electrical parameters, this could be in excess of household current.

12. Numerous studies of the brain-damaging effects of such large doses are cited in my book *Electroshock: Its Brain-Disabling Effects* (New York: Springer, 1979). See, for example, A. I. Rabin, "Persons Who Received More than 100 Electric Shock Treatments," *Journal of Personality* 17 (1948): 42–47; D. I. Templer et al., "Cognitive Functioning and Degree of Psychosis in Schizophrenics Given Many Electroconvulsive Treatments," *British Journal of Psychiatry* 123 (1973): 441–43; and A. Ferraro and L. Roizen, "Cerebral Morphologic Changes in Monkeys Subjected to a Large Number of Electrically Induced Convulsions," *American Journal of Psychiatry* 106 (1949): 278–84.

13. See the advertisement "Informed ECT, at Last," in *Psychiatric News*, September 7, 1990, p. 3.

14. Figures through 1983 are available in Carol Warren, "Electroconvulsive Therapy: 'New' Treatment of the 1980s," *Research in Law, Deviance and Social Control* 8 (1986): 41–55. More recent figures are from the State of California, Department of Mental Health, Statistics and Data Analysis Section, July 20, 1989.
15. See, for example, E. N. Zamora and R. Kaebling, "Memory and Electroconvulsive Therapy," *American Journal of Psychiatry* 122 (1965): 546–54. For a complete review, see Peter Breggin, *Electroshock: Its Brain-Disabling Effects,* 63–70.
16. Also see Lewis Rowland, ed., *Merritt's Textbook of Neurology,* 8th ed. (Philadelphia: Lea and Fibiger, 1989). As with many other observations in this book, the comparison between ECT and closed-head injury did not fully dawn on me until emphasized by a survivor of the treatment.
17. I have reviewed the animal studies in detail in *Electroshock: Its Brain-Disabling Effects.* For short summaries, see Peter Breggin, "Neuropathology and Cognitive Dysfunction from ECT," *Psychopharmacology Bulletin* 22, no. 2 (1986): 476–79; Peter Breggin, "Disabling the Brain with Electroshock," in *Divergent Views in Psychiatry,* ed. M. Dongier and E. Wittkower (Hagerstown, Md.: Harper and Row, 1981); and John Friedberg, "Shock Treatment, Brain Damage, and Memory Loss: A Neurological Perspective," *American Journal of Psychiatry* 134 (1977): 1010–14.

    While psychiatrists tend to deny what shock is doing to their patients, psychologists have sometimes been more open about it. James McConnel, in *Understanding Human Behavior,* 4th ed. (New York: Holt, Rinehart and Winston, 1983), reviews my conclusions that ECT effects are "severe," "catastrophic," and "devastating" and concludes, "Most of the literature on ECT tends to support Breggin's view" (p. 565).
18. See note 13, this chapter.
19. See Peter Breggin, *Electroshock: Its Brain-Disabling Effects.*
20. In Max Rinkel and Harold Himwich, eds., *Insulin Treatment in Psychiatry* (New York: Philosophical Library, 1959), shock advocate Hans Hoff states that the object of ECT is to kill brain cells: "cells that are sick, and new brain cells which are potentially sick have to be destroyed. Otherwise relapses will come. This means that one of the most important things is to see that really every cell which is affected is really destroyed" (p. 222). In 1941 Walter Freeman was given space in the prestigious journal *Diseases of the Nervous System* (vol. 2) to publish an editorial entitled "Brain-Damaging Therapeutics." Freeman postulates, "Among the explanations advanced to account for the success of the various shock methods of therapy in the psychoses, that of actual damage to the brain has not received adequate attention." He declares, "Maybe it will be shown that a mentally ill patient can think more clearly and more constructively with less brain in actual operation." Similarly, in a commentary at the end of an article by F. Ebaugh and others in the 1942 *Transactions of the American Neurological Association* (pp. 35–41), one of America's most influential psychiatrists, Abraham Myerson, speaks of how mental patients have "more intelligence than they can handle and that the reduction of intelligence is an important factor in

the curative process." His remarks are made in a discussion of autopsy material gained from patients who died from electroshock treatment.

21. R. L. Kahn, M. Fink, and E. A. Weinstein, "Relation of Amobarbital to Clinical Improvement in Electroshock," *Archives of Neurology and Psychiatry* 76 (1956): 23–29. In a study of the amobarbital interview method, the authors again make clear that the test is useful as a "diagnostic test for the existence of structural brain disease." This is the test that is correlated with a positive clinical outcome following ECT. The meaning is clear: brain damage is considered an improvement. See R. L. Kahn, M. Fink, and E. Weinstein: "The 'Amytal Test' in Patients with Mental Illness," *Journal of the Hillside Hospital* 4 (1955): 3–13.

22. Fink's articles, which are cited in my 1979 book on shock, include those in the *Journal of the Hillside Hospital* 6 (1957): 197–206; *Archives of Neurology and Psychiatry* 80 (1958): 380–86; and *Diseases of the Nervous System* 19 (1958): 113–18. In his book *Convulsive Therapy: Theory and Practice* (New York: Raven, 1973), Fink again makes clear that the degree of improvement is correlated with brain dysfunction as reflected by psychological tests, brain wave studies, and other criteria (p. 127). He points out that "patients become more compliant and acquiescent with treatment" (p. 139) and also continues to connect improvement with denial, disorientation, brain trauma, cerebral dysfunction, and signs of an organic brain syndrome (p. 165). He also mentions anosognosia, the denial of physical damage after trauma to the brain, as a basis for the improvement. Nonetheless, in public Fink has contested my assertion that shock works by producing damage and dysfunction.

23. Max Fink, "Efficacy and Safety of Induced Seizures (EST) in Man," *Comprehensive Psychiatry* 19 (1978). This quote and several others originally were located by shock survivor Marilyn Rice.

24. For a discussion of anosognosia, see note 1 of this chapter.

25. Russ Rymer, "Electroshock," *Hippocrates*, March/April 1989.

26. See David Remnick, "25 Years of Nightmares: Victims of CIA-Funded Mind Experiments Seek Damages from the Agency," *Washington Post*, July 28, 1985; Lee Hockstander, "Victims of 1950's Mind-Control Experiments Settle with CIA," *Washington Post*, October 5, 1988; Leonard Rubenstein, "The CIA and the Evil Doctor," *New York Times*, November 7, 1988; and a letter by Don Weitz, "Psychiatry Bears Guilt in Brainwashing Tests," *New York Times*, November 26, 1988.

27. See the classic article by A. V. Delgado-Escueta et al., "Management of Status Epilepticus," *New England Journal of Medicine* 306 (1982): 1337–40; or James Bernat and Frederick Vincent, eds., *Neurology: Problems in Primary Care* (Oradell, N.J.: Medical Economics, 1987), which states that status epilepticus is "a true medical emergency."

28. In the *British Journal of Psychiatry* (142 [1983]: 1–8), Larry Squire and Pamela Slater surveyed more than sixty patients long after they had received routine shock treatment. Seven months after ECT, patients reported a median memory loss spanning a period of two years prior to and three months after the shock—a total block of twenty-seven months. Three years

after shock, they reported a smaller gross loss, from six months prior to two months after the ECT. The estimate at seven months is surely more accurate. Brain-injured patients, as described, tend to deny their losses (see note 1 of this chapter). While it's very unlikely that the brain would heal any further after seven months, over the years it would become easier for patients to deny the degree of their memory loss. Despite the tendency toward denial, more than half of the patients (55 percent) surveyed by Squire and Slater felt that they had not regained normal memory function over the years. In a personal discussion with me at the 1985 Consensus Conference on ECT, sponsored by NIMH in Bethesda, Maryland, Squire told me that one patient suffered significant memory losses over a span of ten years; but he said he did not consider it important to mention it in his report.

In *Multiple-Monitored Electroconvulsive Therapy* (Boca Raton, Fla.: CRC Press, 1981), Barry Maletzky reports on a survey of forty-seven patients thirty-six months after his shock program. Thirty-six percent had ongoing or continuing cognitive problems, such as keeping sequences straight and remembering new things: "I have been following this soap opera for five years on TV but now I get confused about who is doing what to whom"; "I couldn't tell my neighbor how to get over to my uncle's house when she was driving me there the other day, but I have been going over there for years" (p. 180).

29. Two groups were studied, one with a mean age of 69.7 years and the other 41.7 years. There were control patients as well. None of them had had ECT for at least three months.
30. Nonetheless, the authors remain strong advocates of ECT.
31. Max Fink, *Convulsive Therapy: Theory and Practice* (New York: Raven, 1973); and Richard Abrams, *Electroconvulsive Therapy* (New York: Oxford University Press, 1988).
32. One controlled study using simulated ECT, by J. Lambourn and D. Gill, "A Controlled Comparison of Simulated and Real ECT" (*British Journal of Psychiatry* 133 [1978]: 514–19), found no difference and concludes, "This cast some doubt on current view of the effectiveness of electro-convulsive therapy in general." Even the often cited shock study, S. Brandon et al., "Electroconvulsive Therapy: Results in Depressive Illness from the Leicestershire Trial" (*British Medical Journal* 288 [1984]: 22–25), presents a bleak picture of ECT efficacy. While the authors emphasize an improvement on the Hamilton depression rating scale at four weeks, their data show absolutely no difference between shocked patients and sham patients at twelve or twenty-eight weeks. Their whole argument rests on the hope of a mere four weeks' relief from depression—the period of maximum brain dysfunction. But even in regard to the alleged improvement during the one-month period, the evidence is flimsy at best, relying on a few borderline test results. Wade Hudson summarizes:

> Whether due to the power of suggestion, the benefit of routine support from nursing staff, spontaneous healing, or a combination of the three, those who received simulated shock treatment improved dramatically,

and on most measures, even 1–3 days right after treatment; [and] they improved as much as did those who had electricity passed through their brains.

33. It's unclear why shock advocates frequently misrepresent the Avery and Winokur paper, but as I discuss in my 1979 book on shock (pp. 130–31), they may have gotten the wrong impression from Fink's citation of the paper in a paragraph misleadingly entitled "ECT and Suicide." On one occasion, a shock doctor tried to use the paper in a radio debate with me to prove the efficacy of shock in preventing suicide, but fortunately I was on the phone from my office and was able to locate the paper to quote it on the air. The Avery and Winokur paper is also misused in the APA task force report, *The Practice of Electroconvulsive Therapy* (1990), p. 53.

34. On many occasions I have referred to this as the shame of my life.

35. One-sided or unilateral shock can be more damaging than the usual bilateral shock, because the electrodes are placed closer together. The electrical current strikes the brain with more concentrated force, doing more intense focal damage. This is demonstrable in brain wave studies. It also is demonstrable in studies that show *increased* damage to the verbal centers when the electrodes are placed on the dominant side. Furthermore, attempts to shock the nondominant side will at times end up directing the full force of the shock inadvertently at the verbal centers. Many left-handers and some right-handers are dominant on the same, rather than the opposite, side of the brain.

The dangerousness of unilateral shock is increased by the fact that it is harder to produce a convulsion with it. So sometimes the current controls on the shock machine are turned up higher to deliver a greater shock, or else more than one shock may be needed to produce a seizure. Often additional ECT treatments are given to achieve the desired level of post-ECT brain dysfunction.

Denial and anosognosia are even more pronounced after damage to the nonverbal, or nondominant, side of the brain. Patients with strokes on that side of the brain will not recognize that they have very obvious ill effects, such as paralyzed limbs. Blakeslee remarks that the rest of the brain has trouble recognizing or communicating about any damage to the nonverbal side. Shock advocates are also well aware that nondominant shock makes their patients less aware of the damage done to them. In his 1988 book *Electroconvulsive Therapy*, Richard Abrams observes that anosognosia is especially "profound and striking" after nondominant shock. Yet shock doctors never admit that this causes patients to report falsely that they have less memory loss or mental dysfunction after nondominant ECT.

36. The relative impact of nondominant shock on nonverbal functions is reviewed in D. Fromm-Auch, "Comparison of Unilateral and Bilateral ECT: Evidence of Selective Memory Impairment," *British Journal of Psychiatry* 141 (1982): 608–13.

37. Margaret McDonald, "FDA Orders Tougher ECT Device Standards," *Psychiatric News*, December 7, 1979.

38. "Reclassification of ECT Devices Delayed," *Psychiatric News*, April 6, 1984.

39. See Rael Jean Isaac, "FDA's Shocking Treatment of a Valuable Device," *Wall Street Journal*, December 5, 1990; and Seth Farber, "US Food & Drug Administration Proposes Giving Electroshock the Rubber Stamp," *Dendron*, October 24, 1990. (See appendix A for the availability of *Dendron*.)

40. M. Boss, "Alte und neue Shocktherapien und Shocktherapeuten," *Zeitschrift fur Neurologie* 173 (1941): 776–82.

41. Rex Dalton, "Psychotherapists Having Sex with Patients May Be Jailed," *San Diego Union*, September 27, 1989.

42. Rex Dalton, "Psychiatrist's Former Patient Tells Story of Abuse," *San Diego Union*, January 1, 1989.

43. Leonard Frank, "Electroshock: Death, Brain Damage, Memory Loss, and Brainwashing," *Journal of Mind and Behavior* 11, nos. 3 and 4 (summer and autumn 1990).

Chapter 10

1. For the "party line" on anxiety, see Sandy Rovner, "High Anxiety: Probing the Most Common Mental Disorder," *Washington Post Health*, May 22, 1990.

2. Peter Breggin, *The Psychology of Freedom: Liberty and Love as a Way of Life* (Buffalo, N.Y.: Prometheus, 1980).

3. For a detailed discussion, see *Diagnostic and Statistical Manual of Mental Disorders (Revised)* (Washington, D.C.: American Psychiatric Association, 1987). The description is excellent but somewhat too rigid in its requirements. It also includes a phenomenon, "numbing of general responsiveness," that frequently is absent. More often people become oversensitive and hyperreactive.

4. See Frank Ochberg, ed., *Post-Traumatic Therapy and Victims of Violence* (New York: Brunner/Mazel, 1988); and Spencer Eth and Robert Pynoos, eds., *Post-Traumatic Stress Disorder in Children* (Washington, D.C.: American Psychiatric Press, 1985).

5. The American Psychiatric Press's *Textbook of Psychiatry* (1988), for example, mentions "growing attention" to the subject and reports that "a number of hypotheses have been put forward that are currently being studied," but none of them are given primacy or any detailed analysis. George Vaillant's review of the causes of alcoholism in the *New Harvard Guide to Psychiatry* (1988) does not even discuss a biological cause for alcoholism. The many findings of biological abnormalities in alcoholics are attributable to toxic effects on the brain, liver, and other organs. When the Supreme Court refused to grant alcoholism the status of disease in Traynor v. Turnage and McKelvey v. Turnage in 1988, a spate of articles pro and con appeared in the press. See Al Kamen, "VA Can Define Alcoholism as 'Willful Misconduct,' " *New York Times*, April 21, 1988; Richard Vatz and Lee Weinberg, "There's a New Skepticism Toward Alcoholism as a Disease," *Washington Post Health*, March 7, 1989; and a letter by Jeffrey Schaler,

"Alcoholism Is Not a Disease," *Washington Post*, October 25, 1988. Also see Herbert Fingarette, *Heavy Drinking: The Myth of Alcoholism as a Disease* (Berkeley: University of California Press, 1988).

6. For a thorough evaluation of genetic studies of alcoholism, see John Searles, "The Role of Genetics in the Pathogenesis of Alcoholism," *Journal of Abnormal Behavior* 97 (1988): 153–67. Even genetic researchers in the field who enter with a strong bias toward positive results are forced to limit their claims to evidence for a "gene effect" in "for the less frequent subtype of alcoholism that is marked by early onset, severe alcohol abuse, and sociopathy." Annabel Bolos et al., "Population and Pedigree Studies Reveal a Lack of Association Between Dopamine D₂ Receptor and Gene in Alcoholism," *Journal of the American Medical Association* 264 (1990): 3156–60. However, even that meager assertion is unproven. Bolos et al. further admit: "On the other hand, familial transmission studies do not support the existence of a single gene in the majority of alcoholics." The phrase "single gene" is something of a euphemism, as the authors cite no evidence for multiple gene influences either.

7. K. Blum et al., "Allelic Association of Human Dopamine D₂ Receptor Gene in Alcoholism," *Journal of the American Medical Association* 263 (1990): 2055–60.

8. Annabel Bolos et al., "Population and Pedigree Studies Reveal a Lack of Association Between the Dopamine D₂ Receptor Gene and Alcoholism," *Journal of the American Medical Association* 264 (1990): 3156–60.

9. "Alcoholism Gene Report Undercut," *Washington Post*, December 26, 1990. The concluding sentence of the study itself is very similar: that their findings are "inconsistent" with a "widespread association" between the receptor gene and alcoholism.

10. Susan Squire, *The Slender Balance* (New York: G. P. Putnam, 1983).

11. J. Polivy and C. P. Herman, "Dieting and Bingeing: A Causal Analysis," *American Psychologist* 40 (1985): 193–201.

12. Hilde Bruch, *Eating Disorders: Obesity, Anorexia Nervosa, and the Person Within* (New York: Basic Books, 1973).

Chapter 11

1. Armand Nicholi, Jr., ed., *The New Harvard Guide to Psychiatry* (Cambridge, Mass.: Harvard University Press, 1988), 523.

2. See any psychiatric textbook or the American Psychiatric Association's task force report: *Benzodiazepine Dependence, Toxicity, and Abuse* (Washington, D.C.: American Psychiatric Association, 1990). These drugs are always discussed as a group, with comparisons mostly focused on the duration of action rather than on the actual effect.

3. Ibid.

4. When it was discovered that benzodiazepines attach to a specific type of receptor in the brain, this was treated as evidence that the drugs have a specifically inhibitory effect on anxiety. In reality the receptors are spread

throughout the gray matter of the human brain. See John Talbott et al., *Textbook of Psychiatry* (Washington, D.C.: American Psychiatric Press, 1988).

5. APA task force report, *Benzodiazepine Dependence, Toxicity, and Abuse* (Washington, D.C.: American Psychiatric Association, 1990), 33.

6. See Russell Noyes, Jr., et al., "Benzodiazepine Withdrawal: A Review of the Evidence," *Journal of Clinical Psychiatry* 49 (1988): 382–89.

7. Since doctors frequently do not pay enough attention to the problem, it is worth pointing to two relevant studies of memory dysfunction. In "The Effect of Diazepam on Patients' Memory" in the *Journal of Clinical Psychopharmacology* 4 (1984): 203–6, William Angus and David Romney find that patients taking routine doses of Valium for a minimum of five days did more poorly on both short-term and long-term memory tests than they had done prior to using the medication. Short-term memory was most severely affected. They warn against combining psychotherapy and minor tranquilizers: "Because of the growing body of evidence that diazepam does impair memory, its use as an adjunct to therapies emphasizing learning should be reconsidered. It is possible that diazepam slows down the very learning that is supposed to take place."

Daljit Mac, Rajiv Kumar, and Donald Goodwin of the University of Kansas Medical Center tested the effect of Ativan on memory in a double-blind study reported in the *Journal of Clinical Psychiatry* 46 (1985): 137–38. They gave one drug dose or placebo in the morning and then tested the volunteers throughout the day. Recall was reduced two hours after drug ingestion. The authors conclude, "These results support findings by other investigators that lorazepam has a deleterious effect on short-term recall of verbal content. This has implications for students and others preparing for tests or doing mental work while taking therapeutic doses of lorazepam."

8. An exception is Jack M. Gorman, *The Essential Guide to Psychiatric Drugs* (New York: St. Martin's Press, 1990). Gorman states: "BuSpar might cause neurological problems (tardive dyskinesia) if taken for many years. In fact, this has not occurred in patients who have taken it, although the drug has been on the market only about three years" (p. 145).

9. See, for example, the December 1990 *Psychiatric Annals*.

10. Indeed, studies have shown no difference between Xanax and Valium in panic disorder. See David Dunner et al., "Effect of Alprazolam and Diazepam on Anxiety and Panic Disorder: A Controlled Study," *Journal of Clinical Psychiatry* 47 (1986): 458–60. Drug "efficacy" compared to placebo was not very impressive.

11. Joe Graedon and Dr. Teresa Graedon, "Nervous Breakdown Can Be Drug Induced," press release for the week of October 30, 1989, from King Features Syndicate (235 East Forty-fifth Street, New York, N.Y. 10017).

12. Chad Carlton, "Xanax: Popular Tranquilizer Creates Anxiety About Abuse, Danger with Alcohol," *Lexington Herald-Leader*, August 26, 1990.

13. Reported in identical eight-page advertisements for Xanax in various psychiatric journals, including the December 1990 issues of *Psychiatric Annals*

and the *American Journal of Psychiatry*. The advertising material is dated October 1990.

14. James C. Ballenger et al., "Alprazolam in Panic Disorder and Agoraphobia: Results from a Multicenter Trial—I: Efficacy in Short-Term Treatment," *Archives of General Psychiatry* 45 (1988): 413–22.

15. The figure of "more than 500" is reported in an advertisement for Xanax in *Psychiatric Annals* (December 1990). For a more complete analysis of the sample size, see Gerald Klerman, "Overview of the Cross-National Collaborative Panic Study," *Archives of General Psychiatry* 45 (1988): 407–12; and James Ballenger et al., "Alprazolam in Panic Disorder and Agoraphobia: Results from a Multicenter Trial," *Archives of General Psychiatry* 45 (1988): 413–22. Klerman reports that the basic study involved 600 patients, only one-half of whom were taking Xanax, and that another study involved 1,100, only one-third of whom were on Xanax. Ballenger et al. more accurately explain that in the basic study, only 481 of the 526 patients in the placebo and drug groups completed three weeks. By the end of the study there were only 226 Xanax patients remaining.

16. J. C. Pecknold et al., "Alprazolam in Panic Disorder and Agoraphobia: Results from a Multicenter Trial—III: Discontinuation Effects," *Archives of General Psychiatry* 45 (1988): 429–37.

17. Russell Noyes, Jr., et al., "Alprazolam in Panic Disorder and Agoraphobia: Results from a Multicenter Trial—II: Patient Acceptance, Side Effects, and Safety," *Archives of General Psychiatry* 45 (1988): 423–28.

18. Reported in an advertisement for Xanax in the December 1990 issue of *Psychiatric Annals*.

19. Rajiv Kumar et al., "Anxiolytics and Memory: A Comparison of Lorazepam and Alprazolam," *Journal of Clinical Psychiatry* 48 (1987): 158–60.

20. See, for example, Lewis Baxter et al., "PET Imaging in Obsessive Compulsive Disorder With and Without Depression," *Journal of Clinical Psychiatry* 51 (suppl., 1990): 61–69. The paper reviews several studies, including their own, in which five of nine patients were "on a variety of antidepressants, benzodiazepines, and neuroleptics," while the remaining were drug-free for only two weeks. The authors speculate that the primary damage is to the striatum. This is the area known to be damaged by the neuroleptics (chapter 4) and possibly by the chemically related tricyclic antidepressants.

21. See chapters 1 and 3 for citations concerning my reform work in preventing the resurgence of psychosurgery in the early 1970s.

Chapter 12

1. J. Larry Brown and Stephen R. Bing, "Drugging Children: Child Abuse by Professionals," in *Children's Rights and the Mental Health Professions*, ed. Gerald P. Koocher (New York: John Wiley, 1976).

2. Spencer Rich, "Child-Abuse Cases Total 2.4 Million," *Washington Post*, June 27, 1990.

3. Nicholas Zill and Charlotte Schoenborn, "Developmental, Learning, and Emotional Problems: Health of Our Nation's Children, United States, 1988," *Advance Data from Vital And Health Statistics*, no. 190 (Hyattsville, Md.: National Center for Health Statistics, 1990). Also see the *Chicago Tribune* report, "Problems Found in 1 of 5 Children," in the *Washington Post*, December 9, 1990.

4. In addition to the books cited in this section, for a recent bibliography of studies on the effect of child abuse on adults, see Janet Surrey et al., "Reported History of Physical and Sexual Abuse and Severity of Symptomatology in Women Psychiatric Patients," *American Journal of Orthopsychiatry* 60 (1990): 412–17. In their own investigation, Surrey et al. found that 64 percent of 140 female psychiatric clinic patients reported a history of physical or sexual abuse and that symptoms were more severe among them than among women who reported no abuse. Also see chapter 14 concerning women and abuse.

5. Similar points are made in an earlier book: David Wolfe, *Child Abuse: Implications for Child Development and Psychopathology* (Newbury Park, Calif.: Sage, 1987).

6. For inflated estimates, also see Diane McGuinness, "Attention Deficit Disorder: The Emperor's New Clothes, Animal 'Pharm,' and Other Fiction," in Seymour Fisher and Roger Greenberg, *The Limits of Biological Treatments for Psychological Distress* (Hillsdale, N.J.: Lawrence Erlbaum Associates, 1989), 161.

7. Psychologist Russell Barkley, director of neuropsychology at the Medical College of Wisconsin, is one of the most often quoted experts in the field. More balanced than Wender, he is author of *Hyperactive Children: A Handbook for Diagnosis and Treatment* (New York: Guilford Press, 1981). Barkley recognizes that "the typical picture of the household in which the hyperactive child resides is one of turmoil" and that the children do better when the parents are helped to improve their skills. But he nonetheless concludes that it is the children, and not the parents, who create these "destructive and aversive family situations." Again like Wender, he finds the children to be especially "energetic, exuberant, bright, inquisitive." If the child has a whole bunch of these traits, Barkley suggests, they may add up to an "explosive" combination. And so the best and the most beautiful run afoul of some families and schools and then are polished off by the mental health professionals.

8. Some of Victor Sanua's publications include: "Standing Against an Established Ideology: Infantile Autism, a Case in Point," *Clinical Psychologist* 40 (fall 1987): 96–100; "The Organic Etiology of Infantile Autism: A Critical Review of the Literature," *International Journal of Neuroscience* 30 (1986): 195–225; "Infantile Autism and Childhood Schizophrenia: Review of the Issues from the Sociocultural Point of View," *Social Science and Medicine* 17 (1983): 1633–51; "Cultural Changes and Psychopathology in Children: With Special Reference to Infantile Autism," *Acta Paedopsychiatrica* 47 (1981): 133–42; "Infantile Autism and Parental Socioeconomic Status: A Case of Bimodal Distribution," *Child Psychiatry and Human Development* 17 (1987): 189–98; and "An International Survey of Mental Health Profes-

sionals on the Etiology of Infantile Autism," in *Frontiers of Infant Psychiatry*, vol. 2, ed. Justin Call et al. (New York: Basic Books, 1985).
9. David Simmonds, "Children's Rights and Family Dysfunction: 'Daddy, Why Do I Have To Be the Crazy One?' " in *Children's Rights and the Mental Health Professions*, ed. Gerald Koocher (New York: John Wiley, 1976). Koocher's book contains a number of valuable chapters.

Chapter 13

1. "Increase in Doctors' Use of Ritalin for School Kids," *San Francisco Chronicle*, October 21, 1988.
2. Carole Wade Offir, "Are We Pushers for Our Own Children?" *Psychology Today*, December 1974.
3. "Physician Warns of Dangers in Drugging Children," *Psychiatric News*, May 7, 1975.
4. See, for example, Timothy Kuehnel and Katherine Slama, "Guidelines for the Developmentally Disabled," in *The Psychiatric Uses of Seclusion and Restraint*, ed. Kenneth Tardiff (Washington, D.C.: American Psychiatric Press, 1984), 93–94; Mina Dulcan, "Treatment of Children and Adolescents," in *Textbook of Psychiatry*, ed. John Talbott et al. (Washington, D.C.: American Psychiatric Press, 1988); R. Plotkin and K. Rigling, "Invisible Manacles: Drugging Mentally Retarded People," *Stanford Law Review* 31 (1979): 637–78; and Peter Breggin, *Psychiatric Drugs: Hazards to the Brain* (New York: Springer, 1983), 12–32.
5. See C. Keith Conners, "Psychopharmacologic Treatment of Children," in Albert DiMascio and Richard Shader, eds., *Clinical Handbook of Psychopharmacology* (New York: Science House, 1970), 285.
6. See the APA task force report, *Treatments of Psychiatric Disorders* (Washington, D.C.: American Psychiatric Association, 1989), 374.
7. In addition to the sources listed for side effects, see the *DSM-III-R* description of psychological and behavioral changes associated with Ritalin dependence, which include "depression," "social isolation," "anergia" (loss of energy), and "anhedonia" (loss of pleasure).
8. For discussions of Ritalin side effects, see John Talbott et al., *Textbook of Psychiatry* (Washington, D.C.: American Psychiatric Press, 1988), 990–93; M. K. Dulcan, "Comprehensive Treatment of Children and Adolescents with Attention Deficit Disorders; the State of the Art," *Clinical Psychology Review* 6 (1986): 539–70; Carol Whalen and Barbara Henker, "The Social Ecology of Psychostimulant Treatment: A Model for Conceptual and Empirical Analysis," in *Hyperactive Children: The Social Ecology of Identification and Treatment*, ed. C. Whalen and B. Henker (New York: Academic Press, 1980); and Richard Scarnati, "An Outline of Hazardous Side Effects of Ritalin (Methylphenidate)," *International Journal of Addictions* 21 (1986):837–41. (Scarnati cites a number of articles documenting psychotic reactions to Ritalin. Mixing Ritalin with other drugs, including antidepressants, can be especially hazardous.) See also Charles Grob and Joseph

Coyle, "Suspected Adverse Methylphenidate-Imipramine Interactions in Children," *Journal of Developmental and Behavioral Pediatrics* 7 (1986): 265–67.

9. Physician Larry Plumlee drew my attention to an irony in a story by Lynda Richardson, "Fairfax Family Battles Legacy of Addiction," *Washington Post*, February 6, 1990, which focuses on a family whose son, Andy, is addicted to a variety of drugs, including cocaine. Larry noticed that Andy had been "prescribed medication for hyperactivity at age 9." Years later, the article reports, the family was told "that his hyperactivity made him predisposed toward addiction." More likely, as Plumlee suggests, the medication for hyperactivity predisposed him to seek out similar drugs later in life. Later in the article we find out that the mother "has taken more than a dozen medications for depression since the family's addiction problems became apparent five years ago." As long as psychiatric drugs are labeled "treatments" while illicit drugs are called "addictions," the public will remain confused. Psychoactive drugs in general help people escape from their feelings and their real-life problems, shift the locus of control outside the individual, and make it physiologically and psychologically difficult for people to go on living without a chemical crutch.

10. See the several sources already listed for Ritalin side effects and the *DSM-III-R* (1987) description of symptoms associated with Ritalin dependency, including "irritability," "attentional disturbances," and "memory problems."

11. James Spotts and Carol Spotts, *Use and Abuse of Amphetamine and Its Substitutes* (Rockville, Md.: National Institute of Drug Abuse, undated, circa 1978).

Chapter 14

1. Quoted in " 'America Facing Its Most Tragic Moment'—Dr. Carl Jung," *New York Times*, September 29, 1912.

2. Sigmund Freud, *New Introductory Lectures on Psychoanalysis* (1932), 183.

3. Kate Millett, in *Sexual Politics* (New York: Ballantine, 1969), is critiquing Freud's view that women are inherently masochistic.

4. Elaine Showalter, *The Female Malady: Women, Madness, and English Culture, 1830–1980* (New York: Pantheon, 1985), 19.

5. Virginia Raymond et al., "Mental Health and Violence Against Women: A Feminist Ex-Inmate Analysis," *Phoenix Rising*, winter 1983. This was a position paper resulting from a workshop at the Tenth Annual International Conference on Human Rights and Psychiatric Oppression, Toronto, May 1982.

6. From an unpublished report presented at the Second International Conference on Psychosurgery, Copenhagen, 1970, by R. F. Hetherington, P. Haden, and W. Craig, of the departments of surgery, psychiatry, and psychology, Kingston Psychiatric Hospital and Queens University, Kingston, Ontario. Cited by Peter Breggin, "The Return of Lobotomy and Psycho-

surgery," *Congressional Record*, February 24, 1972. Reprinted with a new introduction in Rem B. Edwards, *Psychiatry and Ethics* (Buffalo, N.Y.: Prometheus Books, 1982).

7. Most recent data are from California. See chapter 9.

8. This is the final report of the American Psychological Association Task Force on Women and Depression, *Women and Depression: Risk Factors and Treatment Issues* (Washington, D.C.: American Psychological Association, 1990). The editors are Ellen McGrath, Gwendolyn Puryear Keita, Bonnie R. Strickland, and Nancy Felipe Russo. The report was not yet available, so the quotes are from an eight-page promotional flier by the same title.

9. Malcolm Gladwell, "Women and Depression: Culture Called a Key Factor," *Washington Post*, December 6, 1990.

10. Judy Mann, "Our Culture as a Cause of Depression," *Washington Post*, December 7, 1990.

11. Peter Breggin, "Psychiatry and Women," recorded seminar presented at the annual meeting of the National Association for Rights Protection and Advocacy (NARPA), Miami Lakes, Florida. See appendix B for availability.

12. Jeffrey Masson, *Freud: The Assault on Truth. Freud's Suppression of the Seduction Theory* (Boston: Faber and Faber, 1984). Masson also discusses and translates a variety of documents concerning psychiatric abuses, often of a sexual nature, in *A Dark Science: Women, Sexuality and Psychiatry in the Nineteenth Century* (New York: Farrar, Straus and Giroux, 1986).

13. Peachey was the first to point out to me the literature confirming that battered women looked "schizophrenic" on clinical evaluation and psychological testing. See chapter 2.

Chapter 15

1. Cited by Matthew Dumont, "In Bed Together at the Market: Psychiatry and the Pharmaceutical Industry," *American Journal of Orthopsychiatry* 60 (1990): 484–85.

2. "APA Official Actions," *American Journal of Psychiatry* 147 (1990): 1401.

3. "Alprazolam First Drug to Receive FDA Approval for Treatment of Panic Disorder," *Psychiatric News*, January 4, 1991.

4. *American Journal of Psychiatry* 138 (October 1981): 1408.

5. Tina Adler, "Budget Deal Is Sweet to Behavioral Science," *APA Monitor* (American Psychological Association) 21 (December 1990): 1. The report says that NIMH has "almost reached sacred-cow status" in Congress, an enormous tribute to the mental health lobby, led by the psychopharmaceutical complex and joined by the American Psychological Association.

6. The figures are taken from the "Report of the Treasurer," *American Journal of Psychiatry* 143 (1986): 1340, table 2.

7. For criticism of Judd's focus at NIMH, see Tina Adler, "Judd Leaves NIMH, Returns to Old Job," *APA Monitor* 21 (December 1990): 6.

8. See "Neuroleptics to Carry FDA Class Warning," *Psychiatric News*, May 17, 1985. The FDA warning on tardive dyskinesia, which was hammered out in consultations with the drug companies and organized psychiatry, contains no hint of the extraordinary frequency of the disease (see chapter 4). It states that "prevalence of the syndrome appears to be highest among the elderly," and while this is true, it leaves room for the wholly misleading conclusion that it is not very high among all drug-treated persons, including children and young adults.

9. "Two New Psychiatric Drugs," FDA *Drug Bulletin* 20, no. 1 (April 1990): 9.

10. Ibid.

11. The Generic Division of the FDA determines which firms will get into the marketplace with a generic version of a drug when the patent runs out. Charles Chang, an FDA chemist who has pleaded guilty to accepting gifts from the pharmaceutical industry, describes in an affidavit the influence that drug manufactures exert over the FDA. He confesses that "favoritism and special handling of applications were common in the division of generic drugs," involving high-ranking FDA officials. He describes "continuous pressure put on the division, at all levels, by the [pharmaceutical] industry through lobbying, conducted by executives, lawyers, consultants, and occasionally through political channels inside and outside the FDA." He found that "the larger and more sophisticated generic firms received special treatment, primarily through personal contacts within the division."

12. Letter from Lewis Judd, professor and chair, Department of Psychiatry, University of California, San Diego, to Laurie Flynn, executive director, NAMI, November 15, 1990.

13. Rael Jean Isaac and Virginia C. Armat's book, *Madness in the Streets: How Psychiatry and the Law Abandoned the Mentally Ill* (New York: Free Press, 1990), reflects the view of NAMI's leadership. The dust jacket carries endorsements from the past president of NAMI and the current president of the California branch, CAMI. The acknowledgments thank "above all" a CAMI representative. The book supports lobotomy, electroshock, drugs, more severe forms of involuntary treatment, and state mental hospitals. It attacks the patients' rights movement and critics of biopsychiatry.

14. Milt Freudenheim, "Maker of Schizophrenia Drug Bows to Pressure to Cut Cost," *New York Times*, December 6, 1990. While the reduced cost of the drug is hailed as a humanitarian outcome, it really means that many more patients will be *forced* to take a drug that produces a particularly overwhelming lobotomy effect (see chapters 3 and 4).

15. The 1987 GAP report laments that the competition is encroaching on psychiatry: "As a growing number of mental health specialists and other physicians become eligible for third-party reimbursements and the competition for patients increases, it becomes vital for the public to understand the role of psychiatrists" (p. 16). The psychiatrist's claim to the lion's share of the market lies in his medical identity—his or her "special skills in the diagnosis and treatment of mental disorders." If these disorders are not genetic and biological, then psychologists and other nonmedical profes-

sionals could just as well do the diagnosing and treating. In fact, they often provide better services.

Chapter 16

1. The problem with quoting Jung and Freud, as well as many other famous therapists, is that they also had so many horrendous things to say. In *Civilization and Its Discontents* (1930) (trans. James Strachey [New York: W. W. Norton, 1962], 57), Freud called the ethical rule "Thou shalt love thy neighbor as thyself" "this grandiose commandment." In a footnote he quotes Heine: "One must, it is true, forgive one's enemies—but not before they have been hanged."
2. Carter Umbarger, Andrew Morrison, James Dalsimer, and Peter Breggin, *College Students in a Mental Hospital: An Account of Organized Social Contacts Between College Volunteers and Mental Patients in a Hospital Community* (New York: Grune and Stratton, 1962). Also see Peter Breggin, "The College Student and the Mental Patient," in *College Student Companion Program: Contribution to the Social Rehabilitation of the Mentally Ill* (Connecticut State Department of Mental Health and NIMH, 1962).
3. See, for example, Roger Coate and Jerel Rosati, eds., *The Power of Human Needs in World Society* (Boulder, Colo.: Lynne Rienner, 1984); and John Burton, *Conflict Resolution and Provention* (New York: St. Martin's Press, 1990). I am currently working on a book based on similar principles: Peter Breggin, *Beyond Conflict* (tentative) (New York: St. Martin's Press, forthcoming). I believe love is the most thorough method of conflict resolution.
4. The quotations from Pinel and Esquirol are in Thorn Shipley, ed., *Classics in Psychology* (New York: Philosophical Library, 1961).
5. How badly hospitals have treated patients over the past one hundred years is documented in many sources, including Emil Kraepelin, *One Hundred Years of Psychiatry* (New York: Philosophical Library, 1962); and Albert Deutsch, *The Mentally Ill in America*, 2d ed. (New York: Columbia University Press, 1949). That the gross mistreatment continues is documented in the Joint Hearings of the Subcommittee on the Handicapped of the Committee on Labor and Human Resources, *Care of Institutionalized Mentally Disabled Persons*, pts. 1 and 2, April 1–3, 1985 (Washington, D.C.: Government Printing Office).
6. See Loren Mosher and Lorenzo Burti, *Community Mental Health: Principles and Practices* (New York: W. W. Norton, 1989); Loren Mosher, Ann Reifman, and Alma Menn, "Characteristics of Nonprofessionals Serving as Primary Therapists for Acute Schizophrenics," *Hospital and Community Psychiatry* 24 (1973): 391–96; Loren Mosher and Alma Menn, "Community Residential Treatment for Schizophrenia: A Two-Year Follow-up," *Hospital and Community Psychiatry* 29 (1978): 715–23; Susan Matthews et al., "A Non-Neuroleptic Treatment for Schizophrenia: Analysis of the Two-Year Postdischarge Risk of Relapse," *Schizophrenia Bulletin* 5 (1979): 322–33; and Loren Mosher et al., "Milieu Therapy in the 1980s: A Comparison of Two

Residential Alternatives to Hospitalization," *Bulletin of the Menninger Clinic* 50 (May 1986): 229–322.

7. In addition to the studies on family communication cited in this section, several are contained in an excellent compendium: Thomas W. Miller, ed., *Stressful Life Events* (Madison, Conn.: International Universities Press, 1989). It also cites research indicating that so-called schizophrenia can be caused by stress. See chapters 2 and 5 for further discussion of these issues.

8. The national office of the Association for Humanistic Psychology is in San Francisco. The annual conferences, as well as regional meetings, are held in a variety of places around the country.

9. Re-evaluation Co-counseling, *Fundamentals of Co-Counseling Manual* (Seattle: Rational Island, 1962). (Rational Island Publishers, P.O. Box 2081, Main Office Station, Seattle, Washington 98111.) The principles draw on a specific approach to psychotherapy, and the individuals who help each other through these techniques are, by almost any definition, "doing psychotherapy," although they may not be getting paid for it.

About the Author

Peter R. Breggin, M.D., a Harvard College and Case Western Reserve School of Medicine graduate and former teaching fellow at Harvard Medical School, was a full-time consultant for the National Institute of Mental Health before going into the private practice of psychiatry in Bethesda, Maryland, from 1968 to the present. He is the director of the Center for the Study of Psychiatry and Professor (Adjunct) of Conflict Analysis and Resolution at George Mason University, as well as the author of numerous books and articles dealing with psychiatry. Dr. Breggin frequently lectures and gives seminars to lay and professional audiences and appears on national television as an expert on psychiatric issues. He has been a consultant in landmark lawsuits and federal legislation on behalf of patients' rights and psychiatric reform.

Index

Index

Index

Ritalin, 122, 291, 293, 409; addiction to, 161, 306–8; for children, 279, 305; efficacy of, 305, 310–11; forced use of, 312–13; neuroleptics and, 309; side effects of, 303–11, 444nn. 7, 8, 445n.10; use of, 275, 303–8

Roche Laboratories, 90, 201

Rockefeller Foundation, 102

Roerig, 353

Rose, Steven, 92, 96

Rosen, John, 339

Rosenbaum, Jerrold, 166

Rosenhan, D. L., 61, 294–95

Rosenthal, David, 97–98, 105, 106

Rubin, William, 66

Ruby Rogers Advocacy and Drop-In Center, 396

Rudin, Ernst, 102–4

Rush, Benjamin, 108–9

Russell, Diana E. H., 333

Rutter, Michael, 284–85

Ryan, Michael, 43

Rylander, Gosta, 53–54

SAD. See Seasonal affective disorder

Safe havens, 44–45, 139, 384–88, 396, 409; for children, 296

Samant, Sidney, 184

Samuels, S. Jay, 281

Sandoz Pharmaceuticals Corporation, 74, 86, 366; CAMI and, 363; influence of, 353; monitoring by, 429n.9; NAMI and, 86; scholarships from, 363–64

San Francisco Board of Supervisors, hearing by, 187, 215

Sankey, W. H. O., 383–84

Santopolo, Anthony C., 52

Sanua, Victor, 290

Satterfield, James H., 310

Schatzberg, Alan, 74

Schiffman, James, 297, 299n

Schizophrenia, 6, 10, 28, 35, 36, 261, 277, 291; bad blood and, 110; biological basis of, 108, 113–15; brain dysfunction and, 83, 84; children and, 92–93, 97–100, 287, 336; dopamine hypothesis of, 110–12; drug-induced, 87, 394–95; environmental factors of, 36, 85, 96–97, 99, 106, 116–17; genetic basis of, 35, 46, 94, 95, 97–100, 101, 105, 106, 107, 108, 115, 148, 279; humiliation and, 37, 38–39; hypothesis for, 108, 111; labeling, 33; NAMI and, 34; number suffering, 367; overcoming, 25, 42, 60–61, 374, 380; psychiatry and, 36; psychotherapy and, 390–92, 404; reality of, 45; self-fulfilling prophecy of, 44; shame and, 222; spiritual focus of, 22; women and, 324. See also Madness

Schizophrenics, 5, 23–24, 51; brain shrinkage and, 13; chronic, 27, 41, 43, 63; communications of, 23; crisis for, 26–27, 128–29; "primary process" thinking of, 32; sterilization of, 104; treating, 7; treating families of, 391–92

Schmauss, C., 249

Schmeck, Harold, 147

Schmidt, William, 303

Schou, Mogens, 176, 177

Schrag, Peter, 278, 313

Schreibman, Laura, 288, 289

Schulsinger, Fini, 97–98

Schwartz, Ira, 299

Schwartz, John, 362

Schwartzman, A. E., 202

Schweitzer, Albert, 31

Seasonal affective disorder (SAD), 122, 127

Secobarbital. See Seconal; Tuinal

Seconal (secobarbital), 242

Sectral (acebutolol), 259

Sedatives, 154, 162, 241, 243, 244, 246, 255, 265, 309; for children, 300; denial and, 255; depression and, 244; efficacy of, 64; electroshock and, 208; hypnotic, 241–46

Seidenberg, Robert, 32, 236–37, 355

Seizures, 247, 309; electroshock and, 189, 204, 208

Select Committee on Children, Youth and Families (House), 270

Self-defeating personality, 335, 377; women and, 334–35

Self-determination, 38, 93–94, 225, 230, 282, 328, 377, 381, 382; encouraging, 9, 10, 45; lack of, 27

Self-esteem, 94, 291, 310, 381, 385; bolstering, 37; eating disorders and, 238

Self-help, 42; books on, 16, 318; future of, 397–98; groups, 333, 403, 409; programs, 380, 396–97

Serax (oxazepam), 242; withdrawal from, 245

Serentil (mesoridazine), 51

Serotonic neurotransmission: levels of, 142; shutdown, 141–42, 165

Serotonin, 141, 163, 165, 167, 260, 261

Sexual abuse, 43, 44, 135, 200, 226, 298, 334, 446n.12; aftereffects of, 333–34, 336–37; children and, 281; metaphors for, 24; prevalence of, 333–34; by psychiatrists, 339; PTSD and, 229; women and, 34, 239, 271, 443n.4. See also Child abuse

Shader, Richard, 60

Shah, Diane, 172, 173

Shame, 36–40, 46, 93, 129, 232, 334; addiction and, 229; childhood origins of, 225; dealing with, 222–25; eating disorders and, 239; psychospiritual overwhelm and, 39; schizophrenia and, 222; source of, 373

Shelp, Earl, 32–33